IADVL SIG Handbook on
Psoriasis

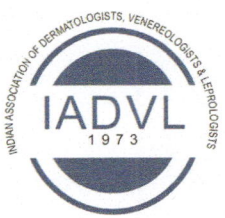

Indian Association of Dermatologists, Venereologists and Leprologists

IADVL SIG Handbook on
Psoriasis

Editors

Sudip Das MD(Derm and Ven) AIIMS New Delhi FRCP(Edinburgh) IFAAD
Professor and Head
Department of Dermatology
Calcutta National Medical College and Hospital
Kolkata, West Bengal, India

Abhishek De MD FAGE SCE(Dermatology) FRCP(Edinburgh) FAAD PhD(Schl)
Associate Professor
Department of Dermatology
Calcutta National Medical College and Hospital
Kolkata, West Bengal, India

Associate Editors

Konakanchi Venkata Chalam MD DVL
Associate Professor
Department of DVL
Government Medical College
Srikakulam, Andhra Pradesh, India

Saurabh Singh MBBS(AIIMS Delhi) MD(AIIMS Delhi) DNB
Additional Professor
Department of Dermatology, Venereology and Leprology
AIIMS Jodhpur, Rajasthan, India
Associate Editor, Indian Journal of Dermatopathology and Diagnostic Dermatology
Assistant Editor, Journal of Cutaneous and Aesthetic Surgery

Forewords
Rajeev Sharma
Vinay Singh

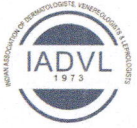

Under the Aegis of IADVL Academy

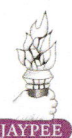

JAYPEE BROTHERS MEDICAL PUBLISHERS
The Health Sciences Publisher
New Delhi | London

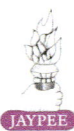 **Jaypee Brothers Medical Publishers (P) Ltd**

Headquarters
EMCA House
23/23-B, Ansari Road, Daryaganj
New Delhi 110 002, India
Landline: +91-11-23272143, +91-11-23272703
+91-11-23282021, +91-11-23245672
E-mail: jaypee@jaypeebrothers.com

Corporate Office
Jaypee Brothers Medical Publishers (P) Ltd.
4838/24, Ansari Road, Daryaganj
New Delhi 110 002, India
Phone: +91-11-43574357
Fax: +91-11-43574314
E-mail: jaypee@jaypeebrothers.com

Overseas Office
JP Medical Ltd.
83, Victoria Street, London
SW1H 0HW (UK)
Phone: +44-20 3170 8910
Fax: +44(0)20 3008 6180
E-mail: info@jpmedpub.com

Website: www.jaypeebrothers.com
Website: www.jaypeedigital.com

© 2025, Jaypee Brothers Medical Publishers

The views and opinions expressed in this book are solely those of the original contributor(s)/author(s) and do not necessarily represent those of editor(s) or publisher of the book.

All rights reserved. No part of this publication may be reproduced, stored or transmitted in any form or by any means, electronic, mechanical, photocopying, recording or otherwise, without the prior permission in writing of the publishers.

All brand names and product names used in this book are trade names, service marks, trademarks or registered trademarks of their respective owners. The publisher is not associated with any product or vendor mentioned in this book.

Medical knowledge and practice change constantly. This book is designed to provide accurate, authoritative information about the subject matter in question. However, readers are advised to check the most current information available on procedures included and check information from the manufacturer of each product to be administered, to verify the recommended dose, formula, method and duration of administration, adverse effects and contraindications. It is the responsibility of the practitioner to take all appropriate safety precautions. Neither the publisher nor the author(s)/editor(s) assume any liability for any injury and/or damage to persons or property arising from or related to use of material in this book.

This book is sold on the understanding that the publisher is not engaged in providing professional medical services. If such advice or services are required, the services of a competent medical professional should be sought.

Every effort has been made where necessary to contact holders of copyright to obtain permission to reproduce copyright material. If any have been inadvertently overlooked, the publisher will be pleased to make the necessary arrangements at the first opportunity.

Inquiries for bulk sales may be solicited at: jaypee@jaypeebrothers.com

IADVL SIG Handbook on Psoriasis / **Sudip Das, Abhishek De**

First Edition: **2025**

ISBN: 978-93-6616-604-9

Printed in India

Contributors

Abhishek De MD
FAGE SCE(Dermatology)
FRCP(Edinburgh) FAAD PhD(Schl)
Associate Professor
Department of Dermatology
Calcutta National Medical
College and Hospital
Kolkata, West Bengal, India

Akshay Sankar Peethambaran MBBS MD(DVL)
Senior Resident
Department of Dermatology
AIIMS Raipur
Chhattisgarh, India

Anupama YG MD DVL
Associate Professor
Department of DVL
Shimoga Institute of Medical Sciences
Shivamogga, Karnataka, India

Anupam Das MD(Dermatology)
Assistant Professor
Department of Dermatology
KPC Medical College and Hospital
Kolkata, West Bengal, India

Apeksha Singh MBBS DVDL DNB
Senior Resident
Department of Dermatology
Calcutta National Medical
College and Hospital
Kolkata, West Bengal, India

Ashish Jacob Mathew
MBBS DNB DM PhD(Univ of Copenhagen)
Professor
Department of Clinical Immunology and Rheumatology
Christian Medical College
Vellore, Tamil Nadu, India

Ayesha Merchant MD
Senior Resident
Department of Dermatology
Grant Government Medical College
Mumbai, Maharashtra, India

Bikash Ranjan Kar MD MNAMS
Professor and Head
Department of DVL
Institute of Medical Sciences and Sum Hospital
Bhubaneswar, Odisha, India

Chinmoy Raj MD
Associate Professor
PG Department of Dermatology
Kalinga Institute of Medical Sciences
KIIT (Deemed-to-be University)
Bhubaneswar, Odisha, India

CR Srinivas MD FRCP(Glasgow)
Professor
Department of Dermatology
Kalinga Institute of Medical Sciences
KIIT (Deemed-to-be University)
Bhubaneswar, Odisha, India

Datta Lokare MBBS
Junior Resident
Department of Dermatology
Grant Government Medical College
Mumbai, Maharashtra, India

Debasmita Behera MD
Professor and Head
PG Department of Dermatology
Kalinga Institute of Medical Sciences
KIIT (Deemed-to-be University)
Bhubaneswar, Odisha, India

Dipra Biswas MBBS MD
Senior Resident
Department of Dermatology, Venereology and Leprology
AIIMS Jodhpur
Jodhpur, Rajasthan, India

Dharshini Sathishkumar MD DDVL
Professor
Department of Dermatology
Christian Medical College
Vellore
Tamil Nadu, India

Disha Chakraborty
Postdoctoral Fellow
Department of Dermatology and Rheumatology
Sacramento VA Medical Center
California, USA

Contributors

Farhat Fatima MBBS MD MRCP SCE
Senior Resident
Department of Dermatology
Calcutta National Medical College and Hospital
Kolkata, West Bengal, India

Kallolinee Samal MD
Assistant Professor
Department of DVL
Institute of Medical Sciences and Sum Hospital
Bhubaneswar, Odisha, India

KA Seetharam MD(DVL)
Professor and Head
Department of DVL
GSL Medical College
Rajamahendravaram,
Andhra Pradesh, India

Kavya Baddireddy DDVL DNB
Civil Assistant Surgeon
Government Hospital for Chest and Communicable Diseases
Andhra Medical College
Visakhapatnam, Andhra Pradesh, India

Kethireddi Susmitha Divya
MD DVL
Assistant Professor
Department of DVL
Andhra Medical College
Visakhapatnam, Andhra Pradesh, India

K Venkatesh MD(DVL)
Senior Resident
Department of DVL
GSL Medical College
Rajamahendravaram,
Andhra Pradesh, India

Lydia Mathew MD DDVL
Associate Professor
Department of Dermatology
Christian Medical College
Vellore, Tamil Nadu, India

Manjeet Naresh Ramteke
MBBS MD(Dermatology, Venereology and Leprosy)
Associate Professor
Department of Dermatology, Venereology and Leprosy
Grant Government Medical College
Mumbai, Maharashtra, India

Shraddha Madanagobalane
MD DNB PhD
Senior Consultant
Dermatologist
Apollo Hospitals Greams Road, Chennai
Helios Advanced Skin Hair and Laser Clinic
Chennai, Tamil Nadu

Neena Khanna MD
Professor and Head
Department of Dermatology
Amrita Institute of Medical Sciences and Research Centre
Faridabad, Haryana, India

Rajesh Kumar MD(AIIMS, New Delhi)
Professor
Department of Dermatology
Grant Government Medical College
Mumbai, Maharashtra, India

Sachin Gupta MBBS(AIIMS, New Delhi) MD DVL (AIIMS, New Delhi)
Senior Resident
Amrita Hospital
Faridabad, Haryana, India

Sambit Chatterjee MBBS
Junior Resident
Department of Dermatology
KPC Medical College and Hospital
Kolkata, West Bengal, India

Sanjeev Handa MD FAMS FAAD FRCP(Edin)
Professor (HAG) and Head
Department of Dermatology, Venereology and Leprology
Postgraduate Institute of Medical Education and Research
Chandigarh, India

Satyaki Ganguly MD(DVL) DNB(DV)
Additional Professor
Department of Dermatology
AIIMS Raipur
Chhattisgarh, India

Saurabh Singh MBBS(AIIMS Delhi) MD(AIIMS Delhi) DNB
Additional Professor
Department of Dermatology, Venereology and Leprology
AIIMS Jodhpur, Rajasthan, India
Associate Editor, Indian Journal of Dermatopathology and Diagnostic Dermatology
Assistant Editor, Journal of Cutaneous and Aesthetic Surgery

Shekhar Neema MD
Professor
Department of Dermatology
Base Hospital
Lucknow, Uttar Pradesh, India

Siddharth Mani
MD(Dermatology)
Assistant Professor
Department of Dermatology
INHS Sanjivani
Kochi, Kerala, India

SK Shahriar Ahmed MBBS MD DNB
Senior Resident
Department of Dermatology
Calcutta National Medical College and Hospital
Kolkata, West Bengal, India

Contributors

Sudip Das MD(Derm and Ven)
AIIMS New Delhi FRCP(Edinburgh)
IFAAD
Professor and Head
Department of Dermatology
Calcutta National Medical
College and Hospital
Kolkata, West Bengal, India

Susmitha Meda MD DVL
Assistant Professor
Department of DVL
Rangaraya Medical College and
Hospital
Kakinada, Andhra Pradesh, India

Sukhdeep Singh MD DNB
Senior Resident
Department of Dermatology,
Venereology and Leprology
PGIMER
Chandigarh, India

Tarun Narang MD MNAMS
FRCP(Edin)
Additional Professor
Department of Dermatology,
Venereology and Leprology
PGIMER
Chandigarh, India

Konakanchi Venkata Chalam
MD DVL
Associate Professor
Department of DVL
Government Medical College
Srikakulam, Andhra Pradesh,
India

Madhumitha Venugopal MD
DVL
Associate Consultant
Department of Dermatology
Kauvery Hospital
Chennai, Tamil Nadu, India

Foreword

Psoriasis, a chronic immune-mediated disorder with significant systemic implications, continues to be a major challenge in dermatology, in terms of both understanding its complex pathogenesis and ensuring optimal patient care. The *"IADVL SIG Handbook on Psoriasis"* represents a remarkable endeavor to bring together the latest scientific insights, clinical expertise, and practical guidance for dermatologists, postgraduate students, and healthcare practitioners.

As the President-Elect of the Indian Association of Dermatologists, Venereologists, and Leprologists (IADVL), it gives me immense pride to introduce this comprehensive handbook, a testament to the unwavering dedication of the Special Interest Group (SIG) on Psoriasis. The editors, Dr Sudip Das and Dr Abhishek De, along with a distinguished panel of contributors, have meticulously curated an invaluable resource that delves into the epidemiology, pathophysiology, clinical subtypes, and latest treatment modalities, including biologics and small-molecule therapies.

Psoriasis extends far beyond its cutaneous manifestations, impacting metabolic health, cardiovascular function, and overall quality of life. Recognizing this, the handbook not only addresses the clinical aspects but also explores the multidimensional burden of psoriasis, emphasizing a holistic, patient-centered approach to management. With the advent of newer immunomodulatory therapies and an expanding understanding of psoriasis endotypes, the book serves as a timely guide to navigating the evolving treatment landscape.

This work underscores IADVL's commitment to fostering academic excellence and advancing dermatological education. I extend my sincere gratitude to the editorial team, the esteemed contributors, and the IADVL Academy for their tireless efforts in bringing this handbook to fruition. I am confident that it will serve as a cornerstone reference for clinicians and researchers alike, ultimately contributing to improved patient outcomes.

Let us continue to push the boundaries of dermatological science and uphold our commitment to excellence in patient care.

Rajeev Sharma MD
President-Elect, IADVL
2024 after President Elect
LM/UP&UK/2251

Foreword

Psoriasis, a complex and often misunderstood skin condition, has remained a challenge not only for those who live with it but also for the medical community striving to provide effective care. Over the years, research has brought us closer to understanding the pathophysiology of psoriasis, but there is always more to learn. The "*IADVL SIG Handbook on Psoriasis*" serves as an invaluable resource, bringing together the latest insights, diagnostic strategies, and treatment modalities in a way that is both accessible and comprehensive.

This book is a culmination of knowledge shared by experts in the field of dermatology, representing a rich collaboration within the Indian Association of Dermatologists, Venereologists, and Leprologists (IADVL). As a dermatology community, we recognize the need for a resource that unifies global advancements in psoriasis care with the unique needs and contexts of our patients in India.

The editors and contributors to this handbook have worked tirelessly and have included their vast experience to ensure that it reflects the latest clinical evidence, practical guidelines, and real-world experiences. The result is a guide that can be used by clinicians at all levels, whether they are just beginning their careers or are seasoned experts seeking the most current and relevant information.

One of the key strengths of this handbook lies in its holistic approach to psoriasis management. From the psychological impact of psoriasis to the most advanced biologic therapies, it addresses the multifaceted nature of this disease. Moreover, it highlights the importance of patient-centered care, emphasizing not only medical treatments but also education, counseling, and support.

I congratulate IADVL Academy and IADVL SIG Psoriasis for supporting various programs to address the evolving challenges of psoriasis management with a focus on evidence-based insights and practical strategies for dermatologists, postgraduate students, and clinicians which have helped in shaping up this handbook. I encourage every healthcare professional involved in the care of psoriasis patients to engage with this handbook. In a world where knowledge is continuously evolving, this book will undoubtedly remain a touchstone for both learning and practice.

With the publication of this comprehensive guide, I am confident that the management of psoriasis will continue to progress, benefiting patients and practitioners alike.

Vinay Singh MD(Gold Medal) Gujarat University
President-Elect 2025 IADVL
President IADVL Delhi State 2021
Director, Vibrance Wellness Vista and
Vibrance Skin Clinic
Delhi-NCR, India

Preface

It is a great pleasure and satisfaction to be the editor of this wonderful "*IADVL SIG Handbook on Psoriasis*". Not only has there been a worldwide increase in the prevalence of psoriasis cases, but the management has also gone through huge changes since our residency days. Metabolic syndromes such as diabetes, obesity, dyslipidemia, and hypertension all have made management of psoriasis challenging day by day. Hence, the disease called psoriasis requires an update on its pathogenesis and management.

It was a wonderful SIG team to work with, now being led by Dr Konakanchi Venkata Chalam, Dr Anupama and Dr Shraddha.

My friends Dr Rajesh, Dr Abhishek, Dr Saurabh and all others contributed to the success and activities of this SIG. We received constant positive encouragement from IADVL EC and Academy in our endeavor. I thank all the authors for their hard work. In short, it is a comprehensive work on psoriasis research and treatment modalities.

Long live IADVL!

Sudip Das

Preface

"Books are the carriers of civilization. Without books, history is silent, literature dumb, science crippled, thought and speculation at a standstill."

—**Barbara W Tuchman**

It is with immense pride, humility, and gratitude that I pen the preface for the "*IADVL SIG Handbook on Psoriasis*". This book, a labor of love, meticulous research, and collective effort, is a testament to the tireless pursuit of knowledge and the unrelenting passion of the dermatology community.

Psoriasis, a multifaceted disease that extends beyond the skin, challenges the diagnostic and therapeutic acumen of dermatologists worldwide. This handbook was conceived to empower clinicians, postgraduate students, and practitioners with the latest evidence-based insights and practical guidance for managing psoriasis. It is a culmination of dedicated teamwork, enriched by the invaluable contributions of experts across the field.

First and foremost, I extend my deepest gratitude to my mentors, guides, and role models who have shaped my journey as a dermatologist and as an academic. My heartfelt thanks go to Professor Kiran Godse, whose guidance during my formative years as a researcher has been nothing short of transformative, and to Professor Raghavendra Rao, whose unwavering encouragement has been a beacon of inspiration. I am equally indebted to Dr Sandipan Dhar and Dr Koushik Lahiri, who have consistently motivated me to strive for excellence in dermatology. Your mentorship has been a source of strength and wisdom.

I owe a profound debt of gratitude to my parents, Nandita Dey and Dwipendra Narayan Dey, for their unwavering belief in my dreams and their sacrifices, enabling me to reach this point in my career. I would like to thank my wife, Dr Aarti Sarda, a brilliant dermatologist and a pillar of support, and to my children, whose smiles brighten my every day. I sincerely thank you for your patience and love as I devoted countless hours to this endeavor.

This book would not have been possible without the unwavering support of the Indian Association of Dermatologists, Venereologists, and Leprologists (IADVL) and the IADVL Academy. I am immensely grateful for their faith in my vision and for providing a platform that celebrates collaboration and academic excellence.

I am especially grateful to my co-editors, Dr Sudip Das, Dr Konakanchi Venkata Chalam, and Dr Saurabh Singh, whose expertise and dedication have helped shape this book into what it is today. I am also deeply thankful to my colleagues in the SIG Psoriasis team, who have enriched the content with their invaluable contributions to various chapters.

This book would not have seen the light of day without the support of our esteemed publisher, Jaypee Brothers Medical Publishers, and the unwavering efforts of Mr Akhilesh Saxena and Mr Sabyasachi Hazra, whose meticulous attention to detail and commitment to quality have ensured that this book meets the highest standards.

Lastly, I dedicate this book to the members of IADVL, whose tireless efforts continue to advance the field of dermatology, and to my patients with psoriasis, who are my greatest teachers. Your courage and resilience inspire me to strive harder every day.

As you journey through the pages of this handbook, I hope you find it a valuable companion in your clinical practice. May it ignite new thoughts, refine your approaches, and, above all, remind us all of the profound privilege we have as dermatologists to transform lives.

"Let us read and let us dance; these two amusements will never do any harm to the world."

—**Voltaire**

With heartfelt gratitude!

Abhishek De

Acknowledgments

The work done in this book has ultimately come to fruition through the efforts, ideas, thoughts, dedication, and invaluable time of many faculties and residents, whom I acknowledge from the core of my heart.

I extend my sincere gratitude to Dr Manjunath Shenmoy, Dr Rajeev Sharma, and Dr Bhumesh Kakatam, the Secretary, for their invaluable support in bringing this book to light. I also extend my heartfelt thanks to IADVL Academic Chairperson, Dr Lalit Kumar, and Dr Sunil Dogra for their significant contributions in making this dream a reality.

I am also indebted to my colleagues, seniors, and residents for making this collective effort successful and worthy. I am grateful to the team of Jaypee Brothers Medical Publishers comprising Ankit Vij (Managing Director), Sabyasachi Hazra (Associate Director—Publishing and Digital Sales), and Akhilesh Saxena (Development Editor), for the tremendous efforts in bringing out this book.

Blessings from the Almighty!

Sudip Das

Contents

1. **Introduction to Psoriasis: Definition, Epidemiology, and Etiology** ... 1
   Anupama YG

2. **Clinical Manifestations of Psoriasis: Plaque, Guttate, Pustular, Erythrodermic, and Inverse Psoriasis** ... 7
   Kethireddi Susmitha Divya, Susmitha Meda

3. **Pathophysiology of Psoriasis: Immune System Dysfunction, Genetics, and Triggers** ... 23
   Bikash Ranjan Kar, Kallolinee Samal

4. **Differential Diagnosis of Psoriasis: Distinguishing Psoriasis from Other Dermatological Conditions** ... 36
   Rajesh Kumar, Ayesha Merchant, Datta Lokare, Disha Chakraborty

5. **Psoriasis: Relation with Probiotics, Prebiotics, and Gut Dysbiosis** ... 51
   Sambit Chatterjee, Anupam Das

6. **Comorbidities Associated with Psoriasis: Cardiovascular Disease, Metabolic Syndrome, and Depression** ... 54
   Sudip Das, Apeksha Singh

7. **Assessment and Scoring of Psoriasis Severity: PASI and Other Scales** ... 65
   Dipra Biswas, Saurabh Singh

8. **Topical Treatments for Psoriasis** ... 72
   KA Seetharam, K Venkatesh

9. **Phototherapy in the Management of Psoriasis** ... 82
   Chinmoy Raj, Debasmita Behera, CR Srinivas

10. **Conventional Systemic Therapies in Psoriasis** ... 100
    Konakanchi Venkata Chalam, Kavya Baddireddy

11. **Small Molecules in Psoriasis** ... 114
    Farhat Fatima, SK Shahriar Ahmed, Sudip Das

12. **Use of Biologics in Psoriasis** ... 121
    Abhishek De, Disha Chakraborty

13. **Combination and Rotational Therapy in the Management of Psoriasis** ... 139
    Lydia Mathew, Dharshini Sathishkumar

Contents

14. **Management of Psoriatic Arthritis: Diagnosis and Treatment Options** — 153
    Ashish Jacob Mathew

15. **Pustular Psoriasis** — 169
    Sudip Das, SK Shahriar Ahmed

16. **Special Considerations in Psoriasis Management: Pregnancy, Children, and Elderly Patients** — 175
    Neena Khanna, Sachin Gupta

17. **Psoriasis and Quality of Life: Impact on Patients' Daily Lives and Mental Health** — 183
    Sanjeev Handa, Sukhdeep Singh, Tarun Narang

18. **Psoriasis and Dermatology Practice: Clinical Pearls and Best Practices for Patient Management** — 189
    Manjeet Naresh Ramteke

19. **Patient Education and Support: Strategies for Improving Patient Adherence and Self-management** — 198
    Satyaki Ganguly, Akshay Sankar Peethambaran

20. **Case Studies in Psoriasis Management: Real-World Applications of Psoriasis Diagnosis and Treatment** — 203
    Shekhar Neema, Siddharth Mani

21. **Novel Therapeutic Targets in Psoriasis: Biologics, Small Molecules, and Cell-based Therapies** — 214
    Shraddha Madanagobalane

22. **Overview of Psoriasis Research Trends** — 234
    Shraddha Madanagobalane

23. **Personalized Medicine in Psoriasis** — 244
    Shraddha Madanagobalane

24. **Advances in Psoriasis Research: Genomics, Proteomics, and Bioinformatics** — 253
    Shraddha Madanagobalane, Madhumitha Venugopal

Index — 261

Introduction to Psoriasis: Definition, Epidemiology, and Etiology

Anupama YG

■ INTRODUCTION

Psoriasis is a chronic skin disorder that affects a substantial proportion of the global population. Despite its prevalence, the condition remains poorly understood. This chapter covers the fundamental aspects of psoriasis, including its definition, epidemiology, and etiology. By understanding these aspects, this chapter lays the groundwork for subsequent discussions on the clinical features, diagnosis, and treatment of psoriasis.

■ DEFINITION

Psoriasis is a common, chronic, immune-mediated inflammatory skin disorder characterized by well-defined, bilaterally symmetrical erythematous plaques with silvery scales present particularly over the extensor surfaces and scalp. It predominantly affects the skin and nails but can also involve the joints, leading to a related condition known as psoriatic arthritis. The association of psoriasis with obesity and metabolic syndrome is well established now. The exact pathogenesis of psoriasis is complex and multifactorial, involving a combination of genetic, immunological, and environmental factors. Understanding the intricate interplay of these factors is crucial for developing effective, personalized treatment strategies. Advances in genetic research, immunology, and our understanding of environmental influences continue to shape the management and therapeutic approaches for this challenging condition.

■ EPIDEMIOLOGY

Global Prevalence

Psoriasis is a common disease affecting approximately 2–3% of the global population.[1] However, its prevalence varies significantly across different regions and populations. For example, the prevalence in the United States and Europe is higher compared to Asian and African populations.[2] In Europe, the prevalence ranges from 0.73 to 2.9%, with the highest rates reported in Scandinavian countries.[3] In India, the prevalence of psoriasis varies from 0.44 to 2.8%.[4] This variation can be attributed to genetic, environmental, and lifestyle differences. Most of the data on prevalence has been derived from hospital-based studies while there are only few well-defined large population-based studies done to find the exact prevalence of this dermatoses in the community.[5,6]

Age and Gender Distribution

Psoriasis can occur at any age, but it typically presents in two peak age groups: Between 15 and 25 years and 50 and 60 years, commonly referred to as type I (early onset) and type II (late onset) psoriasis, respectively.[7] Early-onset psoriasis is generally associated with a stronger genetic component and more severe disease course compared to late-onset psoriasis.[8] Type I psoriasis (hereditary form), which accounts for >75% cases, is human leukocyte antigen (HLA)-associated with a positive family history and has an onset before the age of 40 years. Type II disease (sporadic) is characterized by a later onset, better overall prognosis, and generally no family history or HLA association.

Psoriasis has been reported to occur with almost equal frequency in men and women.[9] But most Indian studies suggest that psoriasis is more common in men.[10-12] However, women often experience a greater psychological impact due to the visibility of the disease and its effects on quality of life.

Ethnic and Racial Differences

Ethnic and racial differences in psoriasis prevalence have been documented, with higher prevalence reported in Caucasians compared to African Americans and Asians.[13] For instance, the prevalence in African American populations in the United States is approximately 1.3%, which is lower than the 3.2% prevalence in Caucasians.[14] Genetic factors, including the frequency of psoriasis-susceptibility alleles, and environmental factors, such as ultraviolet (UV) exposure, may contribute to these differences.[15]

ETIOLOGY

Genetic Factors

Genetic predisposition plays a crucial role in the development of psoriasis. Family studies have demonstrated that having a first-degree relative with psoriasis significantly increases the risk of developing the disease.[16] Twin studies have provided further evidence of the genetic basis, showing higher concordance rates in monozygotic twins compared to dizygotic twins.[17]

The genetic architecture of psoriasis is complex, involving multiple susceptibility loci. The most significant and well-studied genetic locus is the major histocompatibility complex (MHC) on chromosome 6p21, particularly the HLAC*0602 allele, which is strongly associated with psoriasis.[18] Genome-wide association studies (GWAS) have identified over 60 genetic loci associated with psoriasis, implicating various genes involved in immune response, skin barrier function, and inflammatory pathways.[19]

Key genes implicated in psoriasis include *IL23R*, *IL12B*, *TNIP1*, and *TNFAIP3*, among others.[20] These genes are involved in the regulation of immune responses, particularly the IL-23/Th17 (interleukin 23–T helper 17) axis, which plays a central role in the pathogenesis of psoriasis.[21]

Immunological Factors

Psoriasis is primarily driven by dysregulation of the immune system, particularly involving T cells and dendritic cells (DCs). The disease is characterized by an aberrant immune response, with overactivation of the Th1 and Th17 pathways and the release of proinflammatory cytokines such as tumor necrosis factor alpha (TNF-α), IL-17, and IL-23.[22]

The pathogenesis of psoriasis begins with the activation of DCs9 in the skin, which present antigens and secrete cytokines, leading to the differentiation and activation of T cells.[23] Activated T cells migrate to the skin and release cytokines that promote keratinocyte proliferation and inflammation, resulting in the characteristic psoriatic plaques.[24]

The IL-23/Th17 axis is particularly important in psoriasis. IL-23, produced by dendritic cells, promotes the expansion and survival of Th17 cells, which secrete IL-17 and other cytokines that drive inflammation and keratinocyte proliferation.[25] Targeting these cytokines with biologic therapies has been highly effective in managing psoriasis, underscoring their central role in disease pathogenesis.[26]

ENVIRONMENTAL TRIGGERS

While genetic and immunological factors establish the foundation for psoriasis, environmental triggers can precipitate and exacerbate the disease. Common environmental triggers include infections, trauma, medications, and lifestyle factors.

Infections

Infections, particularly streptococcal infections, have long been associated with the onset and exacerbation of psoriasis. Streptococcal throat infections are known to trigger guttate psoriasis, a subtype characterized by small, drop-like lesions.[8] Viral infections, such as human immunodeficiency virus (HIV), can also exacerbate psoriasis, highlighting the role of immune system alterations in disease activity.[27]

Trauma

The Koebner phenomenon, where psoriasis develops at sites of skin injury or trauma, underscores the role of physical factors in disease exacerbation. Trauma can include mechanical injuries, surgical scars, or even minor skin insults like insect bites or tattoos.[28] The usual interval is 7–14 days, but may be as short as 3 days to as long as 3 weeks. The response may be mediated by trauma-induced release of neuropeptides from cutaneous sensory nerve terminals.

Medications

Certain medications can trigger or exacerbate psoriasis. Common culprits include beta blockers, lithium, antimalarials, and nonsteroidal anti-inflammatory drugs (NSAIDs), imiquimod, interferons (IFNs), and angiotensin-converting enzyme (ACE) inhibitors.[29-32] Withdrawal from systemic corticosteroids can also trigger a severe flare of psoriasis.

Lifestyle Factors

Lifestyle factors such as smoking, alcohol consumption, diet, and stress significantly impact psoriasis. Smoking is a well-documented risk factor for both the development and exacerbation of psoriasis, with smokers having a higher risk of more severe disease compared to nonsmokers.[33] Nicotine alters immune responses by directly interacting with T cells and human and/or murine DC, as well as indirectly through brain-immune interactions. In addition, nicotinic cholinergic receptors have been demonstrated on keratinocytes stimulating calcium influx and accelerating cell differentiation. Constant stimulation of these receptors may control keratinocyte adhesion and upward migration in the epidermis.[34]

Alcohol consumption is another lifestyle factor associated with psoriasis. Heavy alcohol use can worsen psoriasis severity and interfere with treatment efficacy.[35] It is thought to impact psoriasis through multiple mechanisms, including immune modulation, liver function impairment, and poor treatment adherence.

Dietary factors can also influence psoriasis. Obesity is a significant risk factor, with studies showing a higher prevalence of psoriasis in obese individuals.[36] Adipose tissue produces proinflammatory cytokines such as TNF-α and IL-6, which may contribute to systemic inflammation and psoriasis exacerbation.[37] Weight loss has been shown to improve psoriasis symptoms and treatment response.[38]

Exposure to sunlight and climate can also affect psoriasis. Phototherapy, using ultraviolet B (UVB) light, is a common and effective treatment for psoriasis. Conversely, cold weather and low humidity can exacerbate psoriasis by drying out the skin and reducing exposure to beneficial UV radiation.[39] Geographic studies have shown higher psoriasis prevalence in regions with less sunlight, supporting the beneficial role of UV exposure in disease management.[40]

Stress is a well-known triggering and exacerbating factor for psoriasis. Stress might induce alterations in the psoriatic lesion by increasing the neuropeptide content with a concomitant decrease in the activity of neuropeptide-degrading enzymes, especially mast cell chymase.[41] An increased beta-endorphin levels, normally observed in psoriatic skin, might affect both substance P (SP)-mediated neurogenic inflammation and transmission of sensory stimuli by its local antinociceptive.[42] Stress management techniques, including relaxation exercises, cognitive–behavioral therapy, and mindfulness, can help reduce disease flares and improve overall well-being.[43]

◼ INTERACTION BETWEEN GENETIC AND ENVIRONMENTAL FACTORS

The interplay between genetic predisposition and environmental triggers is crucial in the onset and progression of psoriasis. While genetic factors provide the underlying susceptibility, environmental factors often determine the timing and severity of disease flares. For instance, carriers of the HLA-C*06:02 allele are more likely to experience psoriasis onset following a streptococcal infection compared to noncarriers.[44] This gene–environment interaction highlights the complexity of psoriasis.

Hormonal Factors

Studies have revealed that psoriasis may remit during pregnancy. The reason may be the increased levels of IL-10 that is a known type-1 immune response inhibitor. However, postpartum period, more often than not, sees an exacerbation. There have been reports of GPP being precipitated during pregnancy. This in turn is implicated on the raised levels of progesterone during the latter half.[45]

Microbiome Factors

The skin microbiome, consisting of various microorganisms, has been found to play a role in psoriasis. Diet and gastrointestinal diseases have an impact on the skin functions. Intestinal dysbiosis increases intestinal permeability and promotes the migration of bacteria, toxins, and metabolites into the bloodstream, reaching skin and joints. Skin dyshomeostasis can induce inflammatory skin disease including psoriasis. Probiotics integration may improve skin condition by reducing inflammation, improving the barrier function, modulating immune activation, and hindering the colonization of harmful bacteria.[46]

◼ CONCLUSION

Psoriasis is a chronic, immune-mediated skin disorder that affects millions of people worldwide. With a global prevalence of 2–3%, psoriasis has a substantial impact on quality of life, mental health, and healthcare systems. Genetic, environmental, and immune system factors contribute to its complex etiology. Understanding the epidemiology and etiology of psoriasis is crucial for emerging effective treatment strategies and improving patient outcomes.

TAKE HOME MESSAGE

- Psoriasis is a chronic skin condition with a global prevalence of 2–3%.
- The etiology of psoriasis includes the interaction of genetic predisposition, environmental triggers and immune system dysregulation.
- Understanding epidemiology and etiology is essential for developing effective treatments and improving patient outcomes.

REFERENCES

1. Parisi R, Symmons DP, Griffiths CE, Ashcroft DM; Identification and Management of Psoriasis and Associated ComorbidiTy (IMPACT) project team. Global epidemiology of psoriasis: a systematic review of incidence and prevalence. J Invest Dermatol. 2013;133(2):377-85.
2. Menter A, Gottlieb A, Feldman SR, Van Voorhees AS, Leonardi CL, Gordon KB, et al. Guidelines of care for the management of psoriasis and psoriatic arthritis. J Am Acad Dermatol. 2008;58(5):826-50.
3. Christophers E. Psoriasis—epidemiology and clinical spectrum. Clin Exp Dermatol. 2001;26(4):314-20.
4. Dogra S, Yadav S. Psoriasis in India: prevalence and pattern. Indian J Dermatol Venereol Leprol. 2010;76(6):595-601.
5. Hellgren L. Psoriasis: The Prevalence in Sex, Age and Occupational Groups in Total Populations in Sweden. Morphology, Inheritance and Association with Other Skin and Rheumatic Diseases. Stockholm: Almquist and Wiksell; 1967.
6. Brandrup F, Green A. The prevalence of psoriasis in Denmark. Acta Derm Venereol. 1981;61:344-6.
7. Tsoi LC, Spain SL, Knight J, Ellinghaus E, Stuart PE, Capon F, et al. Identification of 15 new psoriasis susceptibility loci highlights the role of innate immunity. Nat Genet. 2012;44(12):1341-8.
8. Gudjonsson JE, Elder JT. Psoriasis: epidemiology. Clin Dermatol. 2007;25(6):535-46.
9. Lal S. Clinical pattern of psoriasis in Punjab. Indian J Dermatol Venereol. 1966;32(1):5-12.
10. Verma KC, Bhargava NC. Psoriasis: a clinical and some biochemical investigative study. Indian J Dermatol Venereol Leprol. 1979;45:32-8.
11. Kaur I, Kumar B, Sharma VK, Kaur S. Epidemiology of psoriasis in a clinic from North India. Indian J Dermatol Venereol Leprol. 1986;52:208-12.
12. Sharma T, Sepha GC. Psoriasis—clinical study. Indian J Dermatol Venereol. 1964;30:191-7.
13. Valenzuela F, Silva P, Valdés MP, Papp K. Epidemiology and quality of life of patients with psoriasis in Chile. Actas Dermosifiliogr. 2011;102(10):810-6.
14. Nestle FO, Kaplan DH, Barker J. Psoriasis. N Engl J Med. 2009;361(5):496-509.
15. Gelfand JM, Stern RS, Nijsten T, Feldman SR, Thomas J, Kist J, et al. The prevalence of psoriasis in African Americans: results from a population-based study. J Am Acad Dermatol. 2005;52(1):23-6.
16. Elder JT, Bruce AT, Gudjonsson JE, Johnston A, Stuart PE, Tejasvi T, et al. Molecular dissection of psoriasis: integrating genetics and biology. J Invest Dermatol. 2010;130(5):1213-26.
17. Brandrup F, Holm N, Grunnet N, Henningsen K, Hansen HE. Psoriasis in an unselected series of twins. Arch Dermatol. 1978;114(6):874-8.
18. Strange A, Capon F, Spencer CC, Knight J, Weale ME, Barton A, et al. A genome-wide association study identifies new psoriasis susceptibility loci and an interaction between HLA-C and ERAP1. Nat Genet. 2010;42(11):985-90.
19. Tsoi LC, Spain SL, Knight J, Ellinghaus E, Stuart PE, Capon F, et al. Identification of 15 new psoriasis susceptibility loci highlights the role of innate immunity. Nat Genet. 2012;44(12):1341-8.
20. Capon F, Bijlmakers MJ, Wolf N, Quaranta M, Huffmeier U, Allen M, et al. Identification of ZNF313/RNF114 as a novel psoriasis susceptibility gene. Hum Mol Genet. 2008;17(13):1938-45.
21. Di Meglio P, Villanova F, Nestle FO. Psoriasis. Cold Spring Harb Perspect Med. 2014;4(8):a015354.
22. Lowes MA, Suárez-Fariñas M, Krueger JG. Immunology of psoriasis. Annu Rev Immunol. 2014;32:227-55.
23. Krueger JG, Bowcock A. Psoriasis pathophysiology: current concepts of pathogenesis. Ann Rheum Dis. 2005;64Suppl 2(Suppl 2):ii30-6.

24. Mehta NN, Krueger JG. The immunological basis of psoriasis and its clinical consequences. J Clin Invest. 2014;124(6), 2323-9.
25. Gaffen SL, Lowes MA. IL-17: a key inflammatory cytokine in psoriasis. J Clin Invest. 2008;118(5):1657-65.
26. Papp KA, Langley RG, Lebwohl M, Krueger GG, Szapary P, Yeilding N, et al. Efficacy and safety of ustekinumab, a human interleukin-12/23 monoclonal antibody, in patients with psoriasis: 52-week results from a randomised, double-blind, placebo-controlled trial (PHOENIX 2). Lancet. 2012;371(9625):1675-84.
27. Telfer NR, Chalmers RJ, Whale K, Colman G. The role of streptococcal infection in the initiation of guttate psoriasis. Arch Dermatol. 1992;128(1):39-42.
28. Schon MP, Boehncke WH. Psoriasis. N Engl J Med. 2005;352(18):1899-912.
29. Felix RH, Ive FA, Dahl MG. Cutaneous and ocular reactions to practolol. Br Med J. 1974;4(5940):321-4.
30. Roland MGM, Stevenson CJ. Exfoliative dermatitis and practolol. Lancet. 1972;1:1130.
31. Leonard JC. Letter. Oxprenolol and a psoriasis-like eruption. Lancet. 1975;1(7907):630.
32. Brauchli YB, Jick SS, Curtin F, Meier CR. Association between beta-blockers, other antihypertensive drugs and psoriasis: population-based case-control study. Br J Dermatol. 2008;158(6):1299-307.
33. Wolk K, Mallbris L, Larsson P, Rosenblad A, Vingård E, Ståhle M. Excessive body weight and smoking associates with a high risk of onset of plaque psoriasis. Acta Derm Venereol. 2009;89(5):492-7.
34. Naldi L, Chatenoud L, Linder D, Belloni Fortina A, Peserico A, Virgili AR, et al. Cigarette smoking, body mass index, and stressful life events as risk factors for psoriasis: results from an Italian case-control study. J Invest Dermat. 2005;125(1):61-7.
35. Poikolainen K, Reunala T, Karvonen J. Smoking, alcohol and life events related to psoriasis among women. Br J Dermatol. 1994;130(4):473-7.
36. Jensen P, Zachariae C, Christensen R, Geiker NR, Schaadt BK, Stender S, et al. Effect of weight loss on the severity of psoriasis: a randomized clinical study. JAMA Dermatol. 2014;149(7):795-801.
37. Naldi L. Psoriasis and smoking: links and risks. J Eur Acad Dermatol Venereol. 2012;26(7):813-9.
38. Herron MD, Hinckley M, Hoffman MS, Papenfuss J, Hansen CB, Callis KP, et al. Impact of obesity and smoking on psoriasis presentation and management. Arch Dermatol. 2005;141(12):1527-34.
39. Yosipovitch G, Tang MB. Seasonal changes in the prevalence of psoriasis. Clin Exp Dermatol. 2002;27(8):700-4.
40. Weatherhead SC, Farr PM, Jamieson D. Comparison of narrow-band UV-B phototherapy and UV-B photochemotherapy in the treatment of psoriasis. J Am Acad Dermatol. 2011;65(1):170-1.
41. Harvima IT, Viinamaki H, Naukkavinen A, Paukkonen K, Neittaanmäki H, Harvima RJ, et al. Association of cutaneous mast cells and sensory nerves with psychic stress in psoriasis. Psychother Psychosom. 1993;60(3-4):168-76.
42. Glinski W, Brodecka H, Glinska-Ferenz M, Kowalski D. Neuropeptides in psoriasis: possible role of beta-endorphin in the patho-mechanism of the disease. Int J Dermatol. 1994;33(5):356-60.
43. Zachariae R, Zachariae C, Lei U, Pedersen AF, Zederkopff J. Effect of psychologic intervention on psoriasis: a preliminary report. J Am Acad Dermatol. 2008;59(4):629-35.
44. Nair RP, Stuart PE, Nistor I, Hiremagalore R, Chia NV, Jenisch S, et al. Sequence and haplotype analysis supports HLA-C as the psoriasis susceptibility 1 gene. Am J Hum Genet. 2006;78(5):827-51.
45. Baker H, Ryan TJ. Generalized pustular psoriasis: a clinical and epidemiological study of 104 cases. Br J Dermatol. 1968;80(12):772-93.
46. Celoria V, Rosset F, Pala V, Dapavo P, Ribero S, Quaglino P, et al. The Skin Microbiome and Its Role in Psoriasis: A Review. Psoriasis (Auckl). 2023;13:71-8.

Clinical Manifestations of Psoriasis: Plaque, Guttate, Pustular, Erythrodermic, and Inverse Psoriasis

Kethireddi Susmitha Divya, Susmitha Meda

INTRODUCTION

Psoriasis is a papulosquamous disorder with variable morphology, distribution, severity, and course involving multiple systems. It can present in any age-group with a bimodal distribution. The mean age of onset for the first peak ranges from 15 to 20 years and for the second peak is 55–60 years. The clinical course is marked by relapses and remissions with various triggers like winter season, stress, smoking, alcohol, pregnancy, and drugs like beta blockers, lithium, antimalarials, imiquimod, angiotensin-converting enzyme inhibitors, and interferons. The most common signs of psoriasis are erythema, scaling, and induration. The various patterns of psoriasis are given in the following text **(Box 1)**.

> **BOX 1: Clinical spectrum of psoriasis.**
> - *Generalized*:
>   - Plaque psoriasis
>   - Guttate psoriasis
>   - Erythrodermic psoriasis
>   - Pustular psoriasis
> - *Regional*:
>   - Palmoplantar psoriasis
>   - Scalp psoriasis
>   - Flexural (inverse) psoriasis
>   - Genital psoriasis
>   - Oral mucosa
>   - Ocular
>   - Erythrodermic psoriasis
>   - Nail psoriasis
> - *Rare variants*:
>   - Follicular psoriasis
>   - Linear psoriasis

PLAQUE PSORIASIS

- Chronic plaque psoriasis, also known as psoriasis vulgaris is the most common form of psoriasis in which patients may have sharply circumscribed, round–oval, or nummular (coin-sized) plaques with silvery white scales **(Fig. 1)** characteristically present over the extensor aspects of the extremities, especially the elbows and knees, along with scalp, lower lumbosacral, buttocks, and genital involvement. The umbilicus and the intergluteal cleft are also commonly involved areas. The silvery white scale is due to the reflection of light at the keratin–air interface between layers of skin. The progression of the disease varies from person to person. The lesions usually begin as erythematous macules (flat and <1 cm) or papules, extend peripherally, and coalesce to form plaques of diameter varying from one to several centimeters.
- A zone of hypopigmentation around the lesion known as *Woronoff's ring* **(Fig. 2)**, may be observed in the skin surrounding a psoriatic plaque. Few authors reported association of Woronoff's ring with

Molluscum contagiosum.[1] The reasons proposed for this Woronoff's ring are:
- Interleukin 17 (IL-17) and tumor necrosis factor alpha (TNF-α) increase the proliferation of melanocytes but inhibit melanogenesis.
- Deficiency of prostaglandin E2
- Treatment with corticosteroids/ultraviolet (UV) rays

Zone of immunity locale is the central portion that resolves in a psoriatic plaque and is refractory to the experimental induction of psoriasis.

With a gradual peripheral extension, plaques may develop different configurations as described in **Table 1**.

Few variants of psoriasis develop thick lesions and **Table 2** describes the hyperkeratotic variants of psoriasis.

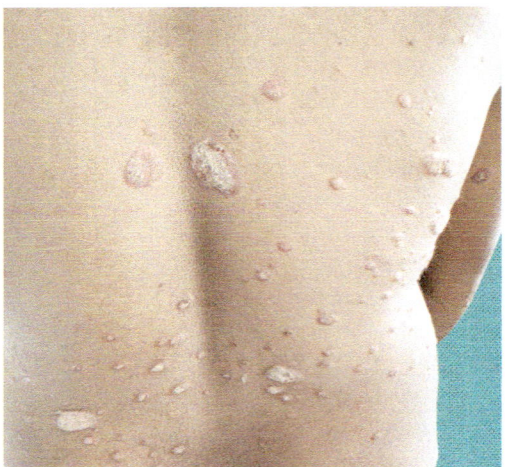

FIG. 1: Psoriasis vulgaris.

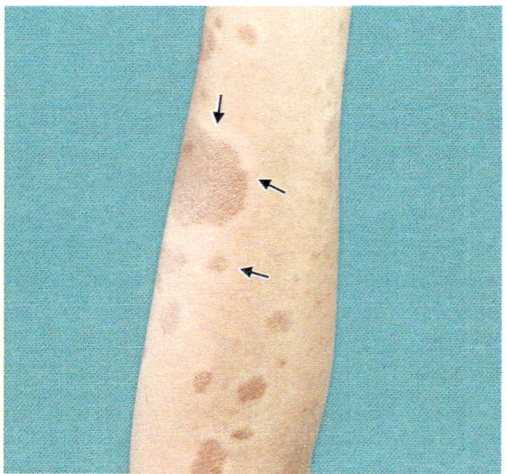

FIG. 2: Woronoff's ring.

TABLE 1: Variants of chronic plaque psoriasis

Variants of chronic plaque psoriasis	Clinical features
Nummular psoriasis	Coin-sized lesions
Annular psoriasis	Ring-like lesions develop with central clearing
Psoriasis gyrata	Curved linear patterns predominate, caused by fusions of annular lesions, resulting in a gyrate appearance
Psoriasis geographica	Large-sized lesions

TABLE 2: Hyperkeratotic variants

Variant	Description	Key features
Elephantine psoriasis	Presents with large, thick, hyperkeratotic plaques on trunk/lower limbs	Dense, heavy scaling; large plaques
Rupioid psoriasis	Small plaques (2–5 cm) with highly hyperkeratotic, conical scales	Heaped-up, peaked scales resembling limpet shells
Ostraceous psoriasis	Hyperkeratotic plaques with concave centers	Resembles oyster shells; thicker borders with central depression
Psoriasis verrucosa	Verrucous papules along psoriatic lesions	• Dome-shaped papules with a keratotic plug • Crater-shaped papules with central depression

CHAPTER 2: Clinical Manifestations of Psoriasis: Plaque, Guttate, Pustular, Erythrodermic, and...

The most common dermoscopic features of the lesions were light, erythematous background; red, dotted vessels in regular distribution **(Figs. 3A and B)**; red globular rings; twisted loops; and glomerular or bushy vessels;[2] diffuse white scales; patchy scale distribution; pigmentary changes; and pearly white structures (PWS).[3]

Auspitz Sign

Auspitz sign **(Fig. 4)** is named after Heinrich Auspitz and is a bedside diagnostic test to confirm psoriasis. The steps in eliciting the Auspitz sign are described in **Flowchart 1**.

The reasons for the Auspitz sign are:
- Parakeratosis, suprapapillary thinning of the stratum malpighii
- Elongation of dermal papillae
- Dilatation and tortuosity of the papillary capillaries

Auspitz sign is neither sensitive as it is absent in inverse, pustular, erythrodermic, and guttate variants of psoriasis, nor specific as it is seen in Darrier's disease and actinic keratosis.[4]

Dermoscopic Auspitz Sign

Appreciation of vascular pattern of regular, dotted vessels and tiny, red blood drops after removal of the scale under dermoscopy is known as dermoscopic Auspitz sign **(Fig. 5)**, which helps in the diagnosis of psoriasis, without actually having to induce bleeding and causing significant pain or discomfort to the patient.[5]

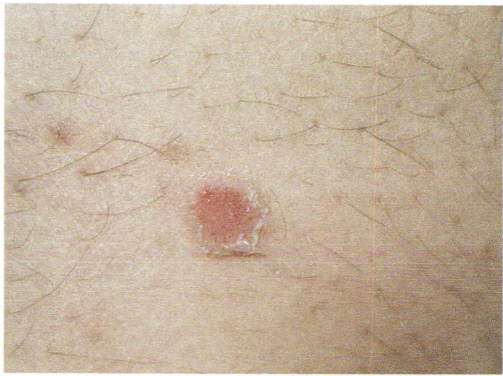

FIG. 4: Auspitz sign showing bleeding points after removal of the Bulkeley's membrane.

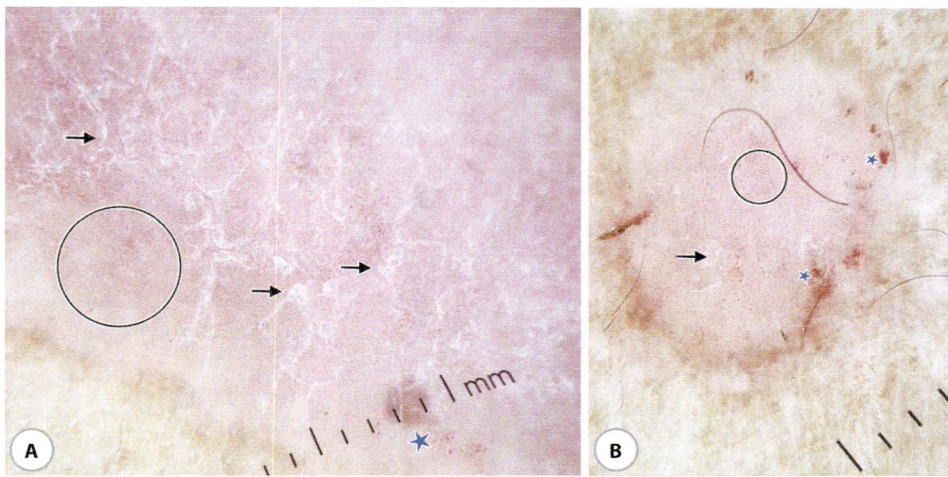

FIGS. 3A AND B: Dermoscopy of psoriasis vulgaris. (A) Regularly arranged red dots (circle), red globules (blue stars) over the pinkish background, white scales (black arrow) (DermLite DL4, nonpolarized mode); and (B) regularly arranged red dots (circle), red globules (blue stars) over a pinkish background, white scales (black arrow) (DermLite DL4, nonpolarized mode, shot with Samsung S22 Plus with 3× magnification).

CHAPTER 2: Clinical Manifestations of Psoriasis: Plaque, Guttate, Pustular, Erythrodermic, and...

> Scraping the lesion with a slide (Grattage test), results in the removal of silvery white scales, which can be easily scraped off from the surface as shaving off the candle wax described as Candle sign or Wax spot phenomenon *(Signe de la tache de bougie)*. This is due to parakeratotic hyperkeratosis

↓

> After the scales are completely scraped off, subsequently a surface membrane is exposed and is seen as a moist red surface called as membrane of Bulkeley which is the stratum mucosum (basement membrane)—this is known as *Sign of the last Hautchen* (last membrane phenomenon)

↓

> The lesion remains dry until this last level is reached which will also come off as a whole through which dilated capillaries at the tip of elongated dermal papillae are torn, leading to multiple pinpoint bleeding points (Auspitz sign)

FLOWCHART 1: Steps in eliciting the Auspitz sign.

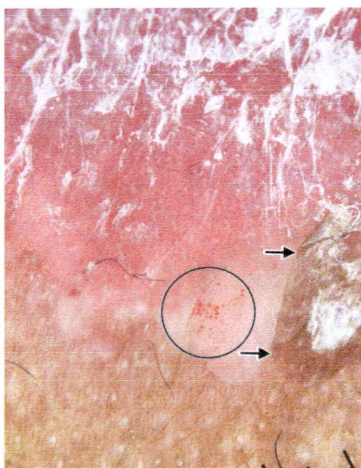

FIG. 5: Dermoscopic Auspitz sign. The scales and Bulkeley's membrane (black arrow) are scrapped to reveal the more clearly visualized dotted vessels seen as red globules [tiny, red blood drops (circle)] (DermLite DL4, nonpolarized mode, shot on Samsung S22 Plus 3× magnification).

Koebner Phenomenon

The appearance of isomorphic lesions along the line of trauma on previously unaffected skin is known as Koebner or isomorphic phenomenon. 11–75% has been the reported incidence of psoriasis demonstrating Koebner response. The psoriatic lesions at the sites with high mechanical tension such as elbows and knees are currently thought to indicate the Koebner phenomenon.

It is most commonly seen in the acute/eruptive stage/progressive stage or when psoriasis is unstable and flaring and is less likely to quiescent or resolving psoriasis. It occurs more frequently in the winter than in the summer.[6] The incubation period from skin injury to the onset of the Koebner phenomenon is not determined. In psoriasis, Koebner phenomenon usually appears within 10–14 days but can also occur as early as 3 days or as late as 2 years.[7]

Various forms of cutaneous injury, such as excoriations, tattoos, friction, trauma, surgical instrumentation, burns, and exposure to UV or irradiation, can induce this phenomenon. More extensive injury may result in more severe skin lesions. The response's severity also varies, and can be categorized into four grades:[7]

1. None
2. Abortive (lesions disappearing spontaneously within about 2 weeks)
3. Minimal (localized lesions near the injury site)
4. Maximal (extensive lesions)

Koebner phenomenon shows an "all or none" reactivity pattern.

Reverse or Negative Koebner Phenomenon

It refers to the disappearance of existing lesions after local trauma. This is due to the pressure, which leads to the occlusion of cutaneous vessels resulting in the clearing of lesions.

Renbök Phenomenon

The disappearance of a primary lesion when a different condition appears concurrently at the same location; Bon et al. observed that a patient with alopecia areata began to show hair growth locally after psoriatic lesions on the scalp and proposed the Renbök phenomenon to describe this phenomenon.[8] Inflammation in psoriasis may antagonize the alopecia areata inflammatory reactions as different T-helper (Th) inflammatory subsets result in the competition between these two immune-related diseases.

Deep Koebner Phenomenon

The flexor tendon pulleys are subjected to very high physical stress, which makes them thickened and contributes to psoriatic arthritis (PsA)-related tenosynovitis and dactylitis and these excessive repair responses in the pulleys support the idea of "deep Koebner" phenomenon in PsA.[9]

■ GUTTATE PSORIASIS

Guttate psoriasis, meaning *"droplet"* in Greek, presents as multiple 2–10 mm erythematous, scaly lesions, ranging from 5 to over 100, with cephalocaudal distribution primarily on the trunk **(Fig. 6)**. In early lesions, the scale is subtle. The face, scalp, and ear lesions tend to be faint and short-lived. Palms and soles are usually spared.

Guttate psoriasis is strongly associated with HLA-Cw6, it typically follows beta-hemolytic streptococcal pharyngeal infection, severe acute respiratory syndrome coronavirus 2 (SARS-CoV-2), or other viral infections such as coxsackievirus.[10] Accounting for 2% of psoriasis cases, it is usually self-limiting in children but may complicate chronic plaque disease in adults.

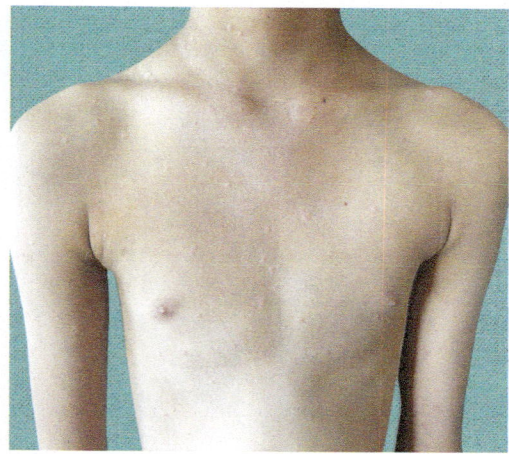

FIG. 6: Guttate psoriasis.

There are three stages of guttate psoriasis:[11]
1. *Mild*: Only a few spots cover about 3% of the skin.
2. *Moderate*: Lesions cover about 3–10% of skin.
3. *Severe*: Lesions cover 10% or more of the body and could cover the entire body.

Dermoscopy of guttate psoriasis[12] shows uniformly distributed red, dotted vessels with bright red, dull red, or pink background on which a diffuse white–gray scales are seen.

■ ERYTHRODERMIC PSORIASIS

Erythrodermic psoriasis (EP) is a severe variant of psoriasis vulgaris, with an estimated prevalence of 1–2.25% among psoriatic patients.[13] Body surface area involvement >90% is known as erythroderma **(Figs. 7A and B)**.

Psoriatic erythroderma can be a result of the progression of chronic plaque psoriasis or unstable psoriasis becoming generalized by factors like sudden withdrawal of oral or potent topical corticosteroids, infections, low calcium, excessive alcohol consumption, medications like lithium, antimalarials,

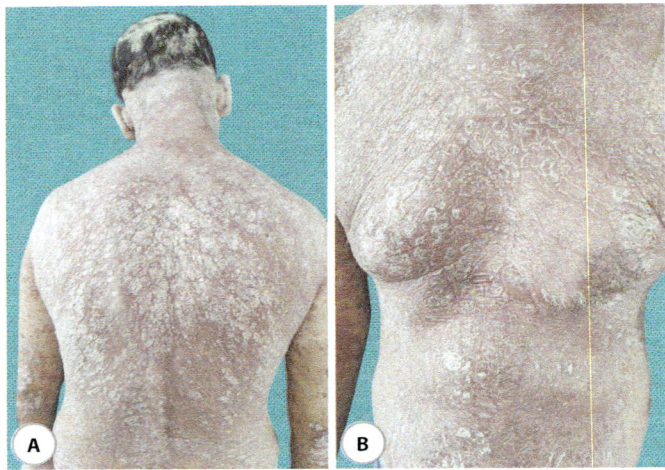

FIGS. 7A AND B: Erythroderma secondary to psoriasis: Erythema and scaling involving (A) the posterior aspect of the trunk and (B) the anterior aspect of the trunk.

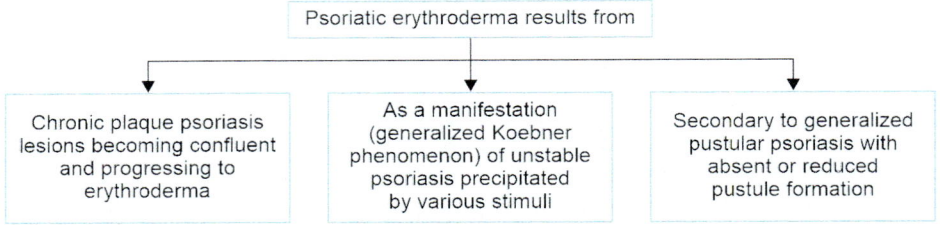

FLOWCHART 2: Pathways leading to psoriatic erythroderma.

etc., or a manifestation of generalized pustular psoriasis (GPP) without pustules **(Flowchart 2)**.

Dermoscopy plays an important role in identifying the cause of erythroderma, as erythroderma secondary to psoriasis can show a regular distribution of red dots on a fairly homogenous, reddish background with white scales **(Fig. 8)**.[14]

Pavithran's nose sign is the sparing of the nose and perinasal skin in patients with erythroderma. *Dermatopathic lymphadenopathy or lipomelanotic reticulosis or Pautrier-Woringer disease* is a generalized and benign enlargement of lymph nodes commonly seen in erythroderma. The complications of erythroderma secondary to psoriasis are described in **Table 3**.

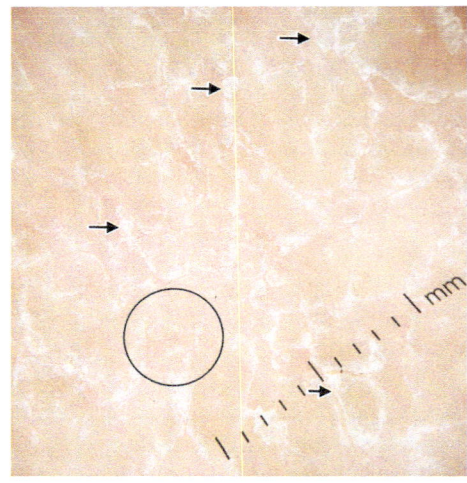

FIG. 8: Dermoscopy of erythroderma secondary to psoriasis showing multiple uniformly arranged red dots on a pinkish background (circle), diffuse white scales (black arrows) (DermLite DL4, nonpolarized mode).

PUSTULAR PSORIASIS

Pustular psoriasis is an immune-mediated variant with systemic association, presenting with multiple sterile pustules on an erythematous background, which can be widespread or localized, are sterile with predominant neutrophilic infiltrate, and are often tender to palpation.[15] Risk factors like sudden withdrawal of systemic steroids, infections, electrolyte imbalance, hypocalcemia (i.e., von Zumbusch subtype), medications (lithium, iodine, penicillin, interferon alpha, etc.), pregnancy (i.e., impetigo herpetiformis), and phototherapy and vaccinations (BCG and H1N1) may result in precipitation of pustular psoriasis.

The pustular psoriasis is divided based on the distribution and morphology of lesions into the following:
- *Generalized*:
  - Acute GPP or von Zumbusch subtype: It is characterized by sudden onset of burning sensation and erythema, on which pustules occur either de novo or over existing psoriatic plaques. The pustules appear in crops, coalescing to form the lake of pus that later exfoliates. Oral mucosal changes include geographic tongue. Apart from other psoriatic nail changes, subungual pustules causing onycholysis, onychomadesis, and destruction of the nail plate are seen in pustular psoriasis.

Generalized pustular psoriasis is associated with systemic symptoms like high-grade fever, severe malaise, and arthralgias. Acute kidney injury as well as cardiovascular shock is precipitated by increased water loss and dehydration. Malabsorption and sudden diffusion of plasma proteins into tissues cause hypoalbuminemia and precipitate hypocalcemia. Arthritis, uveitis, otitis media, and epigastric pain are the other manifestations. Postinflammatory

TABLE 3: Complications of erythroderma secondary to psoriasis

Category	Description	Consequences
Cutaneous impact	Impairment of thermoregulation	Hypothermia
	Reduced sweating due to eccrine duct occlusion	Hyperpyrexia
	Impaired barrier function	Increased percutaneous absorption, requiring caution with topical agents
Cardiovascular impact	High output cardiac failure due to increased blood flow	Tachycardia, high volume collapsing pulse, capillary pulsation, elevated jugular venous pressure (JVP), high pulse pressure, cardiomegaly, systolic murmur
Nutritional impact	Dermatogenic enteropathy	Leading to malabsorption and secondary deficiencies
	Loss of large quantities of epidermal scales (the amount of protein loss may reach up to 9 g/m^2 of body surface area or more whereas the normal exfoliated skin amounts to 500–1,000 mg/day)	Loss of protein, iron, vitamin B12, and folate, causing anemia
	Hypoalbuminemia from protein loss	Limb edema, hypocalcemia
Renal impact	Decreased renal blood flow	Oliguria
Others	Immobility	Deep venous thrombosis and pulmonary embolism

hyperpigmentation, telogen effluvium, and amyloidosis may occur as late sequelae.

- Annular subtype: Characterized by lesions that start with discrete areas of erythema, later becoming edematous and raised with slow central clearing as shown in **(Fig. 9)**; pustules appear on the advancing edge of the lesion, which leaves behind a trail of scales on drying. The systemic symptoms are usually not seen. It may also be a common presentation of pustular psoriasis during infancy and early childhood. Recurrent circinate erythematous psoriasis is a variant without pustulation, but histopathologically spongiform pustules are noticed.
- Exanthematic subtype: It is an acute pustular eruption without any systemic symptoms that resolves after a few days.
- Impetigo herpetiformis: Pustular psoriasis occurring during pregnancy. It is most commonly seen in the third trimester, though cases occurring as early as the first month of gestation have been reported. Remission is seen in the postpartum period. It tends to relapse with subsequent pregnancies, with the disease occurring earlier and being associated with more morbidity in subsequent pregnancies. It may occur de novo or with previous psoriatic history. The lesions start in the inguinal–genital folds and then can progress to involve the whole body, showing a picture similar to GPP. Other constitutional symptoms like fever, arthralgia, malaise, tachycardia, diarrhea, and seizures may be seen. Pustular psoriasis occurring in pregnancy can be classified into two distinct subsets. First, GPP of pregnancy, which is mostly seen in patients who already have a history of pustular psoriasis or psoriasis vulgaris. Here the lesions are more generalized and associated with systemic abnormalities, as seen in GPP. The second variant, which is the true impetigo herpetiformis, occurs for the first time during pregnancy and recurs with each successive pregnancy.

- *Localized*:
  - Acrodermatitis continua of Hallopeau: Pustules affecting the fingers, toes, and nail beds; it usually starts as painful erythema at the tip of the digit, followed by painful pustules around and below the nail bed and matrix, causing onychodystrophy and anonychia. Acrodermatitis continua of Hallopeau is a more aggressive disease with intermittent eruptions without periods of complete remission, a more generalized disease, and progressive worsening of the disease characterized by acro-osteolysis. A more benign form described by Radcliffe and Crocker is termed as dermatitis repens or acropustulosis repens. It is a more localized form characterized by one or a few pustules on fingers and toes, with asymptomatic phases between the flares, and without any permanent structural damage.

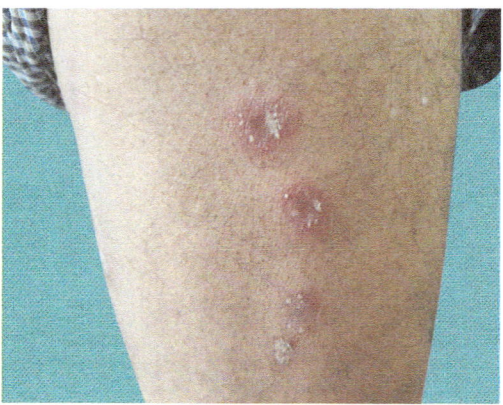

FIG. 9: Pustular psoriasis.

- Palmoplantar pustulosis: Pustules affecting the palms and soles; cigarette smoking is strongly associated. This can be seen as part of SAPHO syndrome.

Dermoscopy of pustular psoriasis shows regular red dots and micropustules on the erythematous background. Bright white superficial scales are seen arranged diffusely over the entire lesion. The distribution of micropustules will be nonfollicular in position as seen in **Figure 10A**. Dermoscopy of nail in pustular psoriasis shows whitish round globules representing micropustules (nonfollicular) over the erythematous background as shown in **Figure 10B**.

PALMOPLANTAR PSORIASIS

Psoriasis characteristically affecting palms and soles is called as palmoplantar psoriasis. It features hyperkeratotic **(Fig. 11)**, pustular, or mixed morphologies. It is a multifactorial variant with genetic and environmental triggers. Environmental triggers include

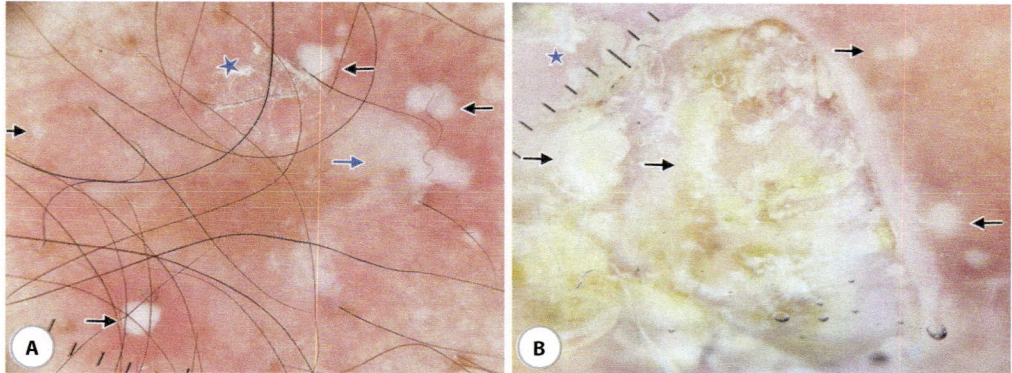

FIGS. 10A AND B: (A) Dermoscopy of pustular psoriasis; whitish, round globules representing micropustules (nonfollicular) (black arrow) over erythematous background, white superficial scales (blue star), few pustules coalesced to form lakes of pus seen as white lacunae (blue star) (DermLite DL4, nonpolarized mode); and (B) dermoscopy of nail in pustular psoriasis; whitish, round globules (black arrow) representing micropustules (nonfollicular) over an erythematous background, scaling (blue star) (DermLite DL4, polarized mode, contact with the gel).

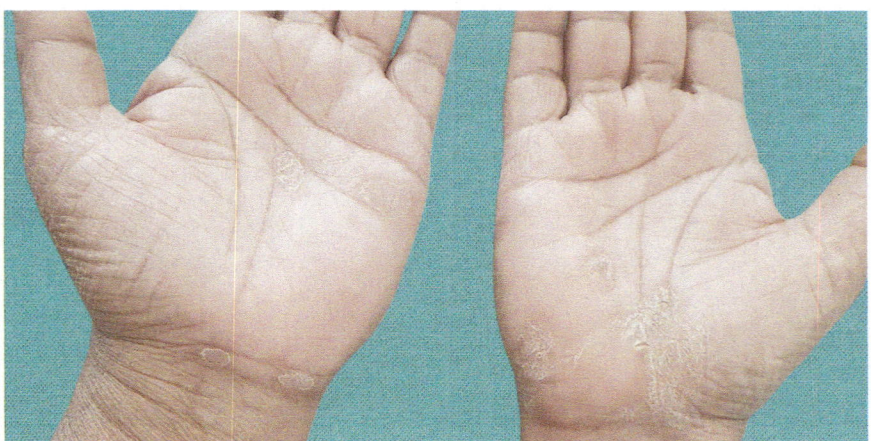

FIG. 11: Palmar psoriasis.

smoking, irritants, friction, and manual or repetitive trauma. Paradoxically, anti-TNF-α agents have been shown to induce palmoplantar eruptions.

Dermoscopy of palmoplantar psoriasis shows regular, dotted vessels **(Fig. 12)**, Yu et al. found that beaded, dotted vessels along sulci cutis is an important finding in psoriasis, which is not seen in palmoplantar eczema.[16]

SCALP PSORIASIS

Scalp psoriasis affects 80% of psoriatic patients, presenting as red, thickened plaques with silvery white scales **(Fig. 13)**, which may be localized or can involve the entire scalp and may extend to the forehead (corona psoriatica), neck, or ears. Itching and flaking are common, causing embarrassment as this is a chronic, relapsing condition. Scaling may pile up and produce an appearance of overlapping roof tiles (pityriasis amiantacea) and may cause temporary localized hair loss in severe cases.

With dermoscopy **(Fig. 14A)**:
- *At low magnification*:
  - Red dots and globules with regular distribution are observed.
  - White/white–silver dry scales are a very frequent finding
  - Hidden hair and signet ring vessels are recently reported signs supporting the diagnosis of psoriasis.
- *At high magnification*:
  - Glomerular vessels arranged into rings or lines
  - Linear looped as seen in **(Fig. 14B)**, lace-like, and comma vessels are other vessel patterns observed.

FLEXURAL (INVERSE) PSORIASIS

This presentation is called "inverse" as lesions are localized to skinfolds and is the reverse of the typical presentation of plaque psoriasis on extensor surfaces. It may also be seen in individuals with plaque psoriasis elsewhere in the body. Common sites of flexural psoriasis are the axilla, groin, under the breasts **(Fig. 15)**, umbilicus, penis, vulva, natal cleft, and around the anus.

Flexural lesions are red, shiny, well-demarcated plaques without scaling and may be confused with candidal intertrigo and dermatophyte infections.

Complications of flexural psoriasis include:
- Constant rubbing due to irritation from heat and sweat
- Secondary fungal infections mostly candidiasis

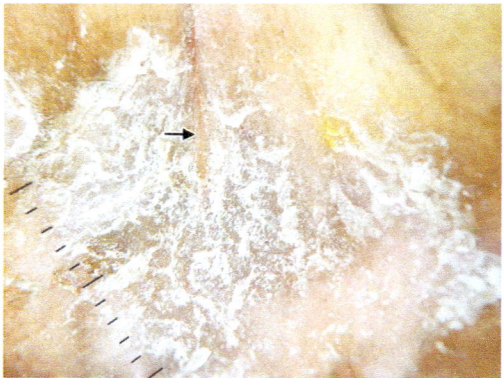

FIG. 12: Beaded, dotted vessels are seen as red dots (black arrow) along sulci cutis (DermLite DL4, nonpolarized mode).

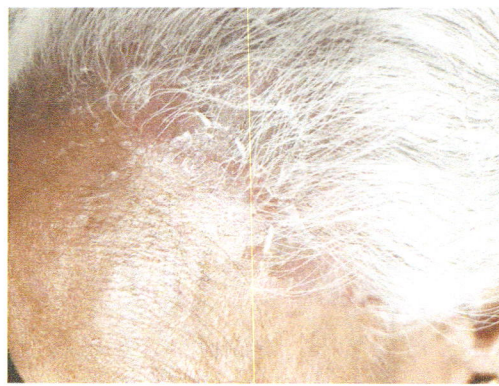

FIG. 13: Scalp psoriasis.

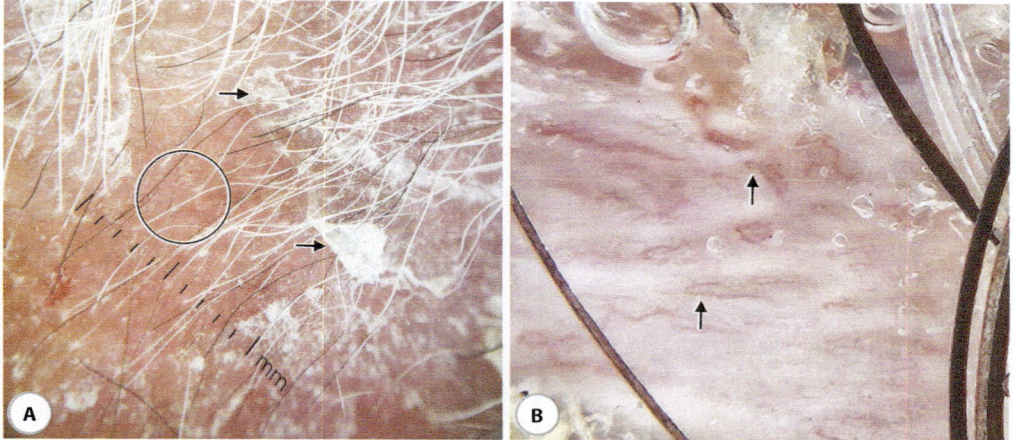

FIGS. 14A AND B: (A) Dermoscopy of scalp psoriasis: (A) Interfollicular, white scales (black arrow), red dots in regular distribution after removal of scales (circle), normal hair shaft (DermLite DL4, nonpolarized mode); and (B) linear, looped vessels (black arrow) (DermLite DL4, polarized mode shot on Samsung S22 Plus 10× magnification).

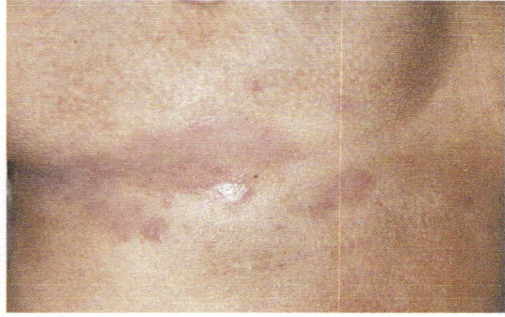

FIG. 15: Flexural psoriasis.

- Lichenification due to repeated scratching, particularly around the anus where fecal material irritates causing increased itching
- Sexual difficulties because of embarrassment and discomfort
- Thinned skin due to long-term overuse of strong topical steroid creams
- *Abramowitz sign*: Redness and maceration of the natal cleft

Low magnification of dermoscopy **(Figs. 16A and B)** shows the "red dots" distributed homogeneously on an erythematous background with less prominent scaling in comparison with chronic plaque psoriasis.

Red dots appear as typical "bushes" of convoluted capillaries at higher magnification.[17]

■ GENITAL PSORIASIS

Psoriasis of the external genitalia and perianal area often presents as well-demarcated, bright red, thin plaques. These usually lack scale, as friction between the skin surfaces rubs it off, but scaling may be seen on the outer aspect of the genital skin, which can be easily scraped off, leaving pinpoint bleeding.

In women, vulval psoriasis appears symmetrical with silvery, scaly patches adjacent to the labia majora and moist, grayish plaques or glossy, red plaques without scaling in the skinfolds.

In men, the shaft of penis, especially the glans **(Fig. 17)**, and corona are involved. In circumcised men, plaques can be scalier than uncircumcised.

Napkin psoriasis in children presents as erythematous plaques with silvery scales and well-defined borders in the nappy area. It usually resolves within a few months to a year but may later generalize into plaque

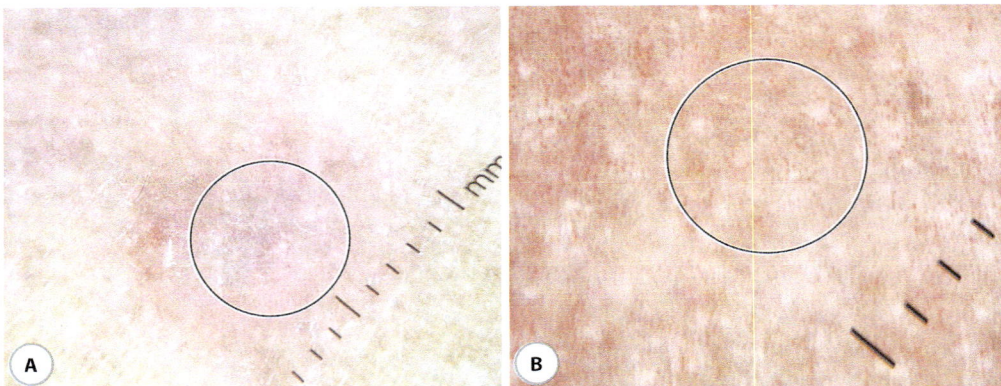

FIGS. 16A AND B: Dermoscopy of flexural psoriasis; (A) regularly arranged red dots, scaling is less prominent when compared to classical psoriatic plaque in extensor surfaces (DermLite DL4, nonpolarized mode); and (B) regularly arranged red dots, scaling is less prominent when compared to classical psoriatic plaque in extensor surfaces (DermLite DL4, polarized mode, contact with the gel and magnified by 3× with Samsung S22 Plus).

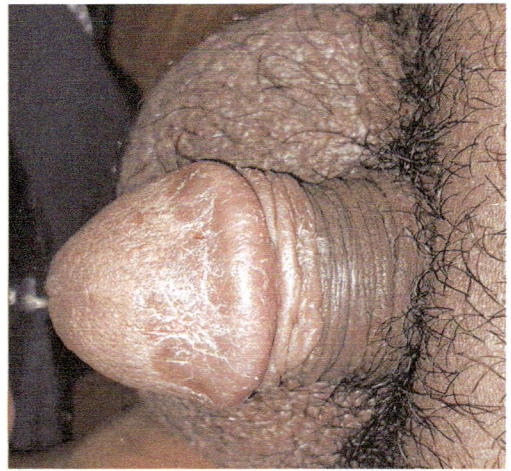

FIG. 17: Genital psoriasis.

psoriasis. The plaques can be itchy, fissured, and painful.[18]

On dermoscopy, homogeneously distributed, dilated, and dotted vessels on an erythematous background are seen.

■ ORAL MUCOSA

The changes in oral mucosa are not very common in psoriasis but are seen in severe variants like pustular psoriasis. Irregular, red patches with raised white borders commonly known as geographic tongue or annulus migrans or erythema migrans or benign migratory glossitis is the most common change observed. Other findings are redness of oral mucosa, ulcers, desquamative gingivitis, and pustules.

■ OCULAR

Common ocular manifestations in psoriasis include blepharitis, dry eyes, conjunctivitis, keratitis, UV-associated cataracts, and retinal pathologies. Blepharitis is the most prevalent, with dry eye, hyperemic conjunctiva, cicatricial entropion, and ectropion also reported. Bilateral cataracts unrelated to steroid use and uveitis, especially acute anterior uveitis in psoriatic arthritis, are also noted.[19]

■ NAIL PSORIASIS

Nail involvement is a visible indicator to predict future joint inflammatory damages and disease activity. Nail psoriasis can manifest clinically as a wide variety of nail changes **(Fig. 18)**, depending upon the part of the nail units involved and the corresponding histopathology, which is described in **Tables 4 and 5**.

Dermoscopic features **(Fig. 19)** of nail psoriasis are dilated hyponychial capillaries, pseudofiber sign, nail plate thickening and crumbling, transverse grooves, fuzzy and mottled lunula, subungual hyperkeratosis, splinter hemorrhages, pitting, onycholysis, salmon patches, leukonychia, and lunular red spots. A recent study defined longitudinal erythema of the nail bed and dilated nail bed capillaries, in addition to peripheral white halos around red spots, dilated nail bed capillaries, and salmon patches, as unique dermoscopic features of nail psoriasis.[20]

■ FOLLICULAR PSORIASIS

Follicular psoriasis affects adults more commonly than children and has no sexual predilection.

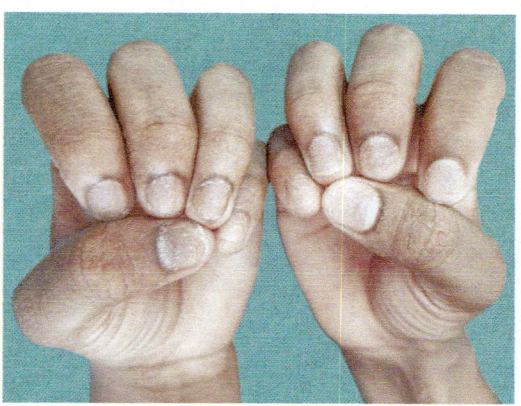

FIG. 18: Nail psoriasis.

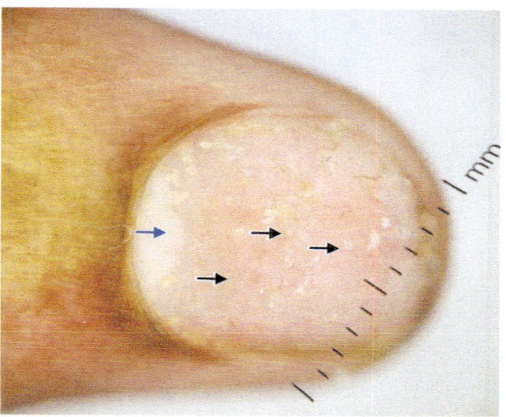

FIG. 19: Dermoscopy of nail psoriasis; pitting (black arrow), fuzzy lunula (blue arrow) (DermLite DL4, nonpolarized mode).

TABLE 4: Nail changes according to the area of involvement	
Nail affected area	**Nail changes**
Proximal nail matrix	• Pitting **(Fig. 19)** • Beau's line, onychorrhexis
Intermediate and distal matrix	Leukonychia
Distal matrix	Erythema of lunula, focal onycholysis, thinned nail plate
Nail bed	Oil drop sign/salmon patch, splinter hemorrhages
Nail bed and hyponychium	Subungual hyperkeratosis, onycholysis
Nail plate	Crumbling and destruction
Proximal and lateral nail folds	Psoriatic changes in skin

TABLE 5: Nail changes with corresponding histological finding	
Clinical signs	**Histological findings**
Pitting	Rapid parakeratotic columns in proximal matrix
Oil drop sign/salmon patch	Exocytosis of leukocytes beneath nail plate
Splinter hemorrhages	Increased capillary damage (fragility) in nail bed
Olfeck phenomenon (brownish red lesion visible through nail plate)	Accumulation of parakeratotic material in nail bed

Among the two clinical subtypes, the adult form commonly affects females and presents as multiple, discrete, follicle-based, hyperkeratotic papules predominantly over the thigh. The second type commonly affects children and presents as asymmetric, grouped, follicular, and keratotic papules predominantly affecting the trunk, axilla, and extensor aspect of limbs **(Fig. 20)**.

Dermoscopic examination reveals **(Figs. 21A to C)** a white-brown background/homogenous area, normal-looking terminal

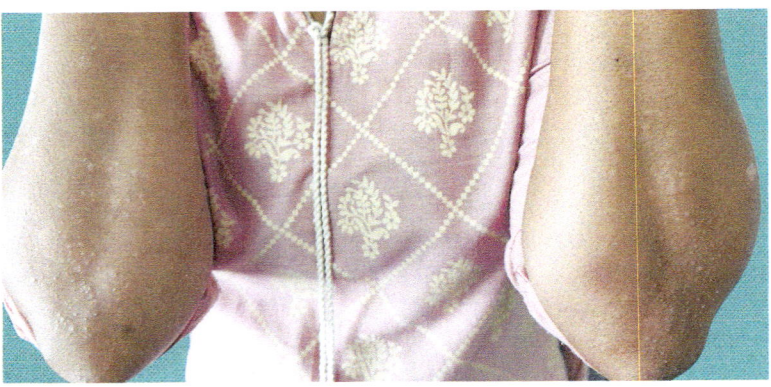

FIG. 20: Follicular psoriasis.

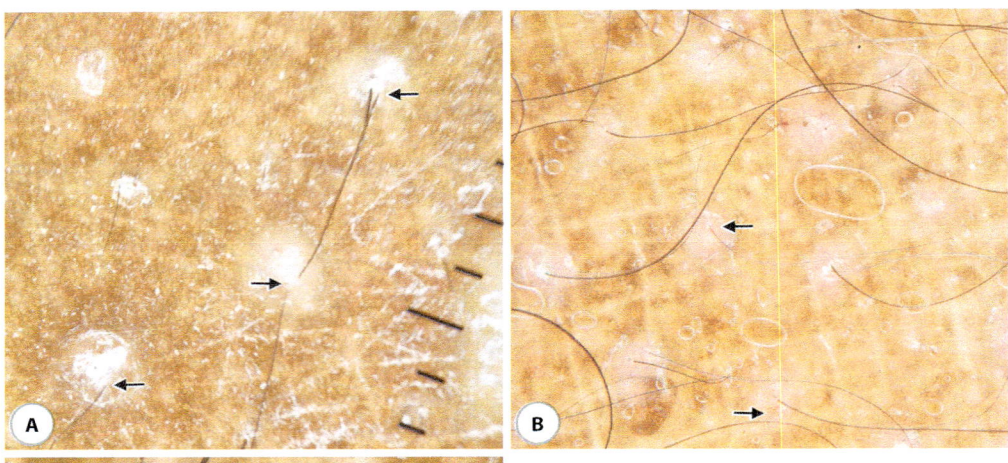

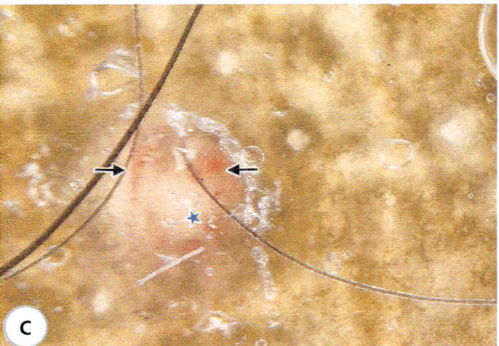

FIGS. 21A TO C: Dermoscopy of follicular psoriasis showing (A) normal-looking terminal hair at the center, perifollicular scales (black arrows) (DermLite DL4, nonpolarized mode DermLite DL4, and magnified by 3× with Samsung S22 Plus); (B) perifollicular homogenous white area with red dots (black arrow) (DermLite DL4, polarized mode, contact with gel and magnified by 3× with Samsung S22 Plus); and (C) the perifollicular homogenous white area (blue star) with red dots and globules (black arrows) (DermLite DL4, polarized mode, contact with the gel and magnified by 10× with Samsung S22 Plus).

hair at the center, perifollicular scaling, multiple red dots/dotted vessels, red globules, twisted red loops, and glomerular vessels/bushy capillaries.[21]

LINEAR PSORIASIS

Linear psoriasis is characterized by a linear distribution of psoriatic lesions along Blaschko's lines. Happle proposed that linear psoriasis results from somatic recombination of a psoriasis-predisposing gene, causing segmental mosaicism.[22] Inflammatory linear verrucous epidermal nevus (ILVEN) and Koebner response of psoriasis over verrucous epidermal nevus are to be differentiated from linear psoriasis.[23] Keratin 10 is low in psoriasis but normal in ILVEN, while involucrin is present in psoriasis but absent in ILVEN.[24]

The dermoscopic patterns in different types of psoriasis are summarized.

CONCLUSION

This chapter briefs about the clinical variants of psoriasis including morphological and distributional patterns. Well-defined erythematous plaques with silvery white scales are the classical features suggesting psoriasis. Grattage test is the bedside diagnostic test to elicit Auspitz sign for confirming psoriasis. Dermoscopy, being a noninvasive tool helps in diagnosing easily. Severe variants like erythrodermic and pustular psoriasis cause skin failure and are potentially fatal.

TAKE HOME MESSAGE

- Psoriasis is a chronic inflammatory skin condition with diverse clinical presentations, including plaque, guttate, pustular, erythrodermic, inverse, etc. Dermoscopy serves as a valuable adjunct, offering insights into characteristic features like white scaling, red dots, etc which aid in distinguishing psoriasis from its mimics. A thorough understanding of the clinical and dermoscopic features ensures better patient outcomes by facilitating early and accurate diagnosis, tailored treatment, and improved quality of life.

REFERENCES

1. Zawar V, Goyal T, Doda D. Woronoff Ring: A Novel Manifestation of Molluscum Contagiosum. Skinmed. 2016;14(5):349-52.
2. Errichetti E, Stinco G. Dermoscopy in general dermatology: A practical overview. Dermatol Ther (Heidelb). 2016;6:471-507.
3. Nwako-Mohamadi MK, Masenga JE, Mavura D, Jahanpour OF, Mbwilo E, Blum A. Dermoscopic Features of Psoriasis, Lichen Planus, and Pityriasis Rosea in Patients With Skin Type IV and Darker Attending the Regional Dermatology Training Centre in Northern Tanzania. Dermatol Pract Concept. 2019;9(1):44-51.
4. Kangle S, Amladi S, Sawant S. Scaly signs in dermatology. Indian J Dermatol Venereol Leprol. 2006;72:161-4.
5. Kaliyadan F. The Dermoscopic Auspitz Sign. Indian Dermatol Online J. 2018;9(4):290-1.
6. Thappa DM. The isomorphic phenomenon of Koebner, Indian J Dermatol Venereol Leprol. 2004;70:187-9.
7. Sanchez DP, Sonthalia S. Koebner Phenomenon. In: StatPearls [Internet]. Treasure Island (FL): StatPearls Publishing; 2024.
8. Bon AM, Happle R, Itin PH. Renbök phenomenon in alopecia areata. Dermatology. 2000;201(1):49-50.
9. Zhang X, Lei L, Jiang L, Fu C, Huang J, Hu Y, et al. Characteristics and pathogenesis of Koebner phenomenon. Exp Dermatol. 2023;32(4):310-23.
10. Gananandan K, Sacks B, Ewing I. Guttate psoriasis secondary to COVID-19. BMJ Case Rep. 2020;13(8):e237367.
11. WebMD. (2024). Guttate Psoriasis Stages. [online] Available from https://www.webmd.com/skin-problems-and-treatments/psoriasis/guttate-psoriasis#1-4 [Last accessed January 2025].
12. Jindal R, Chauhan P, Sethi S. Dermoscopic characterization of guttate psoriasis, pityriasis rosea, and pityriasis lichenoides chronica in dark skin phototypes: an observational study. Dermatol Ther. 2021;34(1):e14631.

13. Boyd AS, Menter A. Erythrodermic psoriasis. Precipitating factors, course, and prognosis in 50 patients. J Am Acad Dermatol. 1989;21(5 pt 1):985-91.
14. Batra J, Gulati S, Sarangal R, Chopra D, Puri S, Kaur R. Utility of Dermoscopy in the Diagnosis of Erythroderma: A Cross-Sectional Study. Indian Dermatol Online J. 2023;14(6):821-8.
15. Tsuchida Y, Hayashi R, Ansai O, Nakajima M, Oginezawa M, Kawai T, et al. Generalized pustular psoriasis complicated with bullous pemphigoid. Int J Dermatol. 2019;58(3):e66-7.
16. Yu X, Wei G, Shao C, Zhu M, Sun S, Zhang X. Analysis of dermoscopic characteristic for the differential diagnosis of palmoplantar psoriasis and palmoplantar eczema. Medicine (Baltimore). 2021;100(5):e23828.
17. Micali G, Lacarrubba F, Musumeci ML, Massimino D, Nasca MR. Cutaneous vascular patterns in psoriasis. Int J Dermatol. 2010;49(3):249-56.
18. Meeuwis KA, de Hullu JA, Massuger LF, van de Kerkhof PC, van Rossum MM. Genital psoriasis: a systematic literature review on this hidden skin disease. Acta Derm Venereol. 2011;91(1):5-11.
19. Kharolia A, Parija S, Moharana B, Sirka CS, Sahu SK. Ocular manifestations in moderate-to-severe psoriasis in India: A prospective observational study. Indian J Ophthalmol. 2022;70(9):3328-32.
20. Yorulmaz A, Artuz F. A study of dermoscopic features of nail psoriasis. Postepy Dermatol Alergol. 2017;34(1):28-35.
21. Behera B, Gochhait D, Remya R, Resmi MR, Kumari R, Thappa DM. Follicular psoriasis—dermoscopic features at a glance. Indian J Dermatol Venereol Leprol. 2017;83:702-4.
22. Happle R. Somatic recombination may explain linear psoriasis. J Med Genet. 1991;28:337.
23. Morag C, Metzker A. Inflammatory linear verrucous epidermal nevus: Report of seven new cases and review of the literature. Pediatr Dermatol. 1985;3:15-8.
24. Vissers WH, Muys L, Erp PE, de Jong EM, van de Kerkhof PC. Immunohistochemical differentiation between inflammatory linear verrucous epidermal nevus (ILVEN) and psoriasis. Eur J Dermatol. 2004;14(4):216-20.

3

Pathophysiology of Psoriasis: Immune System Dysfunction, Genetics, and Triggers

Bikash Ranjan Kar, Kallolinee Samal

■ INTRODUCTION

Psoriasis is a chronic, systemic, recurrent, immune-mediated, hyperproliferative inflammatory skin disease. The typical psoriatic skin lesions are characterized by sharply demarcated, red papules or plaques with silvery white scales over the surface.[1] Although psoriasis etiology remains unknown, it is believed to be multifactorial with numerous contributing components, including genetic susceptibility, environmental triggers, skin barrier disruption, and immune dysfunction.

Immune-related cells, mainly dendritic cells (DCs) and T helper 17 (Th17) cells, along with toll-like receptors (TLRs) and cytokines [interferon alpha (IFN-α), tumor necrosis factor alpha (TNF-α), IFN-γ, interleukin 12 (IL-12), IL-22, IL-23, and IL-17] play a leading role in the pathogenesis of psoriasis.[2]

Genome-wide association studies (GWAS) have shown around 60 psoriasis susceptibility loci, which largely contribute to disease pathophysiology.[2]

■ TRIGGERS

Triggers for psoriasis, including extrinsic and intrinsic risk factors.[2] All these risk factors can trigger both the onset and the recurrence of psoriasis when they persist for a long time in genetically predisposed individuals **(Fig. 1)**. Tissue-resident memory cells (TRMs) in the skin are responsible for psoriasis recurrence at the affected initial sites. In post-treatment resolved psoriatic lesions, CD8+ TRM and CD4+ TRM are retained within the epidermis and dermis, respectively. Triggering events stimulate DCs and Langerhans cells to release IL-23, which binds to IL-23R TRM cell surface, particularly IL-17-producing CD49a CD103+ CD8+ TRM, resulting in the retention of the inflammatory loops in the psoriatic lesion.[3]

■ INFECTIONS[2]

Various microorganisms have been reported as psoriasis triggers and many efforts have been devoted to clarifying their mechanisms. The pathogens that provoke psoriasis are summarized in **Table 1**.

■ SKIN TRAUMA OR PRESSURE[2,4]

Skin trauma or pressure can lead to psoriasis, the Koebner phenomenon (KP). Self-nucleic acids (dsRNA, ssRNA, and DNA), released by damaged keratinocytes (KCs), act as autoantigens to induce the expression of LL-37 and are recognized by plasmacytoid DCs (pDCs) and TLR7 or TLR9, which leads to the secretion of IFN-α. IFN-α from pDCs and IFN-β from KCs promote the maturation of conventional DCs (cDCs), leading to the pathogenesis of psoriasis. Accumulation and reactivation of TRM cells lead to the recurrence of psoriasis at trauma sites. Mechanical stretch activates ATP (adenosine 5'-triphosphate)

CHAPTER 3: Pathophysiology of Psoriasis: Immune System Dysfunction, Genetics, and Triggers

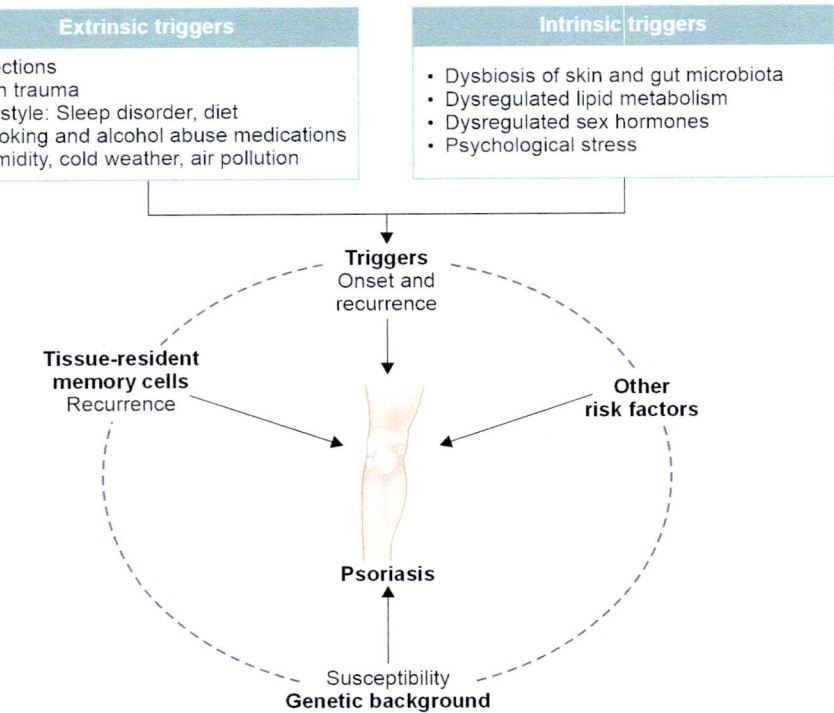

FIG. 1: The extrinsic and intrinsic triggers for the onset and recurrence of psoriasis.[2]

TABLE 1: Infections having a role in the pathogenesis of psoriasis		
Microorganisms	**Route of infection**	**Mechanism of action**
Bacteria		
Streptococcus pyogenes	Tonsil	Streptococcal tonsillitis triggers psoriasis through various mechanisms: • *Molecular mimicry*: The M protein of *S. pyogenes* mimicking human K17, recognized as self-antigen by CD8 T cells • Superantigens of *S. pyogenes* stimulate the release of IL-12 and promote the expression of skin-homing cutaneous lymphocytes associated with CLA+ T cells, migration of IL-17-producing CLA+ T cells to the skin, and expression of psoriasis autoantigens like ADAMTSL5, which is recognized by autoreactive CD8+ T cells in the epidermis • *S. pyogenes* peptidoglycan (PG) is responsible for T cell activation in psoriasis, leading to the proliferation of CD4+ T cells in psoriatic lesions and producing IFN-γ
Staphylococcus aureus	Skin, tonsil	Superantigen toxins of *S. aureus* lead to T-cell independent, enhanced inflammatory skin response in psoriatic subjects, and an increased level of TNF-α mRNA in the psoriatic epidermis may be due to higher expression of HLA-DR in keratinocytes (KCs) by superantigens

Continued

CHAPTER 3: Pathophysiology of Psoriasis: Immune System Dysfunction, Genetics, and Triggers

Continued

Microorganisms	Route of infection	Mechanism of action
Mycoplasma faucium	Oral cavity	Patient with initial guttate and later plaque psoriasis was cutaneously infected with *M. faucium*, which was present intracellularly in the KCs and extracellularly in the upper dermis of the psoriatic lesions
Porphyromonas gingivalis	Oral cavity	Activate human CD14+ monocytes to enhance Th17 differentiation and IL-17 production in vitro
Aggregatibacter actinomycetemcomitans	Oral cavity	Activate human CD14(+) monocytes, enhancing Th17/IL-17 responses
Helicobacter pylori	Digestive tract	Chronic inflammation by *H. pylori* results in the release of IL-6, which induces IL-8 production, which has a vital role in psoriasis
Chlamydophila psittaci	Respiratory transmission	DNA of *C. psittaci* was detected in psoriasis lesions and psoriatic arthritis joint fluids compared to healthy persons
Viruses		Psoriasis is triggered by the viral infection through activating retinoic acid inducible-gene I (*RIG-I*) antiviral signaling, which enhances the expression of IL-23 in the CD11c+ DCs in genetically predisposed individuals, thus leading to the development of psoriasis
Human immunodeficiency virus (HIV)	Maternal–fetal, sexual, transfusion-related transmission	HIV acts as superantigens or as a costimulatory factor in antigen presentation and triggers psoriasis, and HIV infections lead to more IFN-γ release by activated CD8+ T cells. HIV-infected immune cells release neuropeptide substance P, which sets inflammatory and immune responses and enhances the proliferation of KCs
Human papillomavirus	Skin or mucous membranes	A higher prevalence of psoriasis is seen after HPV infections
Hepatitis C virus	Blood transmission	It upregulates INF-γ and other cytokines that enhance susceptibility to psoriasis
Varicella zoster virus	Skin	There are reports of the association of Kaposi varicelliform eruption with psoriasis
Epstein–Barr virus (EBV)	Oral transmission	EBV reactivation is associated with generalized pustular psoriasis
Parvovirus B19	Respiratory transmission	A high prevalence of parvovirus B19 DNA was found in patients with psoriasis
Cytomegalovirus (CMV)	Humoral transmission	Persistent CMV infection correlates with psoriasis severity. Interaction of CMV and psoriasis is mediated by peripheral CD8+ T cells
Zika virus	Arthropod-borne, maternal–fetal, sexual, and transfusion-related transmission	The zika virus triggers generalized pustular psoriasis by activating KC-derived inflammatory mediators and a polyfunctional T-cell-driven cutaneous immune reaction

Continued

CHAPTER 3: Pathophysiology of Psoriasis: Immune System Dysfunction, Genetics, and Triggers

Continued

Microorganisms	Route of infection	Mechanism of action
Coxsackie B	Digestive and respiratory transmission	High antibody titer of coxsackie B virus was associated with psoriasis
Human endogenous retrovirus (HERV)	Skin	HERV sequences of the W, K, and E families were expressed in psoriatic lesions, suggesting a possible role in psoriasis pathogenesis
Chikungunya	Arthropod-borne transmission	RNA virus acts as a superantigen and triggers cellular immunity, thus activating psoriasis
COVID-19	Respiratory transmission	COVID-19 associated with exacerbation of psoriasis. Inflammatory cytokine release is enhanced in SARS-CoV-2-infected patients, and increased granulocyte colony-stimulating factor and TNF-α can lead to psoriasis. There were reports of exacerbation of psoriasis in patients who received COVID-19 vaccines
Fungi		
Candida albicans	Skin	It is frequently associated with intertriginous psoriasis. Superantigens of *C. albicans* lead to the exacerbation of psoriasis. It also triggers the production of cytokines IL-9, IL-17A, and IFN-γ have a role in psoriasis pathogenesis
Malassezia	Skin	*Malassezia* organisms were associated with exacerbation of scalp psoriasis

(COVID-19: coronavirus disease 2019; HLA-DR: human leukocyte antigen DR; IFN-γ: interferon gamma; IL-12: interleukin 12; SARS-CoV-2: severe acute respiratory syndrome coronavirus 2; TNF-α: tumor necrosis factor alpha)

release from KCs and subsequent release of Th17-polarizing cytokines (pro-IL-1β and IL-6). The activated ATP from human KCs activates epidermal Langerhans cells, releasing psoriasis-associated proinflammatory cytokines, antimicrobial peptides (AMPs), and chemokines. Scratch injury to KCs triggers the KP through cytokines or chemokines CCL20 and, to a lesser extent, CXCL8.

■ LIFESTYLES

Smoking[2,5]

There is a dose-dependent effect of smoking intensity and duration on the incidence of psoriasis. Smoking acts as an independent risk factor for the appearance of psoriasis, having many adverse effects on psoriasis patients, including higher Psoriasis Area and Severity Index (PASI) scores, high nail involvement, and the risk of cardiovascular disease development. Nicotine releases inflammatory cytokines that activate innate immune cells, including DCs, macrophages, and KCs. Free radicals formed by smoking initiate protein signaling pathways involved in psoriasis. Smoking also has a role in the upregulation of the expression of psoriasis-associated genes (*HLA-C*06:02, HLA-DQA1*0201,* and *CYP1A1*). A recent study has explained the role of a nicotinic receptor gene, *CHRNA5*, in the pathogenesis and development of psoriasis. Interestingly, smoking also increases the risk of psoriatic arthritis (PsA) in the general population, but smoking appeared to have a protective effect among psoriasis patients, which is known as the "smoking paradox".

Sleep Disorders[2,6]

Sleep disorders and obstructive sleep apnea are associated with an increased risk of psoriasis and PsA. There were data suggestive of an increase in the release of proinflammatory cytokines (IL-1β, IL-6, and IL-12) and a decrease in the production of anti-inflammatory cytokines (e.g., IL-10) in mice having psoriasis with sleep deprivation. Kallikrein-5 and -7 levels were increased in the psoriatic skin in patients with insomnia, which leads to disruption of the epidermal barrier and development of psoriasis. Increased cortisol level in insomnia disrupts epidermal barrier function and enhances proinflammatory cytokine secretion, leading to psoriasis exacerbation.

Dietary Factor[2,7]

Dietary factors like increased gluten intake and sodium chloride (NaCl) intake have a role in the pathogenesis of psoriasis. A 3-month gluten-free diet saw clinical improvements in 73% of psoriatic patients and reduced Ki67 lymphocytes in the psoriatic dermis. High-salt concentration led to activating the p38/MAPK (mitogen-activated protein kinase) pathway that upregulates downstream targets nuclear factor of activated T cells 5 (NFAT5) and serum/glucocorticoid-regulated kinase 1 (SGK1). This upregulated target gene increases the expression of transcription factors RORγt, IL-23R, IL-17A, and IL-17F, further leading to the differentiation of psoriatic Th17 cells from naïve CD4+ T cells. SGK1 has a role in promoting IL-23R expression and stabilizing Th17 cell differentiation through the phosphorylation of *Foxo1*.

Alcohol[8]

Alcohol consumption enhances the severity of psoriasis and decreases treatment effectiveness. Data from the Mendelian randomization study suggest that there was no causal relationship between alcohol intake and psoriasis as well.

Drugs[2]

Multiple drugs like beta blockers, lithium, antimalarial drugs (chloroquine, hydroxychloroquine), imiquimod, IFN-α, β, terbinafine, anti-TNF-α antagonists, anti-PD1 drugs, vascular endothelial growth factor (VEGF) antagonists, bupropion have a role in psoriasis induction or exacerbation of the disease.

■ INTRINSIC FACTOR

Dysbiosis of Skin and Gut Microbiota[2,9,10]

"Gut–skin axis" is a complex interaction between cutaneous and intestinal microbiomes. Data suggest that the close association between dysbiosis of the skin microbiota and gut microbiota leads to the pathophysiology of psoriasis. Common bacterial phylum in psoriatic and healthy skin are Firmicutes and Actinobacteria, respectively. Increased Firmicutes and a corresponding decrease in Actinobacteria were found in psoriatic skin. There is also evidence of higher concentrations of *Corynebacterium* and lower concentrations of *Cutibacterium* psoriatic lesions. *Corynebacterium* species induce an intense IL-23-dependent response and increase cutaneous IL-1β protein level and gamma delta (γδ) T17 cells in the dermis on mouse skin, thus explaining the possible role in the pathogenesis of psoriasis. The gut microbiota dysbiosis leads to a "leaky gut" by increasing intestinal permeability caused by the reduction of the thickness of the mucus layers, disturbing the proliferation and metabolism of intestinal epithelial cells, and decreasing the production of AMPs. The leaky gut eases the translocation of bacteria. It makes a way of exterior antigens from the intestinal lumen to the blood and lymphatic circulations, propelling both local and systemic immune responses. Increased bacterial DNA translocation in patients with intestinal bacteria *Escherichia coli*, *Enterococcus faecalis*, *Shigella fresneli*, and *Prevotella* thus leads to systemic inflammatory response in plaque psoriasis. The microbial metabolites short-chain fatty acids (SCFAs) lead to histone H3 acetylation at the promoter region of the forkhead box P3 (*Foxp3*) locus, which impacts the differentiation of regulatory T (Treg) cells. With specific extracellular pathogens such as *Citrobacter* infection, group 3 innate lymphoid cells (ILC3s) produce IL-22 and IL-17 to maintain mucosal immunity against the pathogens. Probiotic intake has significant beneficial effects in the improvement of psoriasis. "Eubiosis", fecal microbiota transplants from a healthy fecal microbiome to recolonize the gut of the affected patients, may be a possible therapeutic strategy to alleviate the autoimmune disease. Understanding microbiota dysbiosis better is needed to shed light on psoriasis treatments.

Dysregulated Lipid Metabolism[2,11]

Hypertrophic adipocytes in lipid-dysregulated patients release many hormones and cytokines (adipokines), including IL-6, TNF-α, and leptin, which modulate inflammatory cascade. Circulating saturated fatty acids (SFAs) are transferred to the skin and induce myeloid DCs (mDCs) to produce proinflammatory cytokines such as IL-1β. Under the influence of these cytokines, the KCs release chemokines and inflammatory cytokines, which further lead to the recruitment of neutrophils and monocytes to the skin and amplify psoriatic inflammation. SFAs activate DCs that promote Th1/Th17 differentiation, exacerbating psoriatic dermatitis. An increased lipid peroxidation due to the accumulation of reactive oxygen species (ROS) has a role in the Th22/Th17 pathway in psoriasis. High levels of phospholipase A2 (PLA2) in psoriatic lesions produce neolipid skin antigens. These antigens are recognized by the lipid-specific CD1a-reactive T cells and release IL-22 and IL-17A.

Psychological Stress and Other Mental Disorders[2,12]

Stress plays a significant role in the pathophysiology of psoriasis, possibly via the hypothalamic–pituitary–adrenal (HPA) axis, immune pathways, and peripheral nervous system. Psychological stress releases corticotropin-releasing hormone (CRH) from the hypothalamus, releasing the pituitary adrenocorticotropic hormone (ACTH) and the adrenal cortisol.

Corticotropin-releasing hormone promotes suppression of KCs apoptosis and angiogenesis by activating VEGF, mast cells (MCs) activation, and cytokines and chemokines (IL-1, IL-6, IL-31, TNF, and CXCL-8) release.

Stress has a role in the development of neurogenic inflammation by stimulating cutaneous peripheral nerve endings to enhance the secretion of neuropeptides.

Dysregulated Sex Hormones[2,13]

Sex hormones have multiple biological and immunomodulatory effects on the skin. Estrogen may have dual effects on the pathogenesis of psoriasis. Estrogen protects psoriasis by downregulating IL-1β production and proinflammatory role in psoriasis by inducing IL-23.

Existing data suggests a protective role of progestogens in psoriasis.

There is an inverse correlation between total or free testosterone and psoriasis severity.

■ GENETICS

Psoriasis incidence is significantly higher among patients' first- and second-degree relatives compared with the general population,

CHAPTER 3: Pathophysiology of Psoriasis: Immune System Dysfunction, Genetics, and Triggers

and concordance of psoriasis is higher among monozygotic than dizygotic twins.[14] Linkage studies identified nine genomic regions (loci) cosegregated with psoriasis (*PSORS1-9*) in multiplex pedigrees **(Table 2)**.[15]

■ PSORIASIS IN THE GWAS AND POST-GWAS ERA[14]

Genome-wide association studies use extremely advanced microarrays that can proficiently and vigorously genotype millions of genetic markers across the genome. GWAS detected ten loci in psoriasis, including innate immunity genes *DDX58* and *CARD14*. Rare variants in type I IFN signaling genes *IFIH1* and *TYK2* are identified, linking with psoriasis. GWAS data detect novel psoriasis susceptibility locus at *DLEU1* linked to apoptosis **(Fig. 2)**.

Genome-wide association studies identified genes connected with particular adaptive and innate immune pathways.

TABLE 2: Various genomic loci and associated genes in psoriasis mechanism[14]			
Genomic loci	**Chromosome**	**This region contains genes**	**Mechanism of action**
PSORS1 loci	MHC class I on chromosome 6P	Corneodesmosin (*CDSN*) gene	Encodes a desmosomal protein that has a role in keratinocyte cohesion and desquamation; 35–50% of disease inheritance is accounted for by the *PSORS1* gene. *HLA-C*06:02* is now the most likely causal association allele
PSORS2 loci	Chromosomes 17q25	*CARD14* gene	Encodes a nuclear factor-κB (NF-κB) activator and is associated with unusual and common forms of psoriasis
PSORS4 loci	Chromosomes 1q21	Late cornified envelope (*LCE*) genes	Encode stratum corneum proteins have a role in terminal epidermal differentiation, leading to psoriasis susceptibility

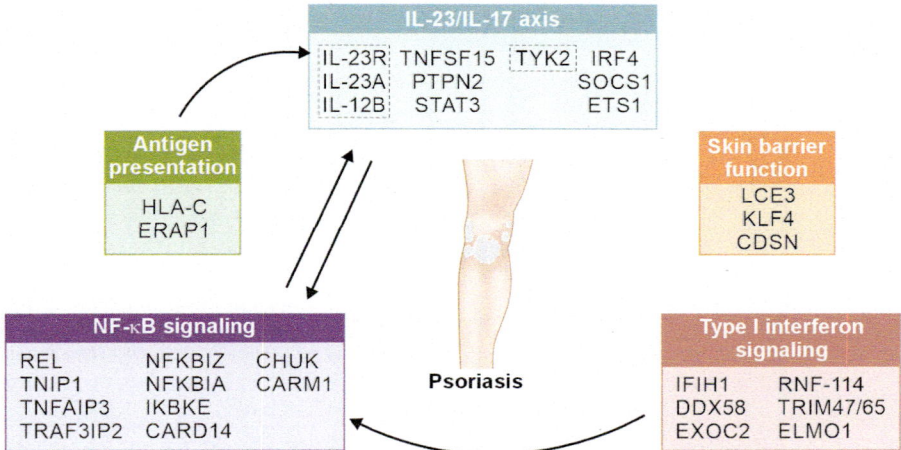

FIG. 2: Biological pathways implicated in psoriasis pathogenesis via genome-wide association studies (GWAS). Candidate causal genes from selected disease-associated loci identified by GWAS. Arrows signify the crosstalk between the immune pathways shown [e.g., interleukin 17 (IL-17) and type I interferon signaling both activate nuclear factor-κB (NF-κB) pathways]. Black dotted boxes: Genes involved in mechanisms currently targeted by psoriasis treatments.[14]

These include genes participating in antigen presentation (*HLA-C*, *ERAP1*), Th17 cell activation (*IL-23R*, *IL-23A*, *IL-12B*, *TRAF3IP2*), innate antiviral immunity/type I IFN signaling (*RNF114*, *IFIH1*), and skin barrier function (*LCE3B/3D*). The coding variants in genes such as *IL-23R*, *TYK2*, and *TNFSF15* uncovered by targeted association analyses further underscore the involvement of the IL-23/Th17 axis in disease pathogenesis.

Data suggest epistasis (gene–gene interactions) contributes to disease inheritance; for instance, the *ERAP1* gene interacts with individuals with the HLA-C risk allele to harbor disease susceptibility.[16]

Missing heritability in genetic studies accounted by epigenetic variation: Differences in gene expression without change in DNA sequence; there are multiple studies aimed to explore the role of epigenetics in psoriasis.[14]

PSORIASIS GENETICS BEYOND THE SUSCEPTIBILITY[14]

Onset: The *HLA-C*06:02* susceptibility allele is associated with earlier disease onset. Environmental risk factors trigger psoriasis onset by modifying the *HLA-C*06:02* gene. Pathogenic contribution of smoking mediated via variants in *CYP1A1*. Gene-specific HLA-B alleles, along with *HLA-B*27*, are associated with higher PsA risk in the presence of psoriasis **(Table 3)**.

Various gene mutations in pustular psoriasis assemble on the dysregulation of IL-36 signaling, thus focusing on IL-36 blockade as an effective treatment strategy regardless of the specific gene mutated.

PATHOPHYSIOLOGY

Brief History

A complex interaction between various cell types and inflammatory cytokines defines psoriasis pathogenesis.

The innate and adaptive immune systems and AMPs (LL-37, defensins, S100 proteins) released from KCs in response to stress are responsible for psoriatic inflammation. Overall, the pathogenesis of psoriasis has an initiation and maintenance phase.[17]

TABLE 3: Gene involved in pustular psoriasis[14]

Gene in pustular psoriasis	Mutation	Mechanism of action
IL-36RN	Autosomal recessive mutation loss in a gene is associated with a severe clinical phenotype of early-onset GPP, characterized by a high risk of systemic involvement	*IL-36RN* encodes the interleukin-36 receptor antagonist (IL-36Ra), which regulates the role of the IL-1 family cytokines IL-36α, β, and γ
AP1S3	Gene defects were associated with 12% of pustular psoriasis cases of European descent	Encodes the σ1 subunit of AP-1 and has a role in the formation of autophagosomes; mutations causing faulty autophagy lead to the accumulation of p62 (an adaptor protein that regulates NF-κB activation) and amplifying IL-36-mediated cutaneous inflammation
CARD14	Deleterious gain-of-function substitution mutation has been detected in GPP	*CARD14* is richly located in keratinocytes and encodes a scaffold protein that, upon oligomerization, regulates TRAF2-dependent initiation of NF-κB signaling

(NF-κB: nuclear factor-kappa B; TRAF2: tumor necrosis factor receptor-associated factor 2)

Initiation Phase[18]

In response to triggers, KCs release AMPs (LL-37, defensins, S100 proteins), which induce DCs. LL37 binds to either DNA or RNA to start the process—the LL37 complexes with DNA to stimulate TLR9 and activate pDCs.

The activated pDCs release type I IFNs (INF-α and IFN-β).

These IFNs act on mDCs to initiate the maturation and differentiation of Th1 and Th17, thus leading to further release of IFN-γ and TNF-α by Th1 cell and IL-17, IL-22, and TNF-α from Th17 cells.

The activated mDCs also migrate to peripheral lymph nodes and directly release inflammatory mediators (TNF-α, IL-23, and IL-12). IL-23 enhances Th17 and Th22 cell survival and proliferation. IL-12 helps in native T cell to Th1 cell differentiation. TNF-α is the primary inflammatory cytokine in psoriasis. DCs are further activated by activated mDCs, which leads to an autoinflammatory loop.

The LL37, when binding to RNA, stimulates TLR7 and TLR8, which leads to the activation of pDCs and mDCs, respectively. LL37 binds to RNA and activates slan+ monocytes, thus releasing TNF-α and IL-23.

B-defensin acts similarly to LL37 and induces self-RNA and self-DNA recognition, thus activating pDCs. S100 acts as a chemoattractant for neutrophil recruitment.

Maintenance Phase[18]

Psoriasis inflammation is mainly maintained by various Th cell subtypes and their cytokines. The TNF-α/IL-23/IL-17 axis is pivotal in the pathogenesis of psoriasis.

The mDCs produce IL-23, which is profoundly found in psoriatic lesions and maintain Th17 cells, a primary source of IL-17.

Besides IL-23-dependent Th17 cells, other IL-23-independent sources of IL-17 are γδ T cells, ILC3s, and natural killer T (NKT) cells.

Interleukin 17 executes inflammation through two different pathways: One is a cytoplasmic adaptor protein ACT1-dependent mechanism, and the other is an ACT1-independent mechanism.

ACT1, along with TNF receptor-associated factor 6 (TRAF6), turns on transcription factor NF-κB, further leading to transcription of inflammatory genes and activation of p38 MAPK. This has a role in the production of cytokines and chemokines in psoriatic lesions.

Janus kinase (JAK) signal transduction pathways and activator of transcription (STAT) pathway independent of ACT1.

The JAKs are protein kinases that transmit signals by attaching them to the intracellular domain of various cytokine receptors. Out of all four members of the JAK family [JAK1, JAK2, JAK3, and tyrosine kinase 2 (TYK2)], signaling of the IL-23 receptor is primarily mediated via TYK2. JAK2 also has a role in the IL-23 receptor signaling pathway.

Cytokine ligand and receptor-mediated binding lead to JAK activation and phosphorylation. An activated JAK forms a homodimer, or heterodimer, by binding with the same family or another family. Dimerization of JAK further leads to STAT binding through a docking site, followed by phosphorylation, activation, and dimerization of STAT. STAT subsequently translocates into the nucleus and thus regulates gene transcription, further propagating the inflammatory pathogenesis of psoriasis. Specifically, STAT1 and STAT3 have pivotal roles in psoriasis pathogenesis. Signals for type I and type II IFNs are propagated through STAT1 via JAK1 and JAK2. This is followed by KC sensitization by IFN-γ and migration of inflammatory cells to psoriatic lesions. Th17 cells induction and differentiation are mediated via STAT3. The JAK2/TYK2 dimer induced by IL-23, or both JAK1/JAK2, and JAK1/TYK2, dimer induced by IL-6 activate STAT3 **(Fig. 3)**.

CHAPTER 3: Pathophysiology of Psoriasis: Immune System Dysfunction, Genetics, and Triggers

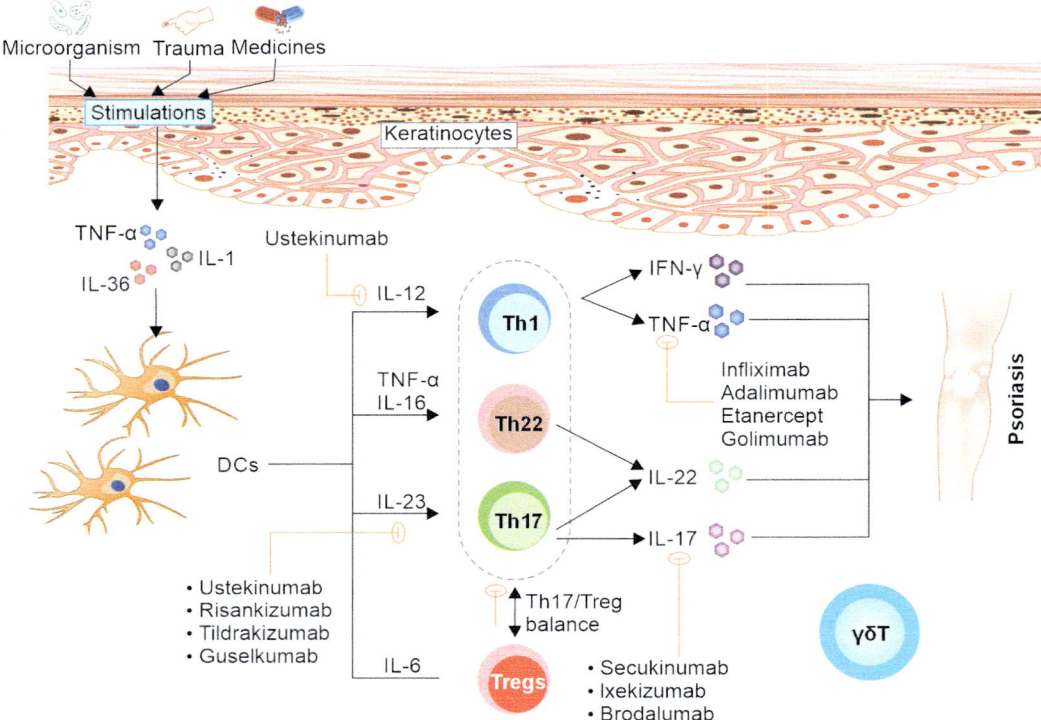

FIG. 3: Overview of psoriasis molecular pathogenesis and targeted therapies.[19]
(DCs: dendritic cells; IFN-γ: interferon gamma; IL-1: interleukin 1; Th17: T helper 17; TNF-α: tumor necrosis factor alpha; Tregs: regulatory T cells)

The immune system comprised of a three-way balance between type 1 (Th1 + IL-C1), type 2 (Th2 + IL-C2), and type 3 (Th17 + IL-C3) immunity, and regulatory cells.

Psoriasis is mainly defined as an IL-17-mediated type 3 dominant disorder along with overproduction of IFN-γ/TNF-α and impairment of regulatory cell function.

■ KEY CYTOKINES IN PSORIASIS[17]

Multiple cytokines are generated in psoriasis lesions. They drive the inflammation and lead to the development of psoriasis lesions. However, IL-23, IL-17, and TNF-α play a pivotal role.

Interleukin 17 in Psoriasis[17]

The IL-17 has six isoforms (IL-17A, IL-17B, IL-17C, IL-17D, IL-17E, and IL-17F). Of them, IL-17A is the main effector cytokine in psoriasis.

The IL-17A works on KCs and produces effects like the release of various inflammatory mediators and rapid abnormal proliferation of KCs.

The combined effect of TNF-α and IL-17A induces the transcription of genes of multiple inflammatory cytokines, like TNF-α, IL-1β, IL-6, and IL-8.

The IL-1β and IL-23 help in IL-17A production in IL-17A-producing cells.

The IL-8 acts as a chemoattractant for neutrophils.

The IL-17A and TNF-α have a role in the release of chemokine C-C-motif ligand (CCL) 20, which is vital for the recruitment of IL-17-producing cells (Th17 cells and γδ T cells).

This inflammatory cascade further amplifies psoriatic inflammation.

The IL-17A, IL-20, and IL-22 lead to the release of IL-19 and IL-36 by KCs, which cause the abnormal proliferation of KCs. The uncontrolled hyperproliferation of KCs leads to epidermal hyperplasia and is the hallmark of psoriasis.

Recent data suggested that IL-23 production is regulated by IL-36 signaling in KCs.

The IL-17F has a biological role similar to IL-17A.

However, the fast and profound therapeutic effects of IL-17A inhibitors on psoriasis lesions are highly suggestive of the significant role of IL-17A in pathogenesis.

The IL-17A is produced mainly by Th17 cells, followed by CD8+ T cells (Tc17), and resident memory T cells (Trms) also produce cytokines.

The innate immune cells (ILC3, γδ T cells, MCs, and neutrophils) may have a role in IL-17A release and thus have a role in the progression of psoriasis lesions.

Interleukin 23 in Psoriasis[17]

Interleukin 23 has two subunits: IL-23p19 (IL-12A) and IL-12/23p40 (IL-12B). Signal transduction via the IL-23 receptor is mediated through JAK.

The principal functions of IL-23 are initiating Th17/Tc17 cell production in the lymph nodes and activating these cells in the skin.

The IL-23 binds to IL-23 receptors on the surface of naïve T cells and, along with the help of other cytokines such as IL-1β, TNF-α, and IL-6, promotes differentiation of naïve T cells to Th17/Tc17 cells in the lymph node.

In the skin, IL-23 activates Th17/Tc17 cells to release IL-17, converts IL-C2 to IL-C3, and activates IL-C3.

The data has found the role of IL-23 in Treg-cell conversion, which has a regulatory function in the inflammatory cascade.

The source of IL-23 in psoriatic lesions are CD11c+ DCs in the dermis, typically called TNF-α and inducible nitric oxide synthase-producing DCs (TIP-DCs), DCs expressing 6-sulfo LacNAc, and DCs expressing macrophage markers CD16. Recently, evidence showed that a subgroup of cDC2 cells expresses IL-12B in psoriasis lesions.

Forkhead Box P3-positive Regulatory T Cell[17]

Forkhead box P3 acts as a critical regulator of transcription of a specific T-cell type, CD4(+) Treg cells. There is unstable *Foxp3* expression in Treg cells in psoriasis, and it is easily transformed into a retinoic acid receptor-related orphan receptor gamma t + IL-17-producing cells by IL-12A. There is impaired Treg cell function in both peripheral blood and skin lesions in psoriasis.

Resident Memory T Cells[17]

CD103 expressing skin Trm marker, CD8+CD103+ Trm cell produces IL-17A in the epidermis of the psoriatic lesion.

■ DANGER SIGNAL FROM KERATINOCYTES[17]

Along with IL-17A, IL-22 leads to the proliferation of KCs by enhancing the release of chemokines (CXCL1, CXCL2, CXCL8, and CCL20) and AMPs.

The AMPs activate DCs and upregulate skin inflammation. CXCL1, CXCL2, and CXCL8 have a role in neutrophil recruitment and lead to neutrophilic microabscess formation.

The CCL20 recruits IL-17A-producing CCR6+ immune cells in the dermis, further amplifying IL-17A-mediated inflammation.

The activation of NF-κB signaling leads to keratin 6 and 16 expression in KCs, which have a role in acanthosis and decreased epidermal turnover time.

■ CONCLUSION

Advanced knowledge in psoriasis immuno-pathogenesis has led to the successful development of new targeted, biological drugs, which caused significant improvements in the clinical picture and patients' quality of life. Even though many parts of the complex psoriasis pathogenesis have been revealed, further research is undoubtedly needed to supplement these findings. In today's era, therapeutic approaches are moving toward precision medicine that respects the patient's biological fingerprint. Accordingly, even more extensive knowledge of immunopathogenesis will be necessary to act on multiple key target sites and achieve maximum results in treating psoriasis and diseases with similar pathogenetic mechanisms.

TAKE HOME MESSAGE

- DCs, Th17 cells, TLRs, and cytokines (IFN-α, TNF-α, IFN-γ, IL-12, IL-22, IL-23, and IL-17) play a leading role in the pathogenesis of psoriasis.
- Both extrinsic factors (infection, skin trauma, life, alcohol, smoking, cold air, humidity, air pollution) and intrinsic factors (skin and gut microbiota dysbiosis, dysregulated lipid metabolism, dysregulated sex hormone, and psychological stress) act as triggers for psoriasis.
- GWAS have shown around 60 psoriasis susceptibility loci contribute to disease pathophysiology.
- Genes participating in antigen presentation, Th17 cell activation, innate antiviral immunity/type I IFN signaling, and skin barrier function have roles in disease pathogenesis.
- IL-36RN, *AP1S3*, *CARD14* genes have a role in the pathogenesis of pustular psoriasis.
- The pathogenesis of psoriasis has an initiation and maintenance phase.
- The TNF-α/IL-23/IL-17 axis is pivotal in the pathogenesis of psoriasis.

REFERENCES

1. Vičić M, Kaštelan M, Brajac I, Sotošek V, Massari LP. Current Concepts of Psoriasis Immunopathogenesis. Int J Mol Sci. 2021;22:11574.
2. Liu S, He M, Jiang J, Duan X, Chai B, Zhang J, et al. Triggers for the onset and recurrence of psoriasis: a review and update. Cell Commun Signal. 2024;22(1):108.
3. Dong C, Lin L, Du J. Characteristics and sources of tissue-resident memory T cells in psoriasis relapse. Curr Res Immunol. 2023;4:100067.
4. Gregorio J, Meller S, Conrad C, Di Nardo A, Homey B, Lauerma A, et al. Plasmacytoid dendritic cells sense skin injury and promote wound healing through type I interferons. J Exp Med. 2010;207(13):2921-30.
5. Pezzolo E, Naldi L. The relationship between smoking, psoriasis, and psoriatic arthritis. Expert Rev Clin Immunol. 2019;15(1):41-8.
6. Hirotsu C, Rydlewski M, Araújo MS, Tufik S, Andersen ML. Sleep loss and cytokines levels in an experimental model of psoriasis. PLoS One. 2012;7(11):e51183.
7. Michaëlsson G, Ahs S, Hammarström I, Lundin IP, Hagforsen E. Gluten-free diet in psoriasis patients with antibodies to gliadin results in decreased expression of tissue transglutaminase and fewer Ki67+ cells in the dermis. Acta Derm Venereol. 2003;83(6):425-9.
8. Brenaut E, Horreau C, Pouplard C, Barnetche T, Paul C, Richard MA, et al. Alcohol consumption and psoriasis: a systematic literature review. J Eur Acad Dermatol Venereol. 2013;27(Suppl 3):30-5.
9. Le ST, Toussi A, Maverakis N, Marusina AI, Barton VR, Merleev AA, et al. The cutaneous and intestinal microbiome in psoriatic disease. Clin Immunol. 2020;218:108537.
10. Quan C, Chen XY, Li X, Xue F, Chen LH, Liu N, et al. Psoriatic lesions are characterized by higher bacterial load and imbalance between Cutibacterium and Corynebacterium. J Am Acad Dermatol. 2020;82(4):955-61.
11. Stolarczyk E. Adipose tissue inflammation in obesity: a metabolic or immune response? Curr Opin Pharmacol. 2017;37:35-40.
12. Rousset L, Halioua B. Stress and psoriasis. Int J Dermatol. 2018;57(10):1165-72.
13. Kanda N, Watanabe S. Regulatory roles of sex hormones in cutaneous biology and immunology. J Dermatol Sci. 2005;38(1):1-7.
14. Dand N, Mahil SK, Capon F, Smith CH, Simpson MA, Barker JN. Psoriasis and Genetics. Acta Derm Venereol. 2020;100(3):adv00030.
15. Capon F, Trembath RC, Barker JN. An update on the genetics of psoriasis. Dermatol Clin. 2004;22:339-347.
16. Genetic Analysis of Psoriasis Consortium & the Wellcome Trust Case Control Consortium 2;

Strange A, Capon F, Spencer CC, Knight J, Weale ME, Allen MH, et al. A genome-wide association study identifies new psoriasis susceptibility loci and an interaction between HLA C and ERAP1. Nat Genet. 2010;42:985-90.
17. Yamanaka K, Yamamoto O, Honda T. Pathophysiology of psoriasis: A review. J Dermatol. 2021;48(6):722-31.
18. Singh R, Koppu S, Perche PO, Feldman SR. The Cytokine Mediated Molecular Pathophysiology of Psoriasis and Its Clinical Implications. Int J Mol Sci. 2021;22:12793.
19. Man AM, Orăsan MS, Hoteiuc OA, Olănescu-Vaida-Voevod MC, Mocan T. Inflammation and Psoriasis: A Comprehensive Review. Int J Mol Sci. 2023;24:16095.

4

Differential Diagnosis of Psoriasis: Distinguishing Psoriasis from Other Dermatological Conditions

Rajesh Kumar, Ayesha Merchant, Datta Lokare, Disha Chakraborty

■ INTRODUCTION

Psoriasis is a chronic inflammatory skin condition marked by the presence of well-defined, erythematous, and scaly plaques. Its onset often follows a bimodal pattern, with peak incidence occurring between the ages of 20–30 and 50–60 years. Diagnosis varies based on clinical presentation but is straightforward when characteristic skin lesions—symmetrical erythematous plaques with scaling—are found on extensor surfaces. Additional indicators of psoriasis may include nail changes, joint symptoms, and lesions in areas such as the gluteal cleft or around the umbilicus. Atypical presentations and variations of psoriasis can pose diagnostic challenges. Common differential diagnoses for plaque psoriasis include atopic dermatitis, nummular dermatitis, lichen simplex chronicus, pityriasis rosea, pityriasis rubra pilaris, and tinea. In uncertain cases, a biopsy may help clarify the diagnosis. Erythematous-psoriasiform eruptions may also result from drug reactions, often presenting as bright red, intensely pruritic lesions accompanied by eosinophilia—features that suggest a drug-induced etiology. Additionally, psoriasis may be confused with mycosis fungoides, which can similarly appear as inflammatory papulosquamous lesions.

Here we explained various differential diagnosis of psoriasis including differential factors such as epidemiology, clinical features, and investigations (biopsy and dermoscopy) **(Table 1)**.

CHAPTER 4: Differential Diagnosis of Psoriasis: Distinguishing Psoriasis from Other...

TABLE 1: Comprehensive differential diagnosis of psoriasis: key factors and distinguishing features

Disease	Epidemiology	Etiopathogenesis	Clinical features

Psoriasis	• *Age*: The mean age is bimodal, peaking between the ages of 15, 20, 55 and 60 years
	• M = F, with a somewhat higher incidence in men
		• Psoriasis is believed to be a T-cell-mediated autoimmune condition, although its exact etiology remains unclear
		• A genetic predisposition is evident in many patients, particularly those from diverse racial and cultural backgrounds, with a strong association with human leukocyte antigen (HLA) such as HLA-CW6
		• A family history further supports this genetic link
		• Psoriatic lesions may be triggered by mechanical, chemical, or radiation-induced trauma
		• Certain medications, including NSAIDs, β-blockers, lithium, chloroquine, and corticosteroids, can aggravate the condition
		• Environmental and lifestyle factors such as winter weather, infections, alcohol consumption, smoking, psychological stress, obesity, and hypocalcemia are also known to exacerbate psoriasis.
			• Psoriasis commonly presents as sharply demarcated, erythematous, scaly plaques that may cause pain or itching
			• Lesions can be round, oval, or irregular in shape and are typically distributed symmetrically, with common involvement of the scalp, intergluteal cleft, and extensor surfaces. Variants such as palmoplantar psoriasis and palmoplantar pustulosis may affect the palms and soles
			• The "Auspitz sign," characterized by pinpoint bleeding upon scraping the dry scales, is a notable clinical feature
			Psoriasis variants include:
			  ○ Pustular psoriasis
			  ○ Erythrodermic psoriasis
			  ○ Guttate psoriasis
			  ○ Plaque psoriasis
			  ○ Inverse psoriasis
			• Nail changes often observed include salmon patches, leukonychia, subungual hyperkeratosis, oil drop signs, and irregular deep pitting

Discoid dermatitis	Nummular dermatitis has a bimodal distribution, ages 15–25 and 50–65 years	The precise cause of nummular dermatitis remains uncertain, though several factors have been implicated: • Xerosis (dry skin) • Contact sensitivity to metals • Reduced cutaneous lipid production • Sensitivity to environmental aeroallergens • Staphylococcal colonization • Frequent hot water bathing and exposure to low-humidity environments • Skin trauma, including the Koebner phenomenon • Rough textiles such as wool and materials associated with breast implantation	Established nummular dermatitis lesions are typically symmetrically distributed, sharply demarcated, round or coin-shaped, and erythematous. These eczematous plaques can range from 1 to 10 cm in size • In later stages, lesions may develop a dry scale and show lichenification • Acute lesions initially present as papules or vesicles that merge to form plaques • Lesions are often associated with mild-to-severe pruritus • The trunk and upper extremities are the most commonly affected sites, followed by the lower extremities

Continued

CHAPTER 4: Differential Diagnosis of Psoriasis: Distinguishing Psoriasis from Other...

Continued

Disease	Epidemiology	Etiopathogenesis	Clinical features
		• Certain medications, such as guselkumab, ribavirin, isotretinoin, retinoids, interferons, antivirals, and gold compounds • Chronic venous stasis	• The scalp and face are usually spared • Postinflammatory pigmentary changes often persist even after lesion resolution.
Pityriasis rosea (PR)	Both men and women have sex, although women have it more frequently • *Age*: It can affect toddlers and older individuals, but it is most common in teens and adults between the ages of 15 and 30 years During the fall and monsoon seasons, there is an increase in occurrence	The exact cause of PR remains unclear, but several factors have been suggested: • Autoimmunity • Atopy (a predisposition to allergic conditions) • Immunizations, including those for COVID-19, hepatitis B, influenza, and BCG • Certain medications, such as NSAIDs, captopril, and gold compounds • PR shows seasonal variation in tropical regions and tends to be more common during the winter months in temperate climates	• Collarette scaling is widespread, and in 25% of cases, the pruritus is severe. The condition starts with a herald patch on the trunk, neck, or proximal extremities, followed by scaly oval plaques grouped along Langer lines, giving the impression of a "Christmas tree" • 1–2 weeks later, a sore throat, gastrointestinal problems, fever, and arthralgia frequently accompany a broad skin eruption with symmetric lesions on the thorax, back, abdomen, and limbs • These secondary lesions, which are dispersed bilaterally and diffusely, are elliptical or oval macules and papules with fine scaling and central wrinkling. Their long axis runs parallel to the lines of tension in the skin.
Pityriasis lichenoides chronica (PLC)	Male predominance of 72.4%.	The pathogenesis of pityriasis lichenoides is believed to involve three primary mechanisms: • Inflammatory response triggered by pathogens • Inflammatory reaction caused by T-cell dysregulation • Hypersensitivity vasculitis mediated by immune complexes	The initial lesion in PLC appears as an erythematous papule that transitions to a reddish-brown hue with a centrally attached, micaceous scale. This scale can be easily removed, revealing a shiny, pinkish-brown surface beneath • Over several weeks, the papule gradually flattens and resolves spontaneously, often leaving behind a hyperpigmented or hypopigmented macule • Individual lesions typically persist for a few weeks • PLC primarily affects the trunk and proximal extremities, though acral and segmental distributions have also been reported • Most lesions are asymptomatic and do not cause significant discomfort

Continued

Continued

Disease	Epidemiology	Etiopathogenesis	Clinical features
Lichen planus (LP)	• Women are more frequently affected than men at a ratio of 1.5:1 • *Age*: Most cases develop between the ages of 30 and 60 years. It is rare in children as they represent <5% of all LP patients.	LP is an idiopathic, T-cell-mediated autoimmune disorder. Its pathogenesis involves an exogenous trigger—such as a virus, medication, or allergic reaction—that alters epidermal self-antigens, leading to the activation of CD8+ T cells and subsequent keratinocyte apoptosis. • *Hepatitis C virus (HCV)*: LP patients are at a significantly higher risk of testing positive for HCV, with a five-fold increased likelihood. • Contact allergies to metals found in dental restorations, such as copper, gold, and mercury, are often linked to oral LP; these lesions may resolve upon removal of the offending metals. • Although drug rechallenge rarely results in lesion recurrence, several medications—including antimalarials, ACE inhibitors, thiazide diuretics, NSAIDs, quinidine, β-blockers, TNF-α inhibitors, and gold—have been associated with the development of LP.	LP typically presents as itchy, violaceous, polygonal, flat-topped papules that are a few millimeters in diameter. This classic form is encapsulated by the "Six P's" of LP: *Purple, Polygonal, Planar, Pruritic, Papules,* and *Plaques*. • The lesions are firm and have a shiny surface, often covered by fine white lines known as *Wickham striae*. • They may appear in various forms, including scattered lesions, plaques, or patterns such as *annular, linear,* or *actinic* (sun-exposed) arrangements. • Like psoriasis, LP displays the *Koebner phenomenon*, where new lesions form at sites of trauma, such as scratching, in response to mechanical irritation. LP typically affects the flexor wrists, dorsal hands, lower back, ankles, and shins. Upon healing, lesions often leave behind a grayish-brown hyperpigmentation due to melanin deposition in the superficial dermis. • *Hypertrophic LP*, a subtype of LP, presents with red, red-brown, or yellow-gray papules and plaques that coalesce to form a thickened or verrucous surface. This form is most commonly found on the shins and ankles, presenting a distinct pattern from the traditional LP appearance. Inverse psoriasis and inverse LP share similarities, primarily affecting intertriginous areas, where the typical lesion appearance is completely altered. In these regions, such as the axillae, limb flexures, inguinal creases, and under the breasts, large erythematous and lichenified lesions appear without clear borders.

Continued

CHAPTER 4: Differential Diagnosis of Psoriasis: Distinguishing Psoriasis from Other...

Continued

Disease	Epidemiology	Etiopathogenesis	Clinical features
			<ul><li>Over half of LP patients experience mucosal involvement, which may be the only symptom present. While it can occur on the *lips, esophagus, glans penis, vulva,* or *vagina*, the *mouth* is the most commonly affected site.</li><li>Oral LP presents in six distinct forms: *reticular, erosive, papular, plaque-like, atrophic,* and *bullous*. LP affecting the *glans penis* often presents in an *annular* shape. In contrast, when LP involves the *vulva* or *vagina* in women, it tends to take on an *erosive* form, which can lead to problematic complications such as *scarring* and *strictures*.</li><li>When LP simultaneously affects both the *female genital* and *oral mucosa*, it is referred to as *vulvovaginal-gingival syndrome*. Approximately 10% of LP patients develop nail involvement, typically affecting multiple nails without significant damage to the surrounding skin. Early signs include *longitudinal ridging* and *nail plate thinning*. As the condition progresses, it can lead to *sandpaper nails (trachyonychia), dorsal pterygium formation, nail matrix scarring*, and potentially *total nail plate loss*.</li><li>*Twenty-nail dystrophy* is a variant of LP where the only visible manifestation is the presence of these nail abnormalities on all twenty nails. This subtype is more common in *children* than in *adults*.</li></ul>The clinical signs of LP affecting the nails include:<ul><li>*Thin nail plates*</li><li>*Longitudinal ridging*</li><li>*Pterygium unguis*</li><li>*Trachyonychia*</li><li>*Onycholysis*</li><li>*Onychorrhexis*</li><li>*Koilonychia*</li><li>*Subungual hyperkeratosis*</li><li>*Chromonychia*</li><li>*Onychomadesis*</li></ul>

Continued

Continued

Disease	Epidemiology	Etiopathogenesis	Clinical features
			Lichen planopilaris (LPP) refers to LP affecting the scalp and other hair-bearing areas. It presents as small, red, follicular papules, and macules at the sites of inflammation, leading to *scarring alopecia*. LPP may appear independently or alongside typical LP lesions elsewhere on the body.
			• *Frontal fibrosing alopecia* is a specific form of LPP that predominantly affects the anterior scalp and eyebrows, typically seen in elderly women. *Lichenoid drug eruption* differs from traditional LP in several ways: • It is more *widespread* and *symmetrical* than classic LP. • Lesions typically appear in *sun-exposed* areas, rather than the usual LP sites • *Wickham striae* are uncommon in drug-induced LP, and the lesions tend to have a more *psoriasiform* or *eczematous* appearance. Diagnosing *drug-induced LP* requires a thorough *medication history* assessment, as there is typically a *latent period* of several months to a year between the initiation of the medication and the onset of lesions.
Tinea corporis	Certain groups, such as *children*, may be more vulnerable to *tinea corporis*. In *prepubertal children*, *tinea capitis* and *tinea corporis* are the most common dermatophytic infections. Children are also more prone to *zoophilic* infections, which are transmitted through direct contact with animals such as *dogs* and *cats*.	Dermatophytoses, or superficial fungal skin infections, occur when dermatophytes adhere to keratinized skin tissue. Over the past 70 years, *Trichophyton rubrum* has been the most commonly implicated species in dermatophyte infections. The main dermatophyte genera responsible for tinea corporis include *Trichophyton, Epidermophyton,* and *Microsporum*, with *T. rubrum* accounting for 80–90% of infections. Other frequently isolated species include *Microsporum audouinii* and *Trichophyton mentagrophytes*. Direct skin contact with contaminated surfaces, animals, or other people's skin is the primary mode of infection transmission.	*Tinea corporis* typically presents as one or more lesions, which are usually *round* or *ovoid* in shape. These lesions appear as patches or plaques on the *exposed skin* of the *neck, trunk,* and/or *extremities*. • The lesions are *annular*, with *elevated erythematous* edges that may be scaly and well-defined, sometimes containing *vesicles*. The degree of inflammation can vary. • As the lesions expand *centrifugally*, the *center* clears and mild residual scaling remains, creating a characteristic "ring" appearance, leading to the common name "ringworm."

Continued

CHAPTER 4: Differential Diagnosis of Psoriasis: Distinguishing Psoriasis from Other...

Continued

Disease	Epidemiology	Etiopathogenesis	Clinical features
	Individuals with *weakened immune systems* are particularly vulnerable to dermatophytic infections. One such infection, *Majocchi granuloma*, is a form of *tinea corporis folliculitis* that affects the deeper dermal layers, distinguishing it from the more superficial typical presentation of tinea corporis.		

Pityriasis rubra pilaris (PRP)	The prevalence of PRP is nearly equal in males and females, although some studies suggest a slight male predominance. PRP can occur at any age, with minor bimodal peaks observed during the first to second and fifth to sixth decades of life.	• The etiology of PRP remains unclear, but several factors and associations have been identified:
		• Drug-induced PRP-like eruptions have been linked to medications, particularly ponatinib and other kinase inhibitors.
		• PRP has been temporally associated with viral infections, vaccinations, trauma, and other illnesses.
		• Inherited PRP, usually presenting before the age of 2, is associated with gain-of-function mutations in the *CARD14* gene, located in the psoriasis susceptibility locus 2 (PSORS2). This gene activates nuclear factor-κB (NF-κB).
		• These CARD14 mutations have also been identified in patients with sporadic adult-onset PRP, highlighting the overlap between PRP and psoriasis.
		• Classical PRP shares similarities with psoriasis, as both are linked to the Th17/IL23 inflammatory pathways.
			• Griffiths (1980) introduced a widely accepted classification system for PRP, categorizing its clinical spectrum into six subtypes based on distribution, lesion characteristics, and age of onset:
			  ◦ *Type I*: Classical adult-onset PRP.
			  ◦ *Type II*: Atypical adult-onset PRP.
			  ◦ *Type III*: Classical juvenile-onset PRP.
			  ◦ *Type IV*: Circumscribed or restricted juvenile-onset PRP.
			  ◦ *Type V*: Atypical juvenile-onset PRP.
			  ◦ *Type VI*: PRP associated with HIV infection.
			• Additionally, CARD14-associated papulosquamous eruption (CAPE) is linked to specific gene mutations.
			• Hallmark features shared across all subtypes include hyperkeratotic follicular papules and palmoplantar hyperkeratosis, forming distinctive red-orange plaques.
			• Localized PRP variants may be only mildly itchy.
			• Widespread PRP, however, is associated with severe pain, intense pruritus, and significantly diminished quality of life, including an elevated risk of suicidal ideation due to the debilitating nature of the condition.

Continued

Continued

Disease	Epidemiology	Etiopathogenesis	Clinical features
Seborrheic dermatitis (SD)	SD exhibits a bimodal prevalence, with peaks occurring: • During the first 3 months of life. • After the fourth decade of life. In patients with HIV/AIDS, SD is notably more prevalent: • Affects approximately 85% of AIDS patients • Present in about 35% of individuals with early HIV infection.	SD is influenced by multiple factors, and its complex nature has led to various theories regarding its etiology and pathophysiology. Key elements include: *Interaction of skin flora and lipids*: The interplay between *Malassezia* spp. (a common component of normal skin flora) and the composition of surface lipids appears to trigger SD. *Individual susceptibility*: Personal predisposition plays a significant role in the condition's development. Notably, neither the quantity of yeast nor the amount of sebum production has been identified as primary contributing factors.	SD is primarily characterized by the distribution of lesions, which typically occur in areas with a high density of sebaceous glands, particularly the face and scalp. *Symptoms*: While SD is often asymptomatic, it may coexist with atopic dermatitis. In contrast, individuals with atypical seborrheic dermatitis (ASD) frequently report burning and itching, especially with scalp involvement, but typically lack a history of atopic dermatitis. *Lesions*: Folliculocentric, salmon-colored papules and plaques. Associated with a fine white scale and a greasy yellow crust. Lesions have ill-defined edges, with less scaling on flexural areas. SD may present in one or multiple locations. The sudden onset of severe SD should raise suspicion for HIV-AIDS, as early recognition and diagnosis can significantly improve long-term outcomes. *Clinical features*: *Common presentations*: Facial redness, scaling, and dandruff. *Darker skin*: Persistent dyschromia, with areas of hyperpigmentation and hypopigmentation.
Lichen simplex chronicus (LSC)	The highest prevalence occurs between middle and late adulthood, peaking between the ages of 30 and 50 years, likely linked to a significant increase in stress during this phase of life. The condition is twice as common in women as in men, with a 2:1 prevalence ratio.	LSC is closely linked to emotional factors, resulting in a repetitive scratching cycle that leads to irritation and the formation of plaques. Commonly affected areas include the scalp, head, neck, hands, arms, and genitalia. *Plaques initiate a vicious cycle*: Emotional stress triggers scratching, which exacerbates stress, causing persistent itching and skin changes. While primarily characterized by itching, LSC may also be associated with atopy, psoriasis, xerosis, or skin barrier disorders.	*Mild variant*: Pityriasis capitis (or sicca) is the mildest form of SD. Primarily affects the scalp and beard area. It presents as light-colored skin flakes on dark clothing, commonly recognized as dandruff. LSC typically manifests as one or more lesions in easily accessible areas, such as the head, neck, arms, scalp, and genitalia. Itching is the predominant symptom, with repetitive scratching causing the formation of plaques and thickened, often pigmented lesions.

Continued

Continued

Disease	Epidemiology	Etiopathogenesis	Clinical features
			The degree of erythema influences the lesion's coloration, which can range from yellow tones to deep reddish-brown, most prominent at the center of the lesion.

Hailey–Hailey disease (HHD)	The onset of the disease occurs in the late teenage years or the third and fourth decades of life.	• Autosomal dominant genodermatosis affects family members with variable expressivity and complete penetrance.
		• 15–30% of patients lack a positive family history due to sporadic mutations or undiagnosed mild cases in relatives.
		• The condition is associated with mutations in the *ATP2C1* gene (located at 3q21–q24), which encodes the Ca^{2+}/Mn^{2+}-ATPase involved in the human secretory pathway.
			• The condition typically affects friction-prone areas such as the neck, axillae, groin, and perineum, with up to 50% of females also experiencing involvement under the breasts.
			• Chronic lesions may progress to erythematous plaques with erosions, painful rhagades (cracks), or moist vegetations.
			• The disease displays a symmetric distribution and is rarely disseminated, though secondary infections may contribute to its spread.
			• Longitudinal leukonychia is present in approximately 70% of patients.
			• Mucosal involvement (mouth, esophagus, vagina, and conjunctiva) is rare.
			• Segmental forms of HHD include:
			  ○ *Type 1*: Affecting localized areas.
			  ○ *Type 2*: Overlapping with conventional HHD lesions, indicative of mosaicism patterns.
			• *Triggers for acute exacerbations*: Trauma, friction, dampness, and infections (notably staphylococcal) can rapidly worsen symptoms.
			• The condition significantly reduces quality of life due to severe itching, pain, and social impact, necessitating comprehensive care approaches

Continued

CHAPTER 4: Differential Diagnosis of Psoriasis: Distinguishing Psoriasis from Other...

Continued

Disease	Epidemiology	Etiopathogenesis	Clinical features

Langerhans cell histiocytosis (LCH)	LCH is a rare condition, with a median diagnostic age of 3 years.
	Incidence in children: Approximately 8.9 per million under age 15 years.
	Incidence in adults: Much rarer, affecting about 0.07 per million annually.
		• LCH origin theories suggest that myeloid-committed hematopoietic progenitors (CD1a/CD207-positive) clonally expand in the bone marrow, differentiating into monocytes that later circulate as Langerhans cells.
		• Further research highlights a link between clonal hematopoiesis (notably TET2 mutations) and the secondary acquisition of a BRAF mutation (or alterations in the MAP kinase pathway) during monocyte differentiation. This essentially amounts to a clonal monocytosis and, upon monocyte release into the circulation, circulating LCH.
			• LCH clinical presentations vary by affected tissues, such as skin, bones, lymph nodes, liver, spleen, or lungs.
			• *Age-related differences*: Children often present with a rash resembling atopic dermatitis or seborrhea, which typically responds poorly to topical treatments.
			• *LCH rash characteristics*:
			  ○ Can manifest as single lesions or widespread involvement.
			  ○ Appears as scaly papules, nodules, or plaques, mimicking SD.
			• *Adult LCH presentation*: Most adults present after age 40 years, often with multisystemic disease.
			• *Identifying features*: Petechiae, bloody crusting, or firmly indurated nodules may help recognize LCH.
			• *Pulmonary LCH (PLCH)*:
			  ○ Almost exclusively affects patients with a history of tobacco use (~90%).
			  ○ Symptoms are often nonspecific, such as cough and exertional dyspnea.
			  ○ May coexist with other conditions, including non-LCH and myeloproliferative diseases.
			• *Hematological, liver, and spleen involvement*: Detailed classifications were provided by Rodriguez-Galindo and Allen in a 2020 study published in *Blood*.
			• *Liver and spleen involvement*: Expansion of the liver and spleen >3 cm below the right and left costal borders, respectively, is indicative of organ involvement in LCH.
			• *Hematopoietic involvement*: At least two cytopenias must be present for hematopoietic involvement.
			• *Disease extent*: Determining whether the disease is single-system or multisystem at diagnosis is essential for guiding treatment decisions.

Continued

CHAPTER 4: Differential Diagnosis of Psoriasis: Distinguishing Psoriasis from Other...

Continued

Disease	Epidemiology	Etiopathogenesis	Clinical features

Secondary syphilis	• *Syphilis incidence*: The incidence of syphilis among women doubled between 2013 and 2017 and increased by 147% from 2016 to 2020.
	• Low- and middle-income countries have been particularly affected.
	• *Sex workers*: The frequency of active syphilis among sex workers worldwide was 10.8% in 2019.
	• *At-risk groups*: Bisexuals and men who have sex with men (MSM) are at higher risk, with factors such as promiscuity and multiple sexual partners playing a significant role in transmission.
	• *Age group*: Primary and secondary syphilis incidence is highest among MSM aged 20–29 years.
		The *Treponema* genus, a spiral-shaped bacteria with an outer phospholipid membrane, belongs to the spirochetal order.
		It has a slow metabolic rate, taking about 30 hours to multiply.
			• *Primary syphilis*: Typically presents as a single, painless vaginal chancre caused by *Treponema pallidum*.
			• Multiple chancres can develop on nongenital areas such as the tonsils, fingers, nipples, and oral mucosa.
			• Inguinal lymphadenopathy (tender or painless) is often present alongside the lesions.
			• *Healing of primary lesions*: Primary syphilis lesions generally heal without scarring if untreated. The incubation period ranges from 10 to 90 days, with a median of 21–25 days.
			• *Progression to secondary syphilis*: If untreated, primary syphilis progresses to secondary syphilis, characterized by hematogenous spread of the bacteria. Broad clinical symptoms, including lymphadenopathy, papulosquamous eruptions (condyloma lata), and a rash on the hands and feet.
			• *Secondary syphilis symptoms*: Common symptoms include headache, myalgia, arthralgia, pharyngitis, hepatosplenomegaly, alopecia, and malaise.
			• *Spontaneous resolution*: Both primary and secondary stages of syphilis often resolve spontaneously, leading to an early or latent phase.
			• In the latent phase, no symptoms are present, but the disease can still be detected via serological testing.
			• *Progression to tertiary syphilis*: If untreated, syphilis may progress to tertiary syphilis, which can involve:
			  ○ Cardiovascular complications, such as aortitis or aneurysms.
			  ○ Late neurosyphilis, including tabes dorsalis and syphilitic paresis.
			  ○ Benign late syphilis, with lesions such as gummas that affect various organs and tissues.

Continued

CHAPTER 4: Differential Diagnosis of Psoriasis: Distinguishing Psoriasis from Other...

Continued

Disease	Epidemiology	Etiopathogenesis	Clinical features
Mycosis fungoides (MF)	*Unknown cause*: Most cases of T-cell lymphoma, including cutaneous T-cell lymphoma (CTCL), have an unidentified cause. *Genetic dysregulation*: The development of CTCL is often associated with: Dysregulation of genes, including cancer-testis genes and B lymphoid tyrosine kinase. Disruptions in key signaling pathways, such as JAK3/STAT and NOTCH1. *Environmental factors*: There is evidence suggesting that chronic cutaneous inflammation, including factors such as chemical exposure or chronic urticaria, may play a role in the development of CTCL.	• *Infectious etiology*: Both CTCL and peripheral T-cell lymphoma (PTCL) have been linked to infectious agents. • *Bacterial associations*: Staphylococcal enterotoxin has been suggested as a potential factor in the development of these lymphomas. • *Viral associations*: Human T-cell leukemia virus (HTLV) 1 and HTLV 2: Particularly linked to adult T-cell lymphoma/leukemia. • *HIV*: Associated with various T-cell lymphomas, including CTCL. • *EBV (Epstein–Barr virus)*: Linked to natural-killer cell/T-cell lymphoma and angioimmunoblastic T-cell lymphoma (AITL). • *Cytomegalovirus* (CMV) and human herpesvirus-8 (HHV-8) have also been implicated in some	• *Early stages of CTCL (specifically mycosis fungoides or MF)*: Initially manifests as macules and patches on the skin, often appearing as benign or nonthreatening, making early diagnosis difficult. • The lesions are typically localized to the skin. • *Progression*: As the disease advances, skin lesions evolve into tumors, plaques, or nodules. • There may also be involvement of lymph nodes (adenopathy) and other organs. • *Common presentation areas*: Lesions are commonly found in areas that are shielded from sunlight, such as the buttocks, groin, and axillae. • *Diagnosis challenges*: Due to the benign nature of early lesions, CTCL (MF) is often misdiagnosed or overlooked in its early stages.
			Sezary syndrome: Arises de novo or as a progression from MF. Characterized by erythroderma (widespread reddening of the skin). Lymphadenopathy (swollen lymph nodes). Presence of Sezary cells (abnormal T-cells) in peripheral blood, skin, and lymph nodes. *SS features*: More aggressive than MF. Higher symptomatic burden and lower remission rates compared to MF. *Precursor lesions*: Certain conditions may precede or evolve into MF, including:

Continued

CHAPTER 4: Differential Diagnosis of Psoriasis: Distinguishing Psoriasis from Other...

Continued

Disease	Epidemiology	Etiopathogenesis	Clinical features
			Clonal dermatitis or cutaneous lymphoid dyscrasias. Follicular mucinosis, lymphoid papulosis, pagetoid reticulosis, and granulomatous slack skin. These conditions can signify early stages or risk factors for the development of MF or SS.
Lupus erythematosus	*Age and gender*: Young to middle-aged females, with females 3–4 times more likely to develop the lesions compared to males.	*Systemic lupus erythematosus (SLE)*: • *Etiology*: The precise cause of SLE is not well understood, but it involves a combination of genetic predisposition and immune dysregulation. • Sunlight exposure is a known trigger for SLE flares, particularly in patients with the underlying genetic and immune factors. • *Drug-induced subacute cutaneous lupus erythematosus (SCLE)*: • Certain medications have been linked to SCLE, including ACE inhibitors. • Anticonvulsants, β-blockers, immune modulators, particularly TNF-α inhibitors. • *SCLE and cancer*: There are case reports suggesting that SCLE can develop in patients with cancer. This suggests a potential association, though the mechanisms remain unclear.	SCLE can indeed present with a variety of skin manifestations that may resemble psoriatic plaques. The clinical types of SCLE are: • *Annular*: These are annular lesions (ring-shaped) with a photosensitive distribution, often seen on sun-exposed areas. • *Papulosquamous*: These lesions resemble psoriatic plaques with scaling and erythema, also found in photosensitive areas, such as the face, chest, and upper extremities. • *Mixed*: A combination of both annular and psoriasiform lesions, often in areas that are commonly exposed to the sun. • *Severe cases*: In some instances, vesiculobullous lesions (blisters or fluid-filled sacs) may develop at the periphery of annular lesions, especially in more severe cases of SCLE.
		• *Genetics of SCLE*: Recent studies have identified several genes that may be linked to SCLE: • *HLA genes*: DQ2, DRw52, DR3, HLA1, B8, and DR3. • *Complement components*: Deficits in C2 and C4 components of the complement system have been associated with SCLE. • *Environmental factors*: Medications and UV radiation are environmental triggers that contribute to the development of SCLE. This reinforces the complex interplay between genetic predisposition and environmental factors in the pathogenesis of SCLE.	

Continued

Continued

Disease	Epidemiology	Etiopathogenesis	Clinical features
			This variety of presentations makes SCLE important to differentiate from other conditions, such as psoriasis or other forms of lupus, especially in patients with a history of sun exposure or medication use.
Parapsoriasis	*Sex*: Male > female *Age*: Fifth decade of life is the most common.	Small plaque parapsoriasis (SPP) is typically considered a reactive process driven primarily by CD4+ T cells. It is characterized by the presence of small, round, well-demarcated plaques that often resemble early stages of MF, but without the typical progression seen in MF. Although some clinicians hypothesize that SPP might be an early or abortive form of T-cell lymphoma, there is no clear evidence (e.g., genetic mutations such as TP53 mutations often seen in other cancers) supporting this hypothesis. On the other hand, large plaque parapsoriasis (LPP) is believed to be a chronic inflammatory disorder that might result from long-term antigen stimulation, possibly due to repeated skin irritation or chronic inflammation. The exact cause remains speculative, but this form is often considered a precursor to MF in some cases.	*In SPP*: • The lesions are well-circumscribed and slightly scaly, with a light salmon color. • Each patch is <5 cm in diameter and often scattered across the trunk and extremities. • A unique form of SPP is the digitate pattern, characterized by palisading, elongated fingerlike patches that follow the dermatome, often most prominent on the lateral thorax and abdomen. *In LPP*: • The lesions are asymptomatic but tend to be larger than 5 cm in size. • They appear as round, oval, or irregularly shaped, with a reddish color and a scaly surface.
		In both conditions, there is no definitive proof of malignant transformation, but they can present a diagnostic challenge due to their clinical similarities to MF. Monitoring and clinical follow-up are generally recommended to track potential changes over time. In LPP, the presence of a dominant T-cell clone—which may account for up to 50% of the T-cell infiltrate—is a key feature. This clone is typically monoclonal, meaning it consists of a single population of T-cells that have undergone expansion, suggesting a degree of clonal proliferation.	

Continued

CHAPTER 4: Differential Diagnosis of Psoriasis: Distinguishing Psoriasis from Other...

Continued

Disease	Epidemiology	Etiopathogenesis	Clinical features
		If the histology appears benign, with no atypical lymphocytes or features of malignancy, the diagnosis is typically LPP. However, if atypical lymphocytes are present, this raises suspicion for a more serious condition, such as CTCL, particularly at the patch stage. This is because atypical lymphocytes are a hallmark of CTCL, and their presence may indicate progression toward a more aggressive form of lymphoma, such as MF or Sezary syndrome (SS).	
		The distinction between benign LPP and patch-stage CTCL can be challenging and requires careful histopathological evaluation, with attention to the presence of atypical lymphocytes, which could signal a more malignant progression.	

(ACE: angiotensin-converting enzyme; AIDS: acquired immunodeficiency syndrome; BCG: bacillus Calmette–Guérin; COVID-19: coronavirus disease 2019; HIV: human immunodeficiency virus; MAP: mitogen-activated protein; NSAIDs: nonsteroidal anti-inflammatory drugs; UV: ultraviolet)

■ CONCLUSION

Classical presentations of psoriasis, such as indurated, erythematous, well defined, scaly plaques on extensors make the diagnosis simple and straight forward. However, cases with atypical presentations can often pose diagnostic challenges. Therefore, clinicians should have an in depth understanding of the epidemiology, etiopathogenesis, clinical features of all the differentials of psoriasis and must integrate these findings with investigations like histopathology, dermoscopy to reach a final diagnosis. Therapeutic responses also play an important role. Hence, in cases wherein patient is not responding to treatment we must reconsider the diagnosis.

Precise differentiation ensues appropriate treatment and prevents unnecessary intervention and progression of disease. Hence, systemic, evidence based approach to the differentials of psoriasis is important in optimizing patient outcome.

TAKE HOME MESSAGE

- Psoriasis has many imitators.
- Clinical presentation and distribution is key.
- Think beyond common variants in cases when there is no response to treatment.
- Histopathology is gold standard for diagnosis.
- Clinico-pathological correlation is important to reach a final diagnosis.
- Dermoscopy plays an important role in aiding the diagnosis.
- Exclude infections first with relevant investigations.
- A stepwise evaluation integrating history, morphology, distribution, supportive investigations, and treatment response will ensure precise differentiation and optimal patient care.

5 Psoriasis: Relation with Probiotics, Prebiotics, and Gut Dysbiosis

Sambit Chatterjee, Anupam Das

■ INTRODUCTION

Psoriasis is a chronic autoimmune T-cell-mediated inflammatory cutaneous condition. It is associated with systemic comorbidities like cardiovascular diseases and metabolic syndrome.[1,2] Recent insights into the pathogenesis of psoriasis have found a link between psoriasis and gut dysbiosis. Studies have also found that probiotics as well as prebiotics can provide benefits to patients.

■ GUT MICROBIOME

The gut microbiome consists of diverse microorganisms, including bacteria, fungi, and viruses, predominantly found in the lower gut. It influences immunity, metabolizes nutrients, and helps in maintaining systemic balance. The gut microbiome affects the skin health by modulating systemic as well as local immune responses.[1-3] Dysbiosis (microbial imbalance) in the gut is linked to chronic inflammatory skin conditions like psoriasis. In psoriasis, there is immune-mediated skin lesions characterized by inflammation and keratinocyte hyperproliferation. Gut dysbiosis in psoriasis patients includes reduced beneficial bacteria like *Faecalibacterium prausnitzii* and increased pathogenic species. These changes influence inflammatory pathways, leading to cytokine production interleukin 17 (IL-17), IL-22, and immune responses, exacerbating skin inflammation.[4,5] Gut bacteria can also influence psoriasis through immune modulation altering T-cell activity. Metabolism of nutrients such as butyrate production enhances gut barrier function decreasing inflammation. Intestinal inflammation and microbial metabolites can exacerbate psoriasis by triggering systemic immune responses.[6,7] Diets like the Mediterranean diet can help in improving symptoms by altering gut microbial diversity as well as reducing inflammation.[7] Some studies have shown that fecal microbiota transplantation (FMT) can help in restoration of microbial balance, decreasing inflammation.[6]

■ ROLE OF PROBIOTICS AND PREBIOTICS

Probiotics and prebiotics restore gut microbiome balance, which can reduce inflammation and help in improving skin barrier function. Studies have suggested that probiotics like *Lactobacillus* and *Bifidobacterium* species alleviated psoriasis symptoms by reducing proinflammatory cytokines and promoting skin healing. Probiotic use has shown promising results in clinical trials; however, further research is necessary to prove their efficacy.[8-10] Modulating the gut microbiome offers a novel approach for managing psoriasis as well as other inflammatory diseases. Probiotics are considered relatively safe with minimal adverse effects, making them a potential adjunct or alternative therapy. A 12-week-long clinical trial was done by Buhaș et al. involving 63 psoriasis patients.[11] The intervention group received probiotics (containing five different *Bacillus* species) and prebiotics along with topical treatment for psoriasis. The control group received topical treatment only. The intervention group showed significant decrease in psoriasis severity [psoriasis area and severity (PASI)] scores as well as improvement in the quality of life [Dermatology Life Quality Index (DLQI)]. There was reduced levels of the proinflammatory cytokines like tumor necrosis factor alpha (TNF-α) and IL-6. There was an increase seen in the levels of anti-inflammatory cytokine IL-10 in the intervention group. The intervention led to positive shifts in the gut microbiota composition including higher diversity and increased beneficial bacterial abundance like *Akkermansia muciniphila* and decreasing inflammation-associated bacteria. Improvements in lipid profiles like decreased low-density lipoprotein (LDL), triglycerides, and uric acid levels were found in the intervention group.[12,13] One of the limitations of this study was that it was a nonrandomized design with a small sample size. Gut microbiota changes were analyzed only in a subset of the intervention group without any comparison with the control group.

The causal relationship between gut microbiota and psoriasis needs more exploration, particularly through large-scale studies as well as animal studies.[14] Probiotics and prebiotics when combined along with standard topical treatment show promising results in improving clinical and systemic outcomes in psoriasis. Further research is needed to confirm these findings and optimize therapeutic strategies.

CONCLUSION

"Gut dysbiosis in psoriasis" refers to an imbalance in the gut microbiome composition of individuals with psoriasis, where the diversity and abundance of certain bacteria are altered compared to healthy individuals, potentially contributing to the development and severity of the skin condition by influencing the immune system and triggering inflammatory responses; research suggests this could be a significant factor in psoriasis pathogenesis, with potential for therapeutic interventions targeting the gut microbiota through probiotics or fecal microbiota transplantation.

TAKE HOME MESSAGE

- Studies have shown that people with psoriasis often exhibit a different gut microbiome composition, with lower diversity and altered ratios of specific bacterial species compared to healthy individuals.
- The gut microbiota plays a crucial role in immune regulation, and changes in its composition can lead to an overactive immune response, contributing to the inflammatory nature of psoriasis.
- Some research suggests that gut dysbiosis might lead to a "leaky gut" where bacteria and their toxins can leak into the bloodstream, triggering systemic inflammation that manifests on the skin as psoriatic lesions.
- Understanding the role of gut dysbiosis in psoriasis opens up possibilities for novel treatments like probiotic supplements, prebiotics to nourish beneficial bacteria, or fecal microbiota transplantation (FMT) to restore a healthier gut microbiome.
- Probiotics and prebiotics may help with psoriasis by restoring the balance of gut bacteria and reducing inflammation.

REFERENCES

1. O'Neill CA, Monteleone G, McLaughlin JT, Paus R. The gutskin axis in health and disease: A paradigm with therapeutic implications. BioEssays. 2016;38:116776.
2. Levkovich T, Poutahidis T, Smillie C, Varian BJ, Ibrahim YM, Lakritz JR, et al. Probiotic bacteria induce a 'glow of health'. PLoS One. 2013;8:e53867.
3. Gloster HM, Gebauer LE, Mistur RL. Cutaneous manifestations of gastrointestinal disease. In: Gloster HM, Gebauer LE, Mistur RL (Eds). Absolute Dermatology Review. Cham: Springer; 2016. pp. 1719.
4. Shah KR, Boland CR, Patel M, Thrash B, Menter A. Cutaneous manifestations of gastrointestinal disease: Part I. J Am Acad Dermatol. 2013;68:189. e121.
5. Thrash B, Patel M, Shah KR, Boland CR, Menter A. Cutaneous manifestations of gastrointestinal disease: Part II. J Am Acad Dermatol. 2013;68:211. e133.
6. Xu Q, Ni JJ, Han BX, Yan SS, Wei XT, Feng GJ, et al. Causal relationship between gut microbiota and autoimmune diseases: A two-sample Mendelian randomization study. Front Immunol. 2021;12: 746998.
7. Neu AK, Pleissner D, Mehlmann K, Schneider R, Puerta-Quintero GI, Venus J. Fermentative utilization of coffee mucilage using Bacillus coagulans and investigation of down-stream processing of fermentation broth for optically pure l(+)-lactic acid production. Bioresour. Technol. 2016;211:398-405.
8. Hidalgo-Cantabrana C, Gómez J, Delgado S, Requena-López S, Queiro-Silva R, Margolles A, et al. Gut Microbiota Dysbiosis in a Cohort of Patients with Psoriasis. Br J Dermatol. 2019;181:1287-95.
9. Zhang X, Shi L, Sun T, Guo K, Geng S. Dysbiosis of Gut Microbiota and Its Correlation with Dysregulation of Cytokines in Psoriasis Patients. BMC Microbiol. 2021;21:78.
10. Schade L, Mesa D, Faria AR, Santamaria JR, Xavier CA, Ribeiro D, et al. The Gut Microbiota Profile in Psoriasis: A Brazilian Case-control Study. Lett Appl Microbiol. 2021;74:498-504.
11. Buhaş MC, Candrea R, Gavrilas LI, Miere D, Tătaru A, Boca A, et al. Transforming Psoriasis Care: Probiotics and Prebiotics as Novel Therapeutic Approaches. Int J Mol Sci. 2023;24:11225.
12. Lin C, Zeng T, Deng Y, Yang W, Xiong J. Treatment of Psoriasis Vulgaris Using Bacteroides Fragilis BF839: A Single-Arm, Open Preliminary Clinical Study. Sheng Wu Gong Cheng Xue Bao. 2021;37:3828-35.
13. Moludi J, Fathollahi P, Khedmatgozar H, Pourteymour Fard Tabrizi F, Ghareaghaj Zare A, Razmi H, et al. Probiotics Supplementation Improves Quality of Life, Clinical Symptoms, and Inflammatory Status in Patients with Psoriasis. J Drugs Dermatol. 2022;21:637-44.
14. Lu W, Deng Y, Fang Z, Zhai Q, Cui S, Zhao J, et al. Potential Role of Probiotics in Ameliorating Psoriasis by Modulating Gut Microbiota in Imiquimod-Induced Psoriasis-Like Mice. Nutrients. 2021;13:2010.

Comorbidities Associated with Psoriasis: Cardiovascular Disease, Metabolic Syndrome, and Depression

Sudip Das, Apeksha Singh

■ INTRODUCTION

Psoriasis is a condition that affects more than only the skin, nails, and scalp. It is frequently accompanied by comorbidities, which reduce working days and increase financial burden. It affects 2% of the population worldwide, irrespective of age, sex or ethnicity,[1] affecting approximately 125 million people worldwide.[1-3] In addition to the much-discussed cardiometabolic diseases, gastrointestinal disorders, chronic kidney diseases, cancer, and infections, there is evidence linking psoriasis to other systemic diseases affecting the skin, reproductive, oral, and ocular systems.

■ PSORIASIS AND METABOLIC SYNDROME ALSO KNOWN AS SYNDROME X

Metabolic syndrome (MetS) and psoriasis have the strongest association. The prevalence of MetS ranges from 20 to 50% in the psoriatic patients, which is higher than the general population. MetS is more frequent in females with psoriasis, patients older than 40 years of age and those with high Psoriasis Area and Severity Index (PASI) scores.[4]

Under current guidelines, revised in 2005 by the National Heart, Lung, and Blood Institute (NHLBI) and the American Heart Association (AHA), MetS is diagnosed when a patient fulfils at least three of the following five criteria:

1. Fasting glucose ≥100 mg/dL
2. Blood pressure ≥130/85 mm Hg
3. Triglycerides ≥150 mg/dL
4. High-density lipoprotein cholesterol (HDL-C) < 40 mg/dL in men or <50 mg/dL in women
5. Waist circumference (WC) ≥ 102 cm (40 inches) in men or ≥88 cm (35 inches) in women [The International Diabetes Federation (IDF) criteria allow the use of a body mass index (BMI) > 30 kg/m² instead of the WC criterion].

■ PATHOPHYSIOLOGY

Metabolic syndrome leads to obesity, which creates a proinflammatory state in the body eventually exacerbating psoriasis. It was first described by GM Reaven in 1988. The main pathophysiology behind MetS is insulin resistance.

Proinflammatory milieu: Cytokines of type 1 helper (Th1) pathway form a common link between the two conditions.

■ METABOLIC SYNDROME AND CHILDHOOD PSORIASIS

A meta-analysis done on children with psoriasis showed that the HDL-C level was significantly decreased and the mean level of

CHAPTER 6: Comorbidities Associated with Psoriasis: Cardiovascular Disease...

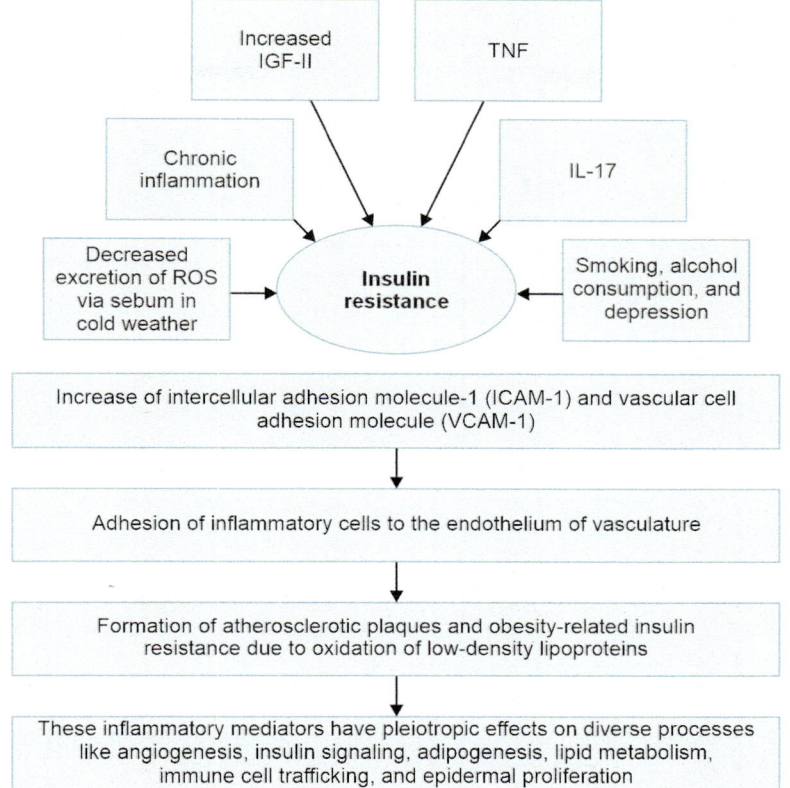

FLOWCHART 1: Moreover, chronic inflammation in psoriasis leads to increased insulin-like growth factor-II (IGF-II), which has a role in epidermal proliferation, atherosclerosis, and lipid metabolism leading to metabolic syndrome (MetS).
(IL-17: interleukin 17; ROS: reactive oxygen species; TNF: tumor necrosis factor)

fasting glucose in children with psoriasis was higher than in healthy children.[5] This may point toward the early stage of MetS in children with psoriasis **(Flowchart 1)**.

■ OBESITY

One independent risk factor for psoriasis is obesity. Higher BMI was reported to enhance the incidence of psoriasis in research on incident psoriasis.[6,7] There is a correlation between an elevated risk of psoriasis and obesity as determined by BMI, WC, waist-to-hip ratio, and weight growth.[8] WC measuring central adiposity is a specific factor affecting psoriatic risk. Tumor necrosis factor alpha (TNF-α) is found to be elevated in the skin and blood of patients with psoriasis. It is also released from adipose tissue in those with obesity **(Flowchart 2)**.

Tumor necrosis factor inhibitors (TNF-i) were linked to a significant increase in body weight when compared to conventional systemic treatments, according to a systematic review and network meta-analysis involving six studies; anti-IL-12/IL-23 or anti-IL-17 biologics, on the other hand, had no effect on an increase in body weight or BMI.[9]

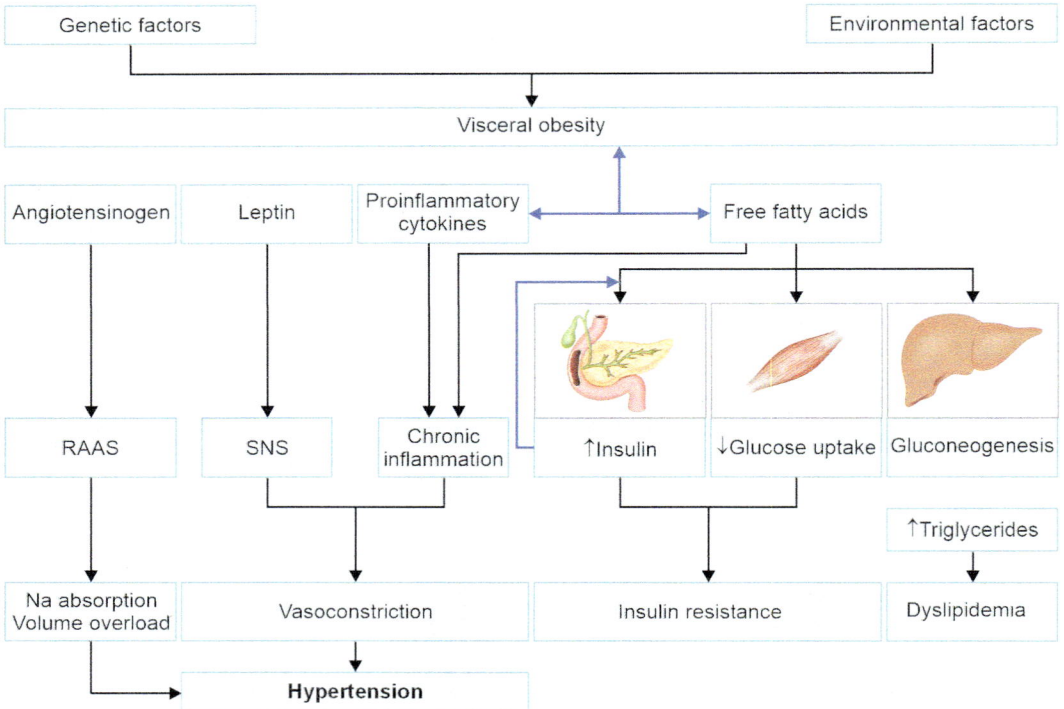

FLOWCHART 2: Pathophysiological dysfunction in metabolic parameters in the body may contribute to skin diseases and vice versa.
(RAAS: renin–angiotensin–aldosterone system; SNS: sympathetic nervous system)

■ HYPERTENSION

Hypertension is more prevalent among patients with versus without psoriasis. The odds of hypertension among patients with psoriasis increased with greater disease severity with odds ratios (ORs) of 1.30 [95% confidence interval (CI) 1.15–1.47] for mild and 1.49 (95% CI 1.20–1.86) for severe psoriasis as defined by treatment patterns.[9]

■ TYPE 2 DIABETES

Ikumi et al. showed that skin severity, blood glucose level, and glycated hemoglobin were highly correlated with psoriasis, mainly via IL-17, in patients with type 2 diabetes. Psoriasis susceptibility loci like PSORS2, PSORS3, and PSORS4 are also associated with loci of susceptibility for MetS, diabetes type 2, familial hyperlipidemia, and cardiovascular disease (CVD).[10]

■ BLOOD LIPIDS

Psoriasis is significantly associated with hypercholesterolemia, hospital-diagnosed hypertension, and hyperlipidemia. Visceral fat was associated with psoriasis, hyper-triglyceridemia, low HDL, and type 2 diabetes, and these associations were linked to serum IL-6, adiponectin, TNF, and insulin resistance.

Psoriasis increases oxidative stress by decreasing the level of folic acid and increased homocysteine levels, eventually leading to an increased level of lipids and cholesterol in the blood.

PSORIASIS AND NONALCOHOLIC FATTY LIVER DISEASE

Gisondi et al. reported that a higher rate of ultrasound-diagnosed nonalcoholic fatty liver disease (NAFLD) (47%) in 130 patients with psoriasis than in 260 healthy controls (28%) matched for age, sex, and BMI.[11] It has been demonstrated that IL-17 plays a role in both psoriasis and NAFLD. The presence of IL-17 and Th17 cells may hasten the transition from mild-to-severe steatohepatitis. In addition to the high frequency of NAFLD in psoriasis, dermatologists should be aware of the potential for steatohepatitis, particularly in cases of severe psoriasis or the presence of MetS symptoms **(Flowchart 3)**.

CARDIOMETABOLIC DISEASE

- CVD is prevalent among patients with psoriasis, especially those with more severe skin disease. The incidence of overall atherosclerotic CVD is higher in psoriasis compared with controls.
- Psoriasis may be an independent risk factor for diabetes and major adverse cardiovascular events (MACE); risk of MACE is greatest among those with severe psoriasis.
- A systematic review and meta-analysis including 24 studies found that psoriasis patients had a higher homocysteine level and a lower folate level.
- Shared pathophysiologic pathways between psoriasis and CVD, including chronic Th1 T-cell- and Th17-mediated inflammation,[12,13] monocyte and neutrophil modulation, increased oxidative stress, endothelial cell dysfunction, increased uric acid[14] angiogenesis.
- In addition, persistent pathophysiologic processes that drive psoriasis (e.g., epidermal hyperproliferation, inflammation,[15] and angiogenesis) may also exert pleiotropic adverse effects on the cardiovascular (CV) system that contribute to atherogenesis.

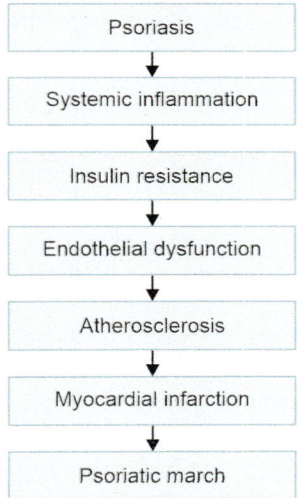

FLOWCHART 3: The idea behind the psoriatic march. Along with causing inflammation on the skin, psoriasis also produces systemic inflammation in the body. This can result in increased insulin resistance, damage to vascular endothelial cells, atherosclerosis, and myocardial infarction. We refer to this series of events as the psoriatic march. In this process, obesity is an exacerbating factor while ongoing systemic medication is a suppressing element.

REDUCTION OF CARDIO-VASCULAR DISEASE RISK BY BIOLOGICS

After receiving biologic therapy for a year in 121 patients who were biologically untreated at baseline, an analysis showed that the treatment was linked to a 6% decrease in the burden of noncalcified plaque ($p = 0.005$) and a 0.03% decrease in necrotic cores. Patients treated with IL-17 inhibitors showed significant reductions in noncalcified coronary plaque burden compared to patients treated with anti-IL-12/IL-23 antibodies or no biologic therapy.[16]

GOUT

A nationwide, population-based, cross-sectional study in Taiwan found gout was associated with psoriasis,[17] and a positive correlation was found between PASI scores and serum uric acid levels in psoriasis patients.

AUTOIMMUNE THYROID DISEASE

Hypothyroidism, hyperthyroidism, and thyroid peroxidase antibody positive may be linked to a higher incidence of psoriatic illness, according to a meta-analysis.[18] Individuals without thyroid problems do not exhibit elevated blood C-reactive protein levels or significantly higher PASI scores than those who do.

MENTAL HEALTH DISEASES

The hazard ratio (HR) of any mental disorder is 1.75 in psoriasis persons compared with the general population, and the main mental disorders reported were as follows: Vascular dementia, schizophrenia, bipolar disorder, unipolar depression, generalized anxiety disorder, and personality disorders.[19] Risk factors include female gender, a younger age of disease onset, those with self-assessment of severe psoriasis, type D personality, younger patients, and those with lesions on sensitive or visible areas.[20]

Depression/Anxiety

Patients with psoriasis had anxiety/depression at rates ranging from 11.52 to 27.00%.[21-23] Comparing psoriasis patients to the referent cohort, they showed a higher likelihood of depression,[21-23] anxiety disorders, co-occurring anxiety and depression, and somatoform disorders.

Sleep Disorders

A systematic review observed an overall 36–81.8% prevalence of obstructive sleep apnea in psoriasis,[24] and psoriasis is also associated with restless legs syndrome, which is a possible sign of autonomic activation in psoriasis.

Newly Reported Mental Comorbidity of Psoriasis

Increased risk of Parkinson disease[25] and migraine, especially migraine with aura was reported in patients with psoriasis; Th17 and proinflammatory cytokines may play a role in the relationship between these two conditions.[26]

CHRONIC KIDNEY DISEASE

Psoriasis and chronic kidney disease (CKD) may be related in both directions. In patients with CKD with anemia, there was a significant correlation between low hemoglobin levels and psoriasis risk.[27] In patients with psoriasis, statin therapy for hyperlipidemia decreased the risk of CKD.

MALIGNANCY

In an extensive review and meta-analysis involving 112 cohort studies, the total cancer prevalence in psoriasis patients was found to be 4.78%.[28] Psoriasis patients had a higher chance of developing keratinocyte cancer, lymphomas, lung cancer, bladder cancer, melanoma, or hematologic cancer. According to reports, individuals with psoriasis receiving systemic treatment had a significantly higher risk of non-Hodgkin lymphoma, skin cancers other than melanoma, and malignancies of the bone and cartilage.[29,30]

FATIGUE

Psoriasis was associated with an elevated risk of chronic fatigue syndrome, which is differentiated by sex and age.[31] Fatigue severity was associated with smoking, pain, and depression, but not with psoriasis severity.

INFLAMMATORY BOWEL DISEASES

The two main gastrointestinal comorbidities of psoriasis are inflammatory bowel diseases (IBDs), which comprise ulcerative colitis (UC) and Crohn's disease (CD), two chronic idiopathic inflammatory disorders. The presence of CD was significantly associated with psoriasis,[32] and psoriasis was associated with an increased risk of CD and UC. These two meta-analyses revealed significant bidirectional associations between psoriasis and IBDs. While psoriasis-CD individuals have mild (early onset) psoriasis but a severe CD phenotype, psoriasis-UC patients may have a higher BMI and fewer skin symptoms than those with psoriasis alone.

INFECTION

Psoriasis is associated with an unremarkable increase in the risk of serious psoriasis severity is a predictor of serious infection risk.[33]

CORONAVIRUS DISEASE 2019

Systemic therapy did not exacerbate coronavirus disease 2019 (COVID-19) in psoriasis, according to a retrospective cohort research conducted in Brazil.[34] In terms of the risk of respiratory tract and severe acute respiratory syndrome coronavirus 2 (SARS-CoV-2) infections, it is not always clear if TNF-i is safer than biologics that target IL-17 and IL-23. Nonbiologic systemic treatments were linked to a higher risk of COVID-19-related hospitalization in patients with moderate-to-severe psoriasis than biologic usage. Established risk variables included older age, male sex, non-white ethnicity, and having comorbidities. Patients with COVID-19 may be more susceptible to mortality if they have a "cytokine storm syndrome".

HEPATITIS B AND C

Hepatitis B or C prevalence did not significantly differ between the psoriasis-affected and nonaffected individuals. Also, among psoriatic patients with chronic viral hepatitis, long-term methotrexate usage may not be linked to a risk of liver cirrhosis.[35]

HUMAN IMMUNODEFICIENCY VIRUS

Severe psoriasis was an independent risk factor for steatosis in patients with human immunodeficiency virus (HIV) infection, and HIV infection was an independent risk factor for the development of psoriasis.

MYCOBACTERIUM

Before beginning biotherapy for psoriasis, it is imperative to detect latent *Mycobacterium tuberculosis* infection since biotherapy has the potential to reactivate the infection. 8.5% of Italian psoriasis patients had latent tuberculosis infection, according to a national investigation. Independent risk variables were male sex, age above 55 years, and starting conventional treatment.

Staphylococcal colonization: A 4.5-fold increase of *Staphylococcus aureus* colonization was found on the patients' skin compared to healthy controls, and 60% was in the nares.

HERPES ZOSTER

The group with moderate-to-severe psoriasis had a considerably higher risk of herpes zoster (HZ), and immunosuppressive medication was linked to this risk.

MUSCULOSKELETAL SYSTEM

Psoriatic Arthritis

Psoriatic arthritis (PsA), which has a strong correlation with psoriasis, develops in about one-third of psoriasis patients. After the commencement of psoriasis, the risk of PsA progressively rises with the length of cutaneous symptoms.

Osteoporosis and Fracture

There is little evidence supporting the association between psoriasis and osteoporosis/osteopenia. Systematic review and meta-analysis including 12 studies concluded that patients with psoriasis/PsA have an increased risk of fractures.

■ SKIN

The most common skin comorbidity associated with psoriasis was onychomycosis, which was followed by rosacea and telangiectasia. According to scores on the Psoriasis Disability Index, Skindex 29, Dermatology Life Quality Index, and other measures, psoriatic patients with skin conditions had a lower quality of life than those without. There have also been reports of vitiligo and bullous illness in conjunction with psoriasis.

Chronic Itch

Women, lower educational attainment, pustular psoriasis, lesions on exposed or sensitive areas, palmoplantar areas, severe illness, disease duration <15 years, and no or few previous systemic therapies were all linked to higher levels of itching.

■ REPRODUCTIVE SYSTEM

Male

Patients with psoriasis had a prevalence of sexual dysfunction (SD) ranging from 40.0 to 55.6%, according to a thorough literature review and meta-analysis that included 28 studies.[36] Risk factors for SD include psychological and physical comorbidities; genital psoriasis, PsA, and anxiety and depression have the largest correlations with SD. Biologic medications are beneficial for improving SD.

Female

Preterm birth, cesarean delivery, (pre)eclampsia, gestational hypertension, and gestational diabetes were among the adverse maternal outcomes that pregnant women with psoriasis had a significantly higher risk of, but not adverse neonatal events.[37]

■ ORAL COMORBIDITIES

In adult patients with psoriasis compared to those without, a positive correlation was observed between both geographical tongue (GT) and fissured tongue, according to a cross-sectional study conducted in a Saudi Arabian hospital.

Patients with GT had statistically higher PASI scores and showed less progress following treatment.

Periodontitis

A meta-analysis encompassing two cohort studies and three case-control studies revealed a statistically significant increased risk of psoriasis in individuals with periodontitis.[38]

Conversely, research revealed a noteworthy elevated risk of periodontitis linked to psoriasis, with the highest risk shown in individuals with severe psoriasis and PsA.

■ TREATMENT

Prior to initiating treatment with any drug for psoriasis, a few tests should always be completed. Prior to beginning cyclosporine therapy, renal function tests must be completed since psoriatic patients have a high incidence of MetS and diabetes mellitus **(Fig. 1)**.

Because apremilast virtually never needs to be monitored while being treated, it has a strong safety record, and it can assist induce

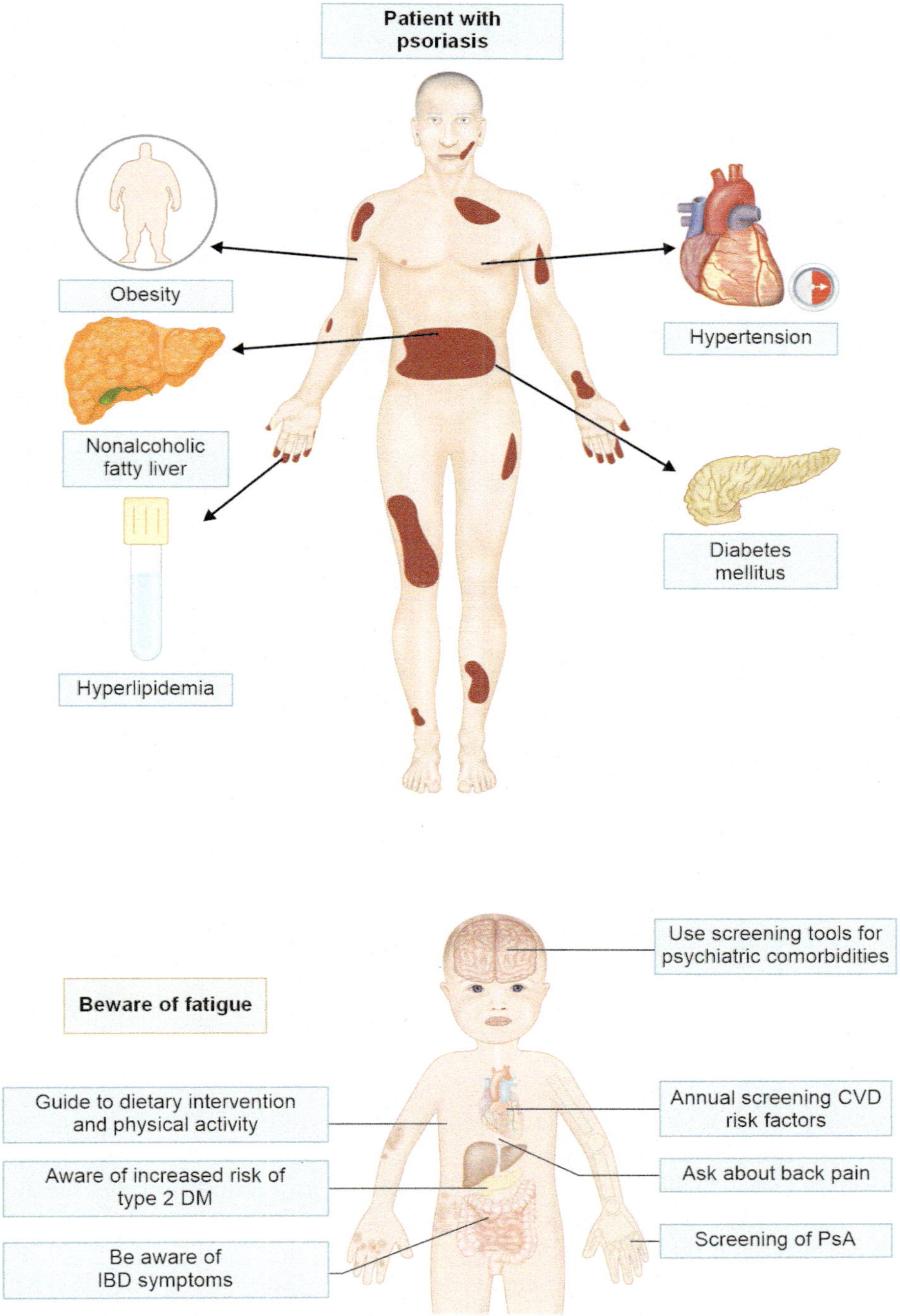

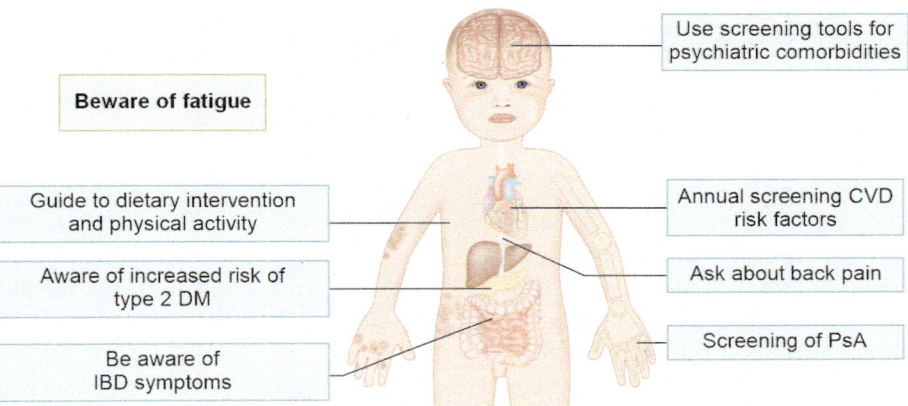

FIG. 1: A brief overview of for the clinician's consideration, regarding psoriasis comorbidities.
(CVD: cardiovascular disease; DM: diabetes mellitus; IBD: inflammatory bowel disease; PsA: psoriatic arthritis)

CHAPTER 6: Comorbidities Associated with Psoriasis: Cardiovascular Disease...

TABLE 1: Adverse effects of drugs used in psoriasis on metabolic syndrome[9]

Systemic drugs used in psoriasis		Adverse effects on metabolic syndrome
Immunomodulators/ immunosuppressors	Methotrexate	Impaired renal and liver function
	Cyclosporine	Dyslipidemia, diabetes, hypertension, impaired renal function
Oral retinoids	Acitretin	Dyslipidemia
Phosphodiesterase 5 inhibitors	Apremilast	None
Biologics	Anti-TNF agents	Obesity
	IL-17 inhibitors	None
	IL-22 and IL-23 inhibitors	None

(IL-17: interleukin 17; TNF: tumor necrosis factor)

TABLE 2: Preferred biologicals in special situations in psoriasis[39]

Class of drugs	Drug/Comorbidity	PsA	CD	CA	Obesity	Atherosclerosis	CHF	MS
TNF-α inhibitors	Etanercept	++	+	–	+	++	–/+	×
	Adalimumab	++	+	–	+	++	–/+	×
	Infliximab	++	++	–	++	++	–/+	×
	Certolizumab	++	++	–	+	++	–/+	×
	Golimumab	++	++	–	+	++	–/+	×
IL-12/ IL-23 inhibitor	Ustekinumab	+	++	+	++	+	++	+
IL-23 inhibitors	Guselkumab	?	?	?/+	++	?	++	?/+
	Tildrakizumab	?	?	?/+	++	?	++	?/+
	Risankizumab	?	?	?/+	?	?	++	?/+
	Mirikizumab	?	?	?/+	?	?	++	?/+
IL-17	Secukinumab	++	++	?/+	++	?	++	+
	Ixekizumab	++	++	?/+	++	?	++	+
	Brodalumab	+	–	?/+	++	?	++	+

(IL-12: interleukin 12; TNF-α: tumor necrosis factor alpha)

weight loss, which is beneficial for both psoriasis and MetS, it is being used more and more for psoriasis profile and helps to induce weight loss, which helps not only in psoriasis but also in MetS. Because anti-TNF drugs have a high safety profile and reduce the risk of new-onset type 2 diabetes in patients receiving conventional treatment, they may be employed in the treatment of psoriasis with concomitant MetS. IL-17, IL-12, and IL-23 is the target of more recent biologicals that are very effective in treating psoriasis; nevertheless, further long-term follow-up data is needed to comment on their involvement in treating psoriasis with accompanying MetS. **Tables 1 and 2** summarizes the negative effects of several psoriasis medications on MetS.

Thus, before initiating a psoriasis patient on long-term treatment with any of the drugs, it is crucial to monitor blood pressure, BMI, WC, look into fasting lipid profile, renal and liver function tests, fasting blood glucose, and get a history of smoking, alcohol consumption, etc.

CONCLUSION

Psoriasis serves as more than a dermatological challenge; it is a systemic disease with profound implications on physical and mental health. Its strong association with conditions such as metabolic syndrome, cardiovascular diseases, and depression necessitates a multidisciplinary approach to care. Understanding the interconnectedness of these conditions is key to designing comprehensive treatment plans that address not only the skin manifestations but also the broader health risks associated with psoriasis. Clinicians should prioritize monitoring for comorbidities, utilizing biologics effectively, and educating patients on lifestyle modifications to mitigate these risks.

TAKE HOME MESSAGE

Psoriasis is not just a skin condition—it is intricately linked to multiple systemic comorbidities that significantly impact a patient's quality of life and overall health. Among these, metabolic syndrome, cardiovascular diseases, and mental health disorders are the most prominent. The shared inflammatory pathways, particularly involving cytokines like IL-17 and TNF-α, underline the interplay between psoriasis and these systemic conditions. Early recognition and integrated management of these comorbidities, alongside effective psoriasis treatment, are critical in improving patient outcomes.

REFERENCES

1. National Psoriasis Foundation. (2022). Psoriasis statistics. [online] Available from https://www.psoriasis.org/cure_known_statistics [Last accessed January 2025].
2. Kurd SK, Gelfand JM. The prevalence of previously diagnosed and undiagnosed psoriasis in US adults: results from NHANES 2003-2004. J Am Acad Dermatol. 2009;60:218-24.
3. Rachakonda TD, Schupp CW, Armstrong AW. Psoriasis prevalence among adults in the United States. J Am Acad Dermatol. 2014;70:512-6.
4. Arnold KA, Treister AD, Lio PA, Alenghat FJ. Association of Atherosclerosis Prevalence With Age, Race, and Traditional Risk Factors in Patients with Psoriasis. JAMA Dermatol. 2019;155(5):622-3.
5. Pietrzak A, Grywalska E, Walankiewicz M, Lotti T, Roliński J, Myśliński W, et al. Psoriasis and metabolic syndrome in children: Current data. Clin Exp Dermatol. 2017;42:131-6.
6. Setty AR, Curhan G, Choi HK. Obesity, waist circumference, weight change, and the risk of psoriasis in women: Nurses' Health Study II. Arch Intern Med. 2007;167(15):1670-5.
7. Kumar S, Han J, Li T, Qureshi AA. Obesity, waist circumference, weight change and the risk of psoriasis in US women. J Eur Acad Dermatol Venereol. 2013;27(10):1293-8.
8. Mehta NN, Yu Y, Pinnelas R, Krishnamoorthy P, Shin DB, Troxel AB, et al. Attributable risk estimate of severe psoriasis on major cardiovascular events. Am J Med. 2011;124:775.e1-6.
9. Agarwal K, Das S, Kumar R, De A. 'Psoriasis and its association with metabolic syndrome'. Indian J Dermatol. 2023;68(3):274-7.
10. Azfar RS, Gelfand JM. Psoriasis and metabolic disease: Epidemiology and pathophysiology. Curr Opin Rheumatol. 2008;20:416-22.
11. Gisondi P, Targher G, Zoppini G, Girolomoni G. Non-alcoholic fatty liver disease in patients with chronic plaque psoriasis. J Hepatol. 2009;51(4):758-64.
12. Armstrong AW, Voyles SV, Armstrong EJ, Fuller EN, Rutledge JC. A tale of two plaques: convergent mechanisms of T-cell-mediated inflammation in psoriasis and atherosclerosis. Exp Dermatol. 2011;20(7):544-9.
13. Wang Y, Gao H, Loyd CM, Fu W, Diaconu D, Liu S, et al. Chronic skin-specific inflammation promotes vascular inflammation and thrombosis. J Invest Dermatol. 2012;132(8):2067-75.
14. Puig JG, Mateos FA, Jiménez ML, Gomez PL, Michán AA, Vázquez JO. Uric acid metabolism in psoriasis. Adv Exp Med Biol. 1986;195(Pt A):411-6.
15. Cheung L, Fisher RM, Kuzmina N, Li D, Li X, Werngren O, et al. Psoriasis Skin Inflammation-Induced microRNA-26b Targets NCEH1 in Underlying Subcutaneous Adipose Tissue. J Invest Dermatol. 2016;136(3):640-8.
16. Elnabawi YA, Dey AK, Goyal A, Groenendyk JW, Chung JH, Belur AD, et al. Coronary artery plaque characteristics and treatment with biologic therapy in severe psoriasis: results from a prospective observational study. Cardiovasc Res. 2019;115(4):721-8.

17. Hu SC, Lin CL, Tu HP. Association Between Psoriasis, Psoriatic Arthritis and Gout: A Nationwide Population-Based Study. J Eur Acad Dermatol Venereol. 2019;33(3):560-7.
18. Khan SR, Bano A, Wakkee M, Korevaar TIM, Franco OH, Nijsten TEC, et al. The Association of Autoimmune Thyroid Disease (Aitd) With Psoriatic Disease: A Prospective Cohort Study, Systematic Review and Meta-Analysis. Eur J Endocrinol. 2017;177(4):347-59.
19. Leisner MZ, Riis JL, Schwartz S, Iversen L, Østergaard SD, Olsen MS. Psoriasis and Risk of Mental Disorders in Denmark. JAMA Dermatol. 2019;155(6):745-7.
20. Lim DS, Bewley A, Oon HH. Psychological Profile of Patients With Psoriasis. Ann Acad Med Singap. 2018;47(12):516-22.
21. Cai Q, Teeple A, Wu B, Muser E. Prevalence and Economic Burden of Comorbid Anxiety and Depression Among Patients With Moderate-To-Severe Psoriasis. J Med Econ. 2019;22(12):1290-7.
22. Oh J, Jung KJ, Kim TG, Kim HW, Jee SH, Lee MG. Risk of Psychiatric Diseases Among Patients With Psoriasis in Korea: A 12-Year Nationwide Population-Based Cohort Study. J Dermatol. 2021;48(11):1763-71.
23. Tian Z, Huang Y, Yue T, Zhou J, Tao L, Han L, et al. A Chinese Cross-Sectional Study on Depression and Anxiety Symptoms in Patients With Psoriasis Vulgaris. Psychol Health Med. 2019;24(3):269-80.
24. Gupta MA, Gupta AK. Psoriasis Is Associated With a Higher Prevalence of Obstructive Sleep Apnea and Restless Legs Syndrome: A Possible Indication of Autonomic Activation in Psoriasis. J Clin Sleep Med. 2018;14(6):1085.
25. Lee JH, Han K, Gee HY. The Incidence Rates and Risk Factors of Parkinson Disease in Patients With Psoriasis: A Nationwide Population-Based Cohort Study. J Am Acad Dermatol. 2020;83(6):1688-95.
26. Capo A, Affaitati G, Giamberardino MA, Amerio P. Psoriasis and Migraine. J Eur Acad Dermatol Venereol. 2018;32(1):57-61.
27. Lee SH, Kim M, Han KD, Lee JH. Low Hemoglobin Levels and an Increased Risk of Psoriasis in Patients With Chronic Kidney Disease. Sci Rep. 2021;11(1):14741.
28. Vaengebjerg S, Skov L, Egeberg A, Loft ND. Prevalence, Incidence, and Risk of Cancer in Patients With Psoriasis and Psoriatic Arthritis: A Systematic Review and Meta-Analysis. JAMA Dermatol. 2020;156(4):421-9.
29. Jensen P, Egeberg A, Gislason G, Thyssen JP, Skov L. Risk of Uncommon Cancers in Patients With Psoriasis: A Danish Nationwide Cohort Study. J Eur Acad Dermatol Venereol. 2018;32(4):601-5.
30. Lee JW, Jung KJ, Kim TG, Lee M, Oh J, Jee SH, et al. Risk of Malignancy in Patients With Psoriasis: A 15-Year Nationwide Population-Based Prospective Cohort Study in Korea. J Eur Acad Dermatol Venereol. 2019;33(12):2296-304.
31. Tsai SY, Chen HJ, Chen C, Lio CF, Kuo CF, Leong KH, et al. Increased Risk of Chronic Fatigue Syndrome Following Psoriasis: A Nationwide Population-Based Cohort Study. J Transl Med. 2019;17(1):154.
32. Eppinga H, Poortinga S, Thio HB, Nijsten TEC, Nuij V, van der Woude CJ, et al. Prevalence and Phenotype of Concurrent Psoriasis and Inflammatory Bowel Disease. Inflamm Bowel Dis. 2017;23(10):1783-9.
33. Takeshita J, Shin DB, Ogdie A, Gelfand JM. Risk of Serious Infection, Opportunistic Infection, and Herpes Zoster Among Patients With Psoriasis in the United Kingdom. J Invest Dermatol. 2018;138(8):1726-35.
34. Lima XT, Cueva MA, Lopes EM, Alora MB. Severe Covid-19 Outcomes in Patients With Psoriasis. J Eur Acad Dermatol Venereol. 2020;34(12):e776-e8.
35. Tang KT, Chen YM, Chang SN, Lin CH, Chen DY. Psoriatic Patients With Chronic Viral Hepatitis Do Not Have an Increased Risk of Liver Cirrhosis Despite Long-Term Methotrexate Use: Real-World Data From a Nationwide Cohort Study in Taiwan. J Am Acad Dermatol. 2018;79(4):652-8.
36. Molina-Leyva A, Salvador-Rodriguez L, Martinez-Lopez A, Ruiz-Carrascosa JC, Arias-Santiago S. Association Between Psoriasis and Sexual and Erectile Dysfunction in Epidemiologic Studies: A Systematic Review. JAMA Dermatol. 2019;155(1):98-106.
37. Xie W, Huang H, Ji L, Zhang Z. Maternal and Neonatal Outcomes in Pregnant Women With Psoriasis and Psoriatic Arthritis: A Systematic Review and MetaAnalysis. Rheumatology (Oxford). 2021;60(9):4018-28.
38. Ungprasert P, Wijarnpreecha K, Wetter DA. Periodontitis and Risk of Psoriasis: A Systematic Review and Meta-Analysis. J Eur Acad Dermatol Venereol. 2017;31(5):857-62.
39. Ahmed SS, De A, Das S, Manchanda Y. Biologics and Biosimilars in Psoriasis. Indian J Dermatol. 2023;68(3):282-95.

7
Assessment and Scoring of Psoriasis Severity: PASI and Other Scales

Dipra Biswas, Saurabh Singh

■ INTRODUCTION

Psoriasis is a disorder known to mankind since ages, having significant morbidity and also affecting the quality of life. Being a chronic disorder it has its own natural history and course, showing variable degrees of involvement and severity in an individual in his lifetime. The therapies for psoriasis often depend on the severity and extent of disease, so it is often important for physician to objectively quantify the disease severity for therapeutic decisions and follow-up. The objective evaluation quality of life in psoriasis is also very important in a therapeutic point of view as well as to assess the response and disease burden on patients. Uniform scoring systems developed in recent times have helped the clinicians worldwide for therapeutic decision-making and follow-up. We will be discussing about the various scoring systems described in literature till date in psoriasis.

■ CLASSIFICATION

Scoring systems in psoriasis can be related to the disease severity, related to the quality of life and patient satisfaction to treatment.

- Validated disease severity scores can be subdivided according to the involvement or morphological type of psoriasis, likewise:
  - *Chronic plaque psoriasis*: PASI (Psoriasis Area and Severity Index), PGA (Physician Global Assessment), IGA (Investigator Global Assessment), BSA (body surface area)
  - *Nail psoriasis*: NAPSI (Nail Psoriasis Severity Index), M-NAPSI (Modified NAPSI), Targeted NAPSI, SNAPS (Severity of Nail Psoriasis Scores)
  - *Pustular psoriasis*: GPPGA (Generalized Pustular Psoriasis Physician Global Assessment Score), GPPASI (Generalized Pustular Psoriasis Area Severity Index), JDA-GPPSI (Japanese Dermatological Association Severity Index of GPP)
  - *Psoriatic arthritis*: DAPSA (Disease Activity Index for Psoriatic Arthritis)
- The life quality index measures can be subdivided into four types:
  i. *Psoriasis-specific*:
     a. Psoriasis Index of Quality of Life (PSORIQoL)
     b. Psoriasis Disability Index (PDI)
     c. Psoriasis Life Stress Inventory (PLSI)
     d. Simplified PASI (SAPASI)
  ii. *Mix quality of life measure*:
     a. Salford Psoriasis Index (SPI)
  iii. *Dermatology-specific*:
     a. Dermatology Life Quality Index (DLQI)
     b. Questionnaire on Experience with Skin Complaints (QES)

iv. *General quality of life measurement scales*:
   a. EuroQoL 5D (EQ-5D)
   b. Subjective Well-being Scale (SWLS)
   c. Short Form 36 (SF-36)

Psoriasis disease-specific activity scores for various forms of psoriasis have been mentioned in the following text.

Chronic Plaque Psoriasis

Psoriasis Area and Severity Index[1]

Psoriasis Area and Severity Index is the most widely accepted and validated scoring system existing in literature for objectively assessing the psoriasis disease severity. It was first introduced by Fredriksson and Petersson in 1987 and from then onward it has become almost the gold standard among the psoriasis disease severity assessment scales.

Calculation of PASI: For the calculation, the BSA has been subdivided into four regions:
1. Head (h)—accounts for 10% of total BSA
2. Upper extremity (u)—accounts for 20% of total BSA
3. Trunk (t)—accounts for 30% of total BSA
4. Lower extremity (l)—accounts for 40% of total BSA

Each area is assessed for Erythema (E), Induration (I) and Scaling (S), then a score of 0 (none) to 4 (very severe) is given according the degree of involvement of the parameters.

The extent of involvement (A) is scored according to **Table 1**.

The formula of PASI being, $PASI = 0.1 (Eh + Ih + Sh) Ah + 0.2 (Eu + Iu + Su) Au + 0.3 (Et + It + St) At + 0.4 (El + Il + Sl) Al$.

The total score of PASI ranges from 0 to 72.

Interpretation of PASI is described in **Table 2**.

A 75% reduction of PASI score from baseline (i.e., PASI 75) is usually taken into consideration of assessing the efficacy of the treatment. Similarly PASI 50, PASI 90, and PASI 100 have also been used in many clinical trials to measure the efficacy outcome.[2]

Limitations of PASI: There may be interperson variability while assessing the BSA, erythema, scaling, and induration, it may vary with the level of experience of the assessor. It often fails to detect the morbidity and quality of life of patients.

Newer developments:

PASI calculator: Online applications are now available to calculate the PASI. The physician has to enter the numericals and the result will be calculated in seconds. The link of the calculator: https://pasi.corti.li/

Low PASI score: In this system, the components are same as classical PASI but the area score has been redesigned to monitor smaller areas. In cases <10% involvement in the anatomical area, a new 4-point scale has been proposed, given in **Table 3**.

TABLE 1: Extent of involvement (A) score in PASI

0	No involvement
1	1–9%
2	10–29%
3	30–49%
4	50–69%
5	70–89%
6	90–100%

TABLE 2: Interpretation of PASI

PASI score	Severity of psoriasis
<5	Mild disease
5–10	Moderate disease
>10	Severe disease

TABLE 3: Low PASI score

Area score	Extent of involvement
0.25	0.1–2.5%
0.5	2.6–5%
0.75	5.1–7.5%
1	7.6–9.9%

This proposed system can precisely document the severity of disease and treatment response.[3]

PASI-high discrimination (PASI-HD): It is proposed in such cases where the extent of involvement is <10% for the given anatomical region. Minute improvements of the severity scoring after therapy will be reflected in this system.[4]

Artificial intelligence-PASI (AI-PASI): To minimize the interobserver variation in PASI, recent image–AI-based assessment model has been proposed where images can be uploaded and by the virtue of deep learning system with the help of virtual image database, the PASI can be calculated by AI. It can calculate PASI in an objective, accurate manner, but yet to be validated.[5] The SkinTeller app is available as a mobile application now.

Physician Global Assessment

Physician Global Assessment is an estimate of the overall psoriasis disease severity in a patient in a given point of time. It takes into consideration of erythema (E), induration (I) and scaling (S) but it does not include the BSA involvement. Many clinical trials use various grading systems, a 5-point[6] to 6-point[7] scoring system for each parameter.

$$PGA = (E + I + S)/3$$

The scoring system is given in **Table 4**.

Many clinical trials use score 0 or 1 as treatment success.

Limitations: PGA does not include the measurement of BSA involved or the anatomical location of the psoriasis. It is very subjective and significant interobserver difference can be seen.

Newer updates:

PGA × BSA composite tool: This was proposed to include the factor of BSA along with PGA for better assessment of the disease and has been compared with PASI being a simple yet effective tool for severity assessment and outcome of therapy measurement.[8]

Investigator Global Assessment

Investigator Global Assessment usually has two variants static IGA and dynamic IGA. Static IGA assesses severity in a point of time, whereas the dynamic IGA is based on the recollection of baseline clinical disease severity. The modified 5-point IGA scale[9] is described in **Table 5**.

The IGA score is simple and easy to use, has high test–retest reliability and good comparability with other scoring systems

TABLE 4: PGA score

PGA score	Clinical severity
0	No disease/clear
1	Almost clear/minimal
2	Mild
3	Moderate
4	Severe
5	Very severe

TABLE 5: Modified 5-point IGA scale

IGA score	Disease severity	Clinical scenario
0	Clear	No signs of psoriasis, postinflammatory pigmentation may be present
1	Almost clear	No thickening, normal or pink coloration
2	Mild	Mild thickening, pink to light red coloration
3	Moderate	Moderate thickening, dull to bright red
4	Severe	Severe thickening, bright to deep red

(high clinical construct variability). It also has moderate agreement with multiple assessors.

Limitations: It is not able to measure the small changes with severity while assessing the treatment outcome. It also does not include the extent of area involved.

Body Surface Area

It is the simplest measure for psoriasis disease severity. It is based on the "Rule of 9" for assessment of burns.[10] The percentage of BSA is given in **Table 6**.

Patient's own palmar area can be considered as 1% of the BSA and total involvement can be calculated using patient's hand areas affected.[11]

It is very simple and crude method to assess the severity.

Limitations: It has high interobserver variation, also the clinical severity like scaling and erythema are not included in this.

Psoriasis disease severity scores for special forms of psoriasis are given in the following text.

Nail Psoriasis

Nail Psoriasis Severity Index[12]

This was proposed by Rich and Scher in 2003 and is a simple, objective score to assess the nail matrix and nail bed severity of involvement. The nail is divided into four quadrants by horizontal and longitudinal imaginary lines. Nail bed disease (oil drop sign/salmon patch, onycholysis, nail bed hyperkeratosis and splinter hemorrhage) and nail matrix disease (pitting, leukonychia, red spots in lunula, nail plate crumbling) of each quadrant is scored in a scale of 0 to 4, on the presence or absence of any of the mentioned clinical points. The score is given separately for nail bed and nail matrix as described in **Table 7**.

A single fingernail has a maximum score of 8 (4 for nail bed features and 4 for nail matrix features). Then the total NAPSI is calculated from the summation of scores of all the fingernails. It ranges from 0 to 80. If the toenails are also included it ranges from 0 to 160.

There is good interobserver agreement for NAPSI. It is used for various clinical trials for the outcome assessment measure.

Modified Nail Psoriasis Severity Index

Modified Nail Psoriasis Severity Index assesses the nail as a whole rather by quadrant, to avoid variability in defining quadrants. Leukonychia, hyperkeratosis, splinter hemorrhages, and red spots in the lunula are scored as either 0 (absent) or 1 (present). Percentage area of onycholysis and oil-drop dyschromia (considered together), number of pits and percentage area of nail plate crumbling: These are scored between 0 and 3, depending on their extent. mNAPSI demonstrated excellent construct validity and interrater reliability.[13]

Targeted Nail Psoriasis Severity Index

Targeted NAPSI assesses the target nail, in which only the worst affected nail in baseline is quantified at follow-up.[14]

TABLE 6: Body area with percentage of BSA	
Body area	Percentage (%) of BSA
Head and neck	9
Upper limb	18
Trunk	36
Anterior leg	18
Posterior leg	18
Genitalia	1

TABLE 7: NAPSI score for nail bed and matrix	
Score	Quadrant of involvement
0	None
1	1/4
2	2/4
3	3/4
4	4/4

Severity of Nail Psoriasis Scores

Severity of Nail Psoriasis Score range from 0 to 40 and takes into consideration the following i.e., presence of pitting, onycholysis, hyperkeratosis and/or severe nail disease in each fingernail, weighing 1 point for each.[15]

Pustular Psoriasis

Generalized Pustular Psoriasis Physician Global Assessment Score[16]

The GPPGA was coined to assess the treatment efficacy of various drugs used for GPP in clinical trials. The clinical components taken into consideration are erythema/redness, scaling/desquamation, and pustules. The calculation is almost similar to PGA, a 5-point score is given for each component according to the severity from clear, almost clear, mild, moderate, and severe. Then the composite mean score is calculated and graded as described in **Table 8**.

Generalized Pustular Psoriasis Area Severity Index[17]

This scoring system has been developed for taking into consideration of the body area involvement while assessing GPP. The calculation is similar to PASI scoring but the induration component is replaced by pustules. The individual components are given scores on a scale of 0–4 according to their severity from clear, almost clear, mild, moderate, and severe. The calculation is similar to PASI and the value ranges from 0 to 72.

Japanese Dermatological Association Severity Index of Generalized Pustular Psoriasis[18]

This scoring system was introduced to include the systemic features along the skin parameters in assessment of GPP. Here, the cutaneous components (overall erythema area, erythema area with pustules, and edema area) are given score on a scale of 0 (none) to 3 (severe). The systemic symptoms are scored based on the clinical/laboratory parameters [pyrexia, white blood cell (WBC) count, serum albumin level and C-reactive protein (CRP) levels] on a scale of 0–2. The laboratory parameter score cutoffs are described in **Table 9**.

Severity classification in JDA-GPPSI scoring system is given in **Table 10**.

The score was initially designed to assess the response of the biologicals used in GPP in Japanese group and the advantage is that this score takes into consideration of the systemic symptoms that usually associated with GPP.

Limitation: The cutoff value of the laboratory parameters are not standardized worldwide, so it lacks global agreement.

Psoriatic Arthritis

Disease Activity Index for Psoriatic Arthritis[19]

The idea of this scoring system was adapted from the scoring system used for rheumatoid arthritis. It consists of five variables: Tender

TABLE 8: Interpretation of GPPGA score

Composite score	GPPGA score	Clinical severity
0	0	Clear
>0 to <1.5	1	Almost clear
1.5 to <2.5	2	Mild
2.5 to <3.5	3	Moderate
≥3.5	4	Severe

TABLE 9: Laboratory parameters and their scores in JDA-GPPSI scoring system

Score	0	1	2
Pyrexia (°C)	<37	37.0 to <38.5	≥38.5
CRP level (mg/dL)	<0.3	0.3 to <7.0	≥7.0
WBC count (/mL)	<10,000	10,000 to <15,000	≥15,000
Serum albumin level (g/dL)	≥3.8	3.0 to <3.8	<3.0

(CRP: C-reactive protein; WBC: white blood cell)

CHAPTER 7: Assessment and Scoring of Psoriasis Severity: PASI and Other Scales

TABLE 10: Severity score in JDA-GPPSI scoring system

Severity	Total score
Mild	0–6
Moderate	7–10
Severe	11–17

and swollen joints (TJC68, SJC66), Patient Global Assessment, patient pain on a visual analog scale (VAS), and CRP.

The score is validated; it has been correlated with radiological disease progression and functional status of the patient.

Quality of Life Scores

Psoriasis-specific Quality of Life Scores
- PSORIQoL
- PLSI
- SAPASI
- PDI

Psoriasis Index of Quality of Life:[20] This scoring tool has 25 items to assess the disease impact on patient's quality of life. It has good construct validity, content validity, and internal consistency as well as reproducibility. It does not have good patient acceptability.

Psoriasis Life Stress Inventory: It evaluates the psychological burden of the patients on coping up with the daily chores in psoriasis patients.

Simplified PASI: It is a simplified form, where the body areas are divided into inequal parts and the effect on self-esteem is assessed if the psoriasis is present on the test areas. This system is quick and easy to use.

Psoriasis Disability Index: This score assesses the impact of psoriasis on the daily life of patients with a 15-item tool.

Mixed Quality of Life Measure

Salford Psoriasis Index: This system takes into consideration of the psychosocial disability, sign, and intervention. The score is validated and reliable.

Dermatology-specific

These scoring systems have been used in other various dermatoses to gauge the quality of life affect. The validated and well accepted scoring systems are:
- DLQI
- QES

General Quality of Life Measurement Scales

These scales are validated and used for quality of life assessment in general, taking into consideration of daily activity, psychological, social, and personal well-being aspects. The scales widely used are:
- EQ-5D
- SWLS
- SF-36

■ CONCLUSION

Among all the scoring systems for clinical severity assessment of chronic plaque psoriasis, PASI score is the most widely used, validated, reliable, reproducible, and time-tested. Other scoring systems like NAPSI, GPPASI, DAPSA are well validated for special form of psoriasis. Among the various quality of life scores, PSORIQoL, SPI, DLQI, SF-36 are reliable, validated, and time-tested.

TAKE HOME MESSAGE

- ❑ Scoring systems in psoriasis primarily serve the purpose of measuring disease severity.
- ❑ They have been developed in order to make measurement more systematic, objective and comparable across different clinical set ups and research studies/trials.
- ❑ They are designed to supplement and bring more uniformity in the clinical decision making and patient counseling but cannot be an alternative to clinical acumen.
- ❑ The applications range from psoriasis vulgaris to its pustular, nail and joint variants.
- ❑ However, the element of subjectivity still remains in most of these systems to a variable extent.

REFERENCES

1. Validity of Outcome Measures. Clinical Review Report: Guselkumab (Tremfya): (Janssen Inc): Indication: For the treatment of adult patients with moderate-to-severe plaque psoriasis who are candidates for systemic therapy or phototherapy. Ottawa: Canadian Agency for Drugs and Technologies in Health; 2018.
2. Carlin CS, Feldman SR, Krueger JG, Menter A, Krueger GG. A 50% reduction in the Psoriasis Area and Severity Index (PASI 50) is a clinically significant endpoint in the assessment of psoriasis. J Am Acad Dermatol. 2004;50(6):859-66.
3. Otero ME, van Geel MJ, Hendriks JCM, van de Kerkhof PCM, Seyger MMB, de Jong EM. A pilot study on the Psoriasis Area and Severity Index (PASI) for small areas: Presentation and implications of the Low PASI score. J Dermatolog Treat. 2015;4;26(4):314-7.
4. Papp KA, Lebwohl MG, Kircik LH, Pariser DM, Strober B, Krueger GG, et al. The Proposed PASI-HD Provides More Precise Assessment of Plaque Psoriasis Severity in Anatomical Regions with a Low Area Score. Dermatol Ther (Heidelb). 2021;11(4):1079-83.
5. Huang K, Wu X, Li Y, Lv C, Yan Y, Wu Z, et al. Artificial Intelligence–Based Psoriasis Severity Assessment: Real-world Study and Application. J Med Internet Res. 2023;25:e44932.
6. Cappelleri JC, Bushmakin AG, Harness J, Mamolo C. Psychometric validation of the physician global assessment scale for assessing severity of psoriasis disease activity. Qual Life Res. 2013;22(9):2489-99.
7. Robinson A, Kardos M, Kimball AB. Physician Global Assessment (PGA) and Psoriasis Area and Severity Index (PASI): why do both? A systematic analysis of randomized controlled trials of biologic agents for moderate to severe plaque psoriasis. J Am Acad Dermatol. 2012;66(3):369-75.
8. Walsh JA, Jones H, Mallbris L, Duffin KC, Krueger GG, Clegg DO, et al. The Physician Global Assessment and Body Surface Area composite tool is a simple alternative to the Psoriasis Area and Severity Index for assessment of psoriasis: post hoc analysis from PRISTINE and PRESTA. Psoriasis (Auckl). 2018;8:65-74.
9. Langley RGB, Feldman SR, Nyirady J, van de Kerkhof P, Papavassilis C. The 5-point Investigator's Global Assessment (IGA) Scale: A modified tool for evaluating plaque psoriasis severity in clinical trials. J Dermatolog Treat. 2015;26(1):23-31.
10. Güler Gürsu K. An experimental study for diagnosis of burn depth. Burns. 1977;4(2):97-103.
11. Lund CC, Browder NC. The Estimation of Areas of Burns. Surg Gynecol Obstet. 1944;79:352-8.
12. Rich P, Scher RK. Nail psoriasis severity index: a useful tool for evaluation of nail psoriasis. J Am Acad Dermatol. 2003;49(2):206-12.
13. Cassell SE, Bieber JD, Rich P, Tutuncu ZN, Lee SJ, Kalunian KC, et al. The Modified Nail Psoriasis Severity Index: Validation of an Instrument to Assess Psoriatic Nail Involvement in Patients with Psoriatic Arthritis. J Rheumatol. 2007;34(1):123-9.
14. Parrish CA, Sobera JO, Elewski BE. Modification of the nail psoriasis severity index. J Am Acad Dermatol. 2005;53(4):745-6.
15. Antony A, Saeed S, Hart D, Nair P, Cavill C, Korendowych E, et al. AB0735 Severity of Nail Psoriasis Score (SNAPS) demonstrates longitudinal construct validity against the Modified Nail Psoriasis Severity Index (MNAPSI) in an observational cohort of patients with psoriatic arthritis. Ann Rheum Dis. 2020;79(Suppl 1):1662.
16. Bachelez H, Choon SE, Marrakchi S, Burden AD, Tsai TF, Morita A, et al. Inhibition of the Interleukin-36 Pathway for the Treatment of Generalized Pustular Psoriasis. N Engl J Med. 2019;380(10):981-3.
17. Burden AD, Choon SE, Gottlieb AB, Navarini AA, Warren RB. Clinical Disease Measures in Generalized Pustular Psoriasis. Am J Clin Dermatol. 2022;23(Suppl 1):39-50.
18. Morita A, Yamazaki F, Matsuyama T, Takahashi K, Arai S, Asahina A, et al. Adalimumab treatment in Japanese patients with generalized pustular psoriasis: Results of an open-label phase 3 study. J Dermatol. 2018;45(12):1371-80.
19. Schoels MM, Aletaha D, Alasti F, Smolen JS. Disease activity in psoriatic arthritis (PsA): defining remission and treatment success using the DAPSA score. Ann Rheum Dis. 2016;75(5):811-8.
20. Bronsard V, Paul C, Prey S, Puzenat E, Gourraud PA, Aractingi S, et al. What are the best outcome measures for assessing quality of life in plaque type psoriasis? A systematic review of the literature. J Eur Acad Dermatol Venereol. 2010;24 Suppl 2:17-22.

Topical Treatments for Psoriasis

KA Seetharam, K Venkatesh

■ INTRODUCTION

For psoriatic individuals with limited disease, such as a few chronic plaque lesions, nail psoriasis, scalp psoriasis, palmoplantar psoriasis, and special instances like psoriasis in infants and human immunodeficiency virus (HIV) patients, local or topical therapy is the primary treatment option. Topical agents are also used adjunctively for resistant lesions in patients with more extensive psoriasis and who are concurrently being treated with either ultraviolet (UV) light or systemic agents. Considering the disease's hyperkeratotic nature, the best way to use any topical therapy is to hydrate the skin first by immersing it in water for a few minutes before applying cream or ointment.

■ EMOLLIENTS

Emollients are the backbone of therapy for psoriasis. They are a valuable first-line treatment because dry skin is common in psoriasis.[1] Emollients are greasy substances that hydrate the stratum corneum by forming a layer over the skin surface, thereby preventing transepidermal water loss and retaining moisture. Emollients help in normalizing hyperproliferation, differentiation, and apoptosis. They have anti-inflammatory effects in addition to improving barrier function. This helps in combating the stresses generated in the skin and Koebner's phenomenon.[2] They help in loosening the adherent hyperkeratotic psoriatic scales and facilitate the penetration of other drugs. The use of liberal bland emollients over a thin layer of topical prescription treatments improves hydration while minimizing treatment costs.

Commonly used agents include liquid paraffin and white soft paraffin. Important effects include reduction in dryness, relief in itching, reduced scaling, and fissuring. The principle of applying them immediately after soaking/bathing and also between treatment periods, as frequently as required, helps in avoiding dryness. The use of urea improves hydration potential and minimizes scaling. However, it is better to avoid in children <2 years.

Emollients can cause a few side effects such as irritant dermatitis, allergic contact dermatitis, fragrance allergy, stinging, cosmetic acne, and pigmentary disorders.[3] These are considered to be safe during pregnancy and lactation as well as for pediatric use.

■ TOPICAL CORTICOSTEROIDS

Topical corticosteroids (TCS) are first-line therapy in mild-to-moderate psoriasis and in sites such as the flexures and genitalia, where other topical agents can induce irritation. Steroids are anti-inflammatory, antiproliferative, immunosuppressive, and vasoconstrictive effects. These applications are easy to apply, nonmessy, and nonirritant.

Topical steroids are effective, fast in relief, and well tolerated. They are very easy to use, cost-effective, and less expensive.[4] They exert the effects through intracellular corticosteroid receptors that regulate gene transcription and inhibiting proinflammatory mediators.

The age of the patient, disease severity, and type and extent of surface area will decide the type of steroid, mild, moderate, or potent, and the vehicle to be used.[5] Low-potency corticosteroids are preferred for use on the face, groin, axillae, on areas with thin skin, and in infants. Higher-potency agents are used on thick chronic plaques. In most other areas or in adult patients, one can usually start mid-potency agents.

Topical corticosteroids are commonly used to treat psoriasis affecting less than 5–10% total body surface area. They are also useful in moderate-to-severe psoriasis, for maintenance therapy after partial clearance with systemic treatment. They can be applied daily in the beginning, slowly tapered after obtaining adequate relief over a period of 2–4 weeks. Initially, we can decrease the potency and then frequency and then maintain with weekend therapy. These can be used as combination therapy along with other topical medicines or systemic treatments. It is preferred not to use >4 weeks continuously. Many randomized controlled studies have shown that topical steroids were safe and effective up to 2–4 weeks in mild-to-severe psoriasis.[6-8] The maximum dose of superpotent topical steroid should not exceed 45 g/week.[9]

Intralesional corticosteroids can be used in some resistant, intensely pruritic plaques and nail lesions of psoriasis. The intramatricial triamcinolone injections are quite effective.[10] It can be used up to 20 mg/mL once in 3–4 weeks. The matrix-induced nail changes such as pitting and leukonychia are more responsive than the nail bed changes like onycholysis and subungual hyperkeratosis.

Cutaneous adverse effects include atrophy, striae, telangiectasia, folliculitis, acneiform eruption, rosacea, contact dermatitis, purpura, and tachyphylaxis. Sudden withdrawal can cause rebound flare. Prolonged use rarely causes adrenal suppression. Prolonged use around the eye can cause intraocular pressure, glaucoma, and cataracts. Systemic side effects can occur on prolonged use of high-potency corticosteroids over a large surface or under occlusion. It is prudent to exercise caution and not to exceed 4 weeks of continuous use. Topical steroids are safe during pregnancy (not exceeding 50–60 g/week).

■ VITAMIN D ANALOGS

The naturally occurring active metabolite of vitamin D3, 1,25-dihydroxyvitamin D3 (calcitriol), and synthetic analogs calcipotriol and 1,24-dihydroxyvitamin D3 (tacalcitol) are effective topically in psoriasis.

They reduce keratinocyte proliferation and enhance differentiation in psoriasis lesions. They act through vitamin D receptors located in the nucleus of keratinocytes. They have an immunomodulatory effect by inhibiting T-cell proliferation in response to interleukin-1 (IL-1) and decrease T-cell infiltration and keratinocyte intracellular adhesion molecule-1 (ICAM-1) expression in treated plaques.[11]

Calcipotriol is available as a 0.005% cream or ointment to treat stable plaque psoriasis and as a 0.005% solution for chronic, moderately severe scalp psoriasis.[11] Calcipotriol and calcipotriene are the same. Calcipotriol is the international nonproprietary name (INN) and calcipotriene is the United States Adapted name (USAN).

Calcipotriene cream and solution should be applied twice daily, whereas calcipotriene ointment may be applied either once or twice daily. Though the clinical response may be seen as early as 2–3 weeks, one should wait to see 8–10 weeks to get the optimum therapeutic effect. Patients should be counseled regarding this to avoid unnecessary modifications in the treatment.

Combining calcipotriol monotherapy applied in the morning with a potent TCS applied in the evening for 2 weeks was superior to either drug used twice daily. Combinations of calcipotriol and potent steroid like clobetasol are very effective. Salicylic acid should not be used along with calcipotriol as it degrades calcipotriol. Calcipotriol can be used along with UVB, PUVA, acitretin, methotrexate (MTX), and cyclosporine, which increases the efficacy. It is very effective in flexural psoriasis. It has shown 99% effective in a study by Duweb et al.[12]

Calcipotriol may cause local irritation, in 20% of patients, and can be particularly difficult on the face, and intertriginous areas. Calcitriol and tacalcitol have better tolerability in sensitive areas as compared to calcipotriene and therefore serve as better options in these areas. Hypercalciuria and hypercalcemia are rare side effects as <1% is absorbed. Vitamin D analogs are contraindicated in patients already suffering from hypercalcemia.[9] Patients with renal impairment need to be observed carefully.[9] It may occur rarely if the maximum dose of 100–150 g/week is exceeded.[13]

Calcipotriene is 100–200 times less calcemic than the parent compound (calcitriol) and was approved by the Food and Drug Administration (FDA) in 1993. A twice-daily application is recommended, which should not be >150 g/week to avoid the risk of hypercalcemia. A close monitoring of serum or 24-hour urinary calcium in children is necessary, if >100 g/week is applied.

Tacalcitol is both well tolerated and effective in treating moderate, persistent plaque psoriasis.[14] It has been used in combination with PUVA, UVB, and with cyclosporine.[15] Calcitriol (3 μg/g) is as effective as calcipotriol (50 μg/g), while showing a significantly better safety profile.[16] Newer vitamin D analogs including maxacalcitol, paricalcitol, and becocalcidiol are being studied for the treatment of psoriasis. These drugs appear to be promising for treating plaque psoriasis.

■ DITHRANOL

Dithranol or anthralin (popularly also known as araroba powder or Goa powder) is chemically 1,8-dihydroxy-9-anthrone. It is a naturally occurring substance found in the bark of the araroba tree in South America. It can also be synthesized from anthrone. The use of dithranol for the treatment of psoriasis was first described by Unna in 1916. Dithranol has been approved for the treatment of persistent plaque psoriasis. It is mostly used on plaques that are resistant to conventional treatments. It can be combined with UVB phototherapy with good results (the Ingram regimen). Dithranol paste (0.05–1%) is applied at night on the lesions, and it was removed in the morning, exposed to UVB irradiation, followed by warm-water bath and emollients. Many modifications were there with this regimen including short contact therapy of dithranol keeping it for 30 minutes, followed by UVB.

Dithranol inhibits the thymidine incorporation and thus the DNA synthesis in epidermal cells.[17] It also binds to mitochondrial DNA and inhibits various enzymes.

It also inhibits polymorphonuclear leukocytes (PMNL) migration and mitogen-stimulated mononuclear cell proliferation in psoriatic lesions. The reactive oxidants produced are immunosuppressive, mediating the effect of dithranol.[18] Anthralin has a methylene group, which takes oxygen from the skin and forms an anthraquinone, and binds to the skin. This oxidation causes irritation and burning, and the bound anthraquinone causes staining.

Dithranol has high efficacy and practically no systemic toxicity. Skin irritation is the most prevalent side effect of anthralin, and it is dose-dependent. To overcome this, low-strength anthralin preparations (0.01–0.1%) incorporated in petrolatum or zinc paste and applied once daily have been used in plaque-type psoriasis.[19] Anthralin also stains lesional and adjacent skin, hair, nails, clothing, and other objects, with which the patients come into contact and it is temporary. Patients need to be counseled about this.

Triethanolamine applied after the removal of anthralin prevents staining and irritation by neutralizing any anthralin residue remaining on the skin. Stains on household items can be removed with chlorine bleach. If the psoriatic plaques are well defined, using an agent like zinc oxide paste helps protect the surrounding normal skin. Short contact therapy has been developed to reduce staining and irritation.[20] It involves the application of higher strengths of anthralin (1–2%) in petrolatum to the psoriatic plaques, which was allowed to remain for half an hour.[20] After this, the anthralin was removed by using olive oil.

Even higher concentrations (2–4%) could also be applied to the skin lesion for about 1 hour and then washed off.[21] This facilitated penetration of anthralin through the affected epidermis, which is about five times faster than the penetration through the uninvolved skin.[22] In rare instances, high concentrations of dithranol can induce burning, perilesional irritation, and pigmentation.[23,24]

Pretreatment of skin lesions with corticosteroids has been found to reduce dithranol-induced erythema. The irritation potential is also reduced by alternate corticosteroid and dithranol administrations. Coal tar is another drug tried in combination with dithranol. Its effect on depressing epidermal DNA synthesis[25] can further be boosted by combination with anthralin.[26] Further, the addition of coal tar to anthralin suppresses anthralin-induced erythema.[27] Combined tar–anthralin therapy was found to be less irritating in the first 3 weeks of treatment than anthralin alone.[28]

Various other agents have also been evaluated. Urea (10%) has also been used in combination with dithranol (1%), with an aim to shorten the duration of treatment. The combination of topical dithranol and oral retinoids enhances the response to traditional dithranol alone. The combination of PUVA and dithranol gives better results than either of them alone.[29]

TARS

The coal tar products are used in the treatment of psoriasis for more than 100 years. In 1925, Goeckerman introduced the use of crude coal tar and UV light for the treatment of psoriasis. Tar is prepared by destructive distillation of coal and is composed of >10,000 compounds. It is known that the more the product is purified, the lesser is its efficacy. The specific activity of its individual constituents may not be known. Isoquinoline may possibly be the important antipsoriatic agent in coal tar.[30]

Tar inhibits epidermal DNA synthesis, reducing mitotic activity in the basal layers of epidermis. Some components probably also have anti-inflammatory activity. It has been shown that the antipsoriatic activity of tar is boosted when combined with ultraviolet radiation (UVR) in the Goeckerman regimen or with UVR and anthralin in the Ingram regimen. Salicylic acid (2–5%) is often added because it enhances the absorption of the coal tar by its keratolytic effect. The conventional regimen of Goeckerman involved the application of black crude coal tar (1–5%) for 24 hours, followed by the removal of excess tar with mineral oil and exposure to narrow-band UVB (NBUVB) light.

Tar therapy has the advantage of being one of the safest treatments for psoriasis, resulting in long-term remission. It is quite useful in chronic plaque psoriasis, and the remissions are longer lasting. It is quite effective and safe in comparison with other psoriatic medications. It can be used for widespread recalcitrant psoriasis among pregnant women, children, and immunocompromised individuals.

Tar causes malodor, folliculitis, irritation and pigmentation. It should not be applied over the face and flexural areas to avoid irritation. Tar's smell, appearance, and staining of clothes are other major disadvantages. Experimental studies in animals and studies of industrial tar exposure have shown that tar can induce skin cancer.[31-33]

However, psoriatic skin is intrinsically resistant to the development of cancer because of lower cutaneous levels of aryl hydrocarbon hydroxylase.[34,35] Coal tar preparations are used either alone or in combination with other agents such as salicylic acid and topical steroids.

SALICYLIC ACID

Salicylic acid is used in the treatment of hyperkeratotic psoriatic lesions mostly as 2–10% ointment applied twice daily. In a concentration <2%, salicylic acid generally acts as a keratoplastic agent, whereas above 3% it behaves as a keratolytic. Salicylic acid leads to desquamation of corneocytes through two pathways. It decreases the intercellular cohesion of the horny cells by dissolving the intercellular cement material. Moreover, it lowers the pH of the stratum corneum, thereby increasing hydration, which results in reduced scaling and softening of the plaques, thereby improving the absorption of other agents. Therefore, salicylic acid is often combined with other topical therapies such as corticosteroids and coal tar.

Topical salicylic acid decreases the efficacy of UVB phototherapy, and systemic absorption can occur, particularly in patients with abnormal hepatic or renal function and when applied to >20% of the body surface area. The serious side effect in such a case scenario is salicylism or even death; however, this can be diligently avoided if the skin area treated is small, the concentration is less than 7–10%, or the frequency of application is twice daily or less. The clinical manifestations of salicylism include hallucinations, nausea, tinnitus, and dyspnea.

VITAMIN A ANALOGS

Tazarotene is a nonisomerizable, receptor-specific, third-generation retinoid (vitamin A derivative). It is useful in limited plaque psoriasis. Tazarotene selectively binds to beta and gamma retinoic acid receptors on the cell surface of keratinocytes and is transported to the nucleus, altering the transcription of genes in keratinocytes. This results in decreasing inflammation, reduced epidermal proliferation, and normalizing keratinocyte differentiation.

Tazarotene is available as a cream and gel (0.05% and 0.1%, respectively).[36] The clinical efficacy is seen as early as the first week of treatment. The beneficial effects are maintained up to 12 weeks after cessation of therapy. It is available as a 0.1% and 0.05% gel and once-a-day application is generally advocated. Tazarotene's potency is comparable to that of mid- to high-potency corticosteroids and weaker than that of ultra-high-potency corticosteroids. The only side effect is mild irritation (retinoid dermatitis). It is prominent, especially when the drug is used alone, particularly in higher concentrations.[37] It is more useful in palmoplantar psoriasis and nail psoriasis.

Tazarotene should not be administered to pregnant or lactating women or women not practicing adequate contraception. The most common side effect is localized irritation. Cream form and low concentration, alternate-day application, and short contact (30–60 minutes) therapy may reduce irritation. TCS or calcipotriol in combination with tazarotene also improves efficacy and minimizes symptoms.

Tazarotene should not be used in sensitive areas like face, flexures, and genitals. The FDA has issued a caution regarding the use of tazarotene and exposure to sunlight, and it should be applied at night and advised to use sunscreens during the daytime.[9]

CHAPTER 8: Topical Treatments for Psoriasis

It may be used either alone or in combination with UVB and/or steroids.[38,39] The drug's efficacy can be enhanced by combining it with a TCS or UVB therapy. Tazarotene 0.1% gel, used in combination with mometasone furoate 0.1% cream, was more effective than calcipotriol ointment used twice daily, or mometasone furoate 0.1% cream used twice daily.

TOPICAL CALCINEURIN INHIBITORS

Tacrolimus is a macrolide antibiotic, derived from the bacteria *Streptomyces tsukubensis*. By binding to immunophilin (FK506 binding protein), it creates a complex that inhibits calcineurin, thus blocking both T-lymphocyte signal transduction and IL-2 transcription. Pimecrolimus is also a calcineurin inhibitor and works in a manner similar to tacrolimus. Both these drugs are currently licensed for use only in moderate-to-severe atopic dermatitis. They are used off-label in psoriasis.

Tacrolimus 0.1% ointment to be safe and effective for psoriasis involving areas with thinner skin, that is face or intertriginous areas, in children and adults. Their advantage is that unlike TCS they are selective, unlikely to be absorbed systemically and do not produce skin atrophy making them more suitable for long-term use.

Pimecrolimus cream 1% has been found to be safe and effective for inverse psoriasis,[40,41] These drugs can be used in combination therapy. Both 1% pimecrolimus and 0.005% calcipotriol might be appropriate for patients with intertriginous psoriasis, for whom the long-term application associated adverse effect profile may be offset by occasional or intermittent rescue therapy with these drugs.[40]

The primary adverse effect of these medications is a mild burning sensation at the application site for a very short time. The boxed warning in the package mentions a theoretical risk of increased cutaneous lymphoma on prolonged systemic use. Several studies did not show any increased incidence of lymphoma on topical use of both these agents. These drugs may produce flushing with ingestion of alcohol.[42,43]

JANUS KINASE INHIBITORS

Tofacitinib, a Janus kinase 1 (JAK1) and JAK3 inhibitor has been found effective in mild-to-moderate psoriasis by blocking signaling of multiple cytokines implicated in immune response and inflammation. It has a direct effect on dysregulated keratinocytes, reduction of inflammatory infiltrations, and normalization of the IL-23/T-helper 17 (Th17) axis.[44]

In a 12-week trial, 2% tofacitinib twice daily application has shown greater efficacy than vehicle at the end of 8 weeks, but at 12th week, there was no significant difference.[45,46] It relieves pruritus as early as 2nd day. Application site pain, nasopharyngitis, and upper respiratory tract infection were noticed in few patients. There were no serious adverse reactions leading to discontinuation of therapy. It is also effective in resistant nail psoriasis.

Topical ruxolitinib 1% and 2% cream has reduced lesional severity scores and lesion areas at the end of 4 weeks. No JAK inhibitors are approved so far for topical use in psoriasis.

PHOSPHODIESTERASE TYPE-4 INHIBITORS

Phosphodiesterase type-4 (PDE4) is an enzyme prominently expressed in immune cells, where it participates in the breakdown of cyclic adenosine monophosphate (cAMP), a crucial intracellular messenger in various signal transduction pathways.[46] The overexpression of PDE4 in psoriatic skin favors the synthesis of proinflammatory cytokines and the proliferation of immune cells; conversely, suppression of PDE4 elevates cAMP levels, resulting in reduced

TOPICAL ROFLUMILAST

Topical roflumilast has a higher potency compared to other PDE4 inhibitors (25–300 times more than apremilast or crisaborole depending on the comparator and PDE4 isoform).

Food and Drug Administration approved topical roflumilast cream 0.3% for plaque psoriasis, for children >6 years and adults.[48] Various studies have shown the positive results with roflumilast achieving an Investigator Global Assessment score of clear or almost clear at 8 weeks in phase III studies.

TOPICAL CRISABOROLE

Crisaborole has anti-inflammatory properties and is found useful in the treatment of facial, anogenital, and intertriginous psoriasis. It does not produce skin atrophy like topical steroids.

The 2% crisaborole ointment for 8 weeks showed significant clinical improvement with lesional clearance in >70% of the participants.[49] It was also effective in palmoplantar psoriasis with significant sustained improvement with minimal adverse events.

FUTURE MOLECULES

Aryl Hydrocarbon Receptor Modulators

Tapinarof is a aryl hydrocarbon receptor (AhR) modulator with the capability to inhibit the differentiation of Th17 cells and reduce the proinflammatory cytokines. It also regulates protein expression to promote skin barrier normalization.[50]

This leads to an overall decrease in skin inflammation. It restores the dysfunctional skin barrier by inducing the expression of essential skin barrier proteins, such as filaggrin and loricrin, along with other crucial components. Enhancement of the antioxidant response mediated by nuclear factor E2-related factor 2 (Nrf2), which is a transcription factor, regulates the defenses against oxidative stress.

It is available as 1% cream formulation specifically designed to be administered once daily to manage plaque psoriasis. In May 2022, the US FDA approved tapinarof for treating plaque psoriasis in adults aged 18 years and older. A phase IIa trial (NCT01098721) which conducted in 61 patients initially showed a significant improvement in disease extension, with almost 80% of the affected body surface being cleared at week 12, compared with patients receiving placebo, who presented worsening of the affected areas.[51]

PROACTIVE MANAGEMENT

Proactive treatment is using optimal topical management of psoriasis during maintenance. It refers to topical treatment of areas that are clinically in remission, but are usually involved in recurrence. Twice weekly treatment of these areas will reduce clinical recurrences. It can be used with any of the topical agents. The common ones are using topical steroids twice weekly and using calcipotriol two times a week. It reduces recurrences and adverse effects.

CONCLUSION

Topical treatments are useful in milder localized forms of psoriasis. It can be used as supportive therapies in moderate-to-severe psoriasis. Emollients are the mainstay. Topical corticosteroids, salicylic acid, vitamin D analogs, tar preparations are useful in the topical management.

CHAPTER 8: Topical Treatments for Psoriasis

> **TAKE HOME MESSAGE**
> - Topical treatments are useful in milder localized forms of psoriasis.
> - Emollients are the back bone of topical therapy.
> - Topical corticosteroids are first-line therapy in mild-to-moderate psoriasis and are are easy to apply, non-messy, and non-irritant.
> - Dithranol (0.05–1%) has been approved for the treatment of persistent plaque psoriasis. Short contact therapy of dithranol keeping it for 30 minutes, followed by UVB is more effective.
> - Tar therapy has the advantage of being one of the safest treatments for psoriasis. The antipsoriatic activity of tar is boosted when combined with UVR in the Goeckerman regimen or with UVR and anthralin in the ingram regimen.
> - Vitamin D analogs reduce keratinocyte proliferation and enhances differentiation in psoriasis lesions.
> - Tazarotene is effective but should not be used in sensitive areas like face, flexures and genitals.
> - Newer molecules like tofacitinib, roflumilast are being used now effectively, and robust evidence is building up now.
> - Proactive management with topical steroids and calcipotriol two times a week reduce recurrences and adverse effects.

REFERENCES

1. Torsekar R, Gautam MM. Topical Therapies in Psoriasis. Indian Dermatol Online J. 2017;8(4):235-45.
2. Fluhr JW, Cavallotti C, Berardesca E. Emollients, moisturizers, and keratolytic agents in psoriasis. Clin Dermatol. 2008;26:380-6.
3. Nola I, Kostović K, Kotrulja L, Lugović L. The use of emollients as sophisticated therapy in dermatology. Acta Dermatovenerol Croat. 2003;11:80-7.
4. Gottlieb AB. Therapeutic options in the treatment of psoriasis and atopic dermatitis. J Am Acad Dermatol. 2005;53(1 Suppl 1):S3-16.
5. Rosso JD, Friedlander SF. Corticosteroids: options in the era of steroid-sparing therapy. J Am Acad Dermatol. 2005;53(1 Suppl 1):S50-8.
6. Bernhard J, Whitmore C, Guzzo C, Kantor I, Kalb RE, Ellis C, et al. Evaluation of halobetasol propionate ointment in the treatment of plaque psoriasis: report on two double-blind, vehicle-controlled studies. J Am Acad Dermatol. 1991;25(6 Pt 2):1170-4.
7. Gottlieb AB, Ford RO, Spellman MC. The efficacy and tolerability of clobetasol propionate foam 0.05% in the treatment of mild to moderate plaque-type psoriasis of nonscalp regions. J Cutan Med Surg. 2003;7(3):185-92.
8. Lebwohl M, Sherer D, Washenik K, Krueger GG, Menter A, Koo J, et al. A randomized, double-blind, placebo-controlled study of clobetasol propionate 0.05% foam in the treatment of nonscalp psoriasis. Int J Dermatol. 2002;41(5):269-74.
9. Ahmed SK, Manchanda Y, De A, Das S, Kumar R. Topical therapy in psoriasis. Indian J Dermatol. 2023;68:437-45.
10. Grover C, Bansal S, Nanda S, Reddy BS. Efficacy of triamcinolone acetonide in various acquired nail dystrophies. J Dermatol. 2005;32(12):963-8.
11. Murdoch D, Clissold SP. Calcipotriol. A review of its pharmacological properties and therapeutic use in psoriasis vulgaris. Drugs. 1992;43(3):415-29.
12. Duweb GA, Eldebani S, Alhaddar J. Calcipotriol cream in the treatment of flexural psoriasis. Int J Tissue React. 2003;25(4):127-30.
13. Dwyer C, Chapman RS. Calcipotriol and hypercalcemia. Lancet. 1991;338:764-5.
14. Lecha M, Mirada A, López S, Artés M; T.O.P. Research Group. Tacalcitol in the treatment of psoriasis vulgaris: the Spanish experience. J Eur Acad Dermatol Venereol. 2005;19(4):414-7.
15. Brazzelli V, Barbagallo T, Prestinari F, Rona C, De Silvestri A, Trevisan V, et al. Non-invasive evaluation of tacalcitol plus PUVA versus tacalcitol plus UVB–NB in the treatment of psoriasis: "right-left intra-individual pre/post comparison design". Int J Immunopathol Pharmacol. 2005;18(4):755-60.
16. Zhu X, Wang B, Zhao G, Gu J, Chen Z, Briantais P, et al. CHAPTER 31: Psoriasis 1191 An investigator-masked comparison of the efficacy and safety of twice daily applications of calcitriol 3 microg/g ointment vs. calcipotriol 50 microg/g ointment in subjects with mild to moderate chronic plaque-type psoriasis. J Eur Acad Dermatol Venereol. 2007;21(4):466-72.

17. Swanbeck G, Lidén S. The inhibitory effect of dithranol on DNA synthesis. Acta Derm Venereol. 1966;46:278-80.
18. Müller K. Antipsoriatic and proinflammatory action of anthralin. Implications for the role of oxygen radicals. Biochem Pharmacol. 1997;53(9):1215-17.
19. Marley WM, Hernandez AD, Josephs JA, Dawkins L. The effectiveness of low strength anthralin in psoriasis. A paired comparison study. Arch Dermatol. 1982;118(11):906-8.
20. Schaefer H, Farber EM, Goldberg L, Schalla W. Limited application period for dithranol in psoriasis: preliminary report on penetration and clinical efficacy. Br J Dermatol. 1980;102(5):571-3.
21. Wiegrebe W, Plumier E, Mayer KK, Runne U, Schultz-Amling W, Rosmarinowski J, et al. Experimental contribution to the dithranol—brown problem. Arch Dermatol Res. 1985;277(2):153-5.
22. Schwarz T, Gsachnait F. Anthralin minute entire skin treatment. A new outpatient therapy for psoriasis. Arch Dermatol. 1985;121(12):1512-5.
23. Runne U, Kunze J. Short duration (minutes) therapy with dithranol for psoriasis: a new outpatient regimen. Br J Dermatol. 1982;106(2):135-9.
24. Chattopadhyaya SP, Aggarwal SK, Arora PN, Agarwal S. 'Minutes' therapy in psoriasis. Indian J Dermatol Venereol Leprol. 1987;53:155-7.
25. Walter JF, Stoughton RB, De Quoy PR. Suppression of epidermal proliferation by ultraviolet light, coal tar and anthralin. Br J Dermatol. 1978;99(1):89-96.
26. Lowe NJ, Wortzman MS, Breeding J, Koudsi H, Taylor L. Coal tar phototherapy for psoriasis reevaluated: erythemogenic versus suberythemogenic ultraviolet radiation with a tar extract in oil and crude coal tar. J Am Acad Dermatol. 1983;8(6):781-9.
27. Schulze HJ, Sterry W, Merk H, Steigleder GK. Suppression of dithranol induced irritation by tar. Arch Dermatol Res. 1984;276:253.
28. Schulze HJ, Schaudin S, Mahrle G, Steigleder GK. Combined tar–anthralin versus anthralin treatment lowers irritancy with unchanged antipsoriatic efficacy: modification of short contact therapy and Ingram therapy. J Am Acad Dermatol. 1987;17(1):19-24.
29. Carabott FM. Hawk JLM. PUVA therapy of psoriasis: an improved dose schedule. Photochem Photobiol. 1986;43:23.
30. Foreman MI, Taylor M, Clark C, Devitt H, Hanlon G, Kelly I, et al. Isoquinoline is a possible antipsoriatic agent in coaltar. Br J Dermatol. 1985;112(3):323-8.
31. Yamagiwa K, Ichikawa K. Experimental study of the pathogenesis of carcinoma. J Cancer Res. 1917;3:1-29.
32. Shabad LM, Khesina AJ, Linnik AB, Serkovskaya GS. Possible carcinogenic hazards of several tars and of locacorten-tar ointment (spectro-fluorescent investigations and experiments in animals). Int J Cancer. 1970;6(2):314-8.
33. Gotz H. Tar keratosis. In: Andrade R, Gumport SL, Popkin GL, Rees TD (Eds). Cancer of the Skin. Philadelphia: WB Saunders; 1976. pp. 492-523.
34. Maughan WZ, Muller SA, Perry HO, Pittelkow MR, O'Brien PC. Incidence of skin cancer in patients with atopic dermatitis treated with coal tar. J Am Acad Dermatol. 1980;3(6):612-5.
35. Jacobs PH, Farber EM, Nall ML. Psoriasis and skin cancer. In: Farber EM, Cox AT (Eds). International Symposium on Psoriasis. New York: Yorke Medical Books; 1977. pp. 350-2.
36. Krueger GG, Drake LA, Elias PM, Lowe NJ, Guzzo C, Weinstein GD, et al. The safety and efficacy of tazarotene gel, a topical acetylenic retinoid, in the treatment of psoriasis. Arch Dermatol. 1998;134(1):57-60.
37. Weinstein GD. Tazarotene gel: efficacy and safety in plaque psoriasis. J Am Acad Dermatol. 1997;37(2 Pt 3):S33-8.
38. Lowe NJ. Optimizing therapy: tazarotene in combination with phototherapy. Br J Dermatol. 1999;140 Suppl 54:8-11.
39. Lebwohl MJ, Breneman DL, Goffe BS, Grossman JR, Ling MR, Milbauer J, et al. Tazarotene 0.1% gel plus corticosteroid cream in the treatment of plaque psoriasis. J Am Acad Dermatol. 1998;39(4 Pt 1):590-6.
40. Gribetz C, Ling M, Lebwohl M, Pariser D, Draelos Z, Gottlieb AB, et al. Pimecrolimus cream 1% in the treatment of intertriginous psoriasis: a double-blind, randomized study. J Am Acad Dermatol. 2004;51(5):731-8.
41. Kreuter A, Sommer A, Hyun J, Bräutigam M, Brockmeyer NH, Altmeyer P, et al. 1% Pimecrolimus, 0.005% calcipotriol, and 0.1% betamethasone in the treatment of intertriginous psoriasis: a double-blind, randomized controlled study. Arch Dermatol. 2006;142(9):1138-43.
42. Elidel® (pimecrolimus) Cream, 1% [package insert]. [online] Available from https://www.accessdata.fda.gov/drugsatfda_docs/label/2014/021302s018lbl.pdf [Last accessed January 2025].
43. Protopic® (tacrolimus) [package insert]. [online] Available from https://www.accessdata.fda.gov/drugsatfda_docs/label/2011/050777s018lbl.pdf [Last accessed January 2025].
44. Merola JF, Elewski B, Tatulych S, Lan S, Tallman A, Kaur M. Efficacy of tofacitinib for the treatment of nail psoriasis: two 52-week, randomized, controlled phase 3 studies in patients with moderate-to-severe plaque psoriasis. J Am Acad Dermatol. 2017;77(1):79-87.e1.

45. Papp KA, Bissonnette R, Gooderham M, Feldman SR, Iversen L, Soung J, et al. Treatment of plaque psoriasis with an ointment formulation of the Janus kinase inhibitor, tofacitinib: a Phase 2b randomized clinical trial. BMC Dermatol. 2016;16(1):15.
46. Torres T, Puig L. Apremilast: A Novel Oral Treatment for Psoriasis and Psoriatic Arthritis. Am J Clin Dermatol. 2018;19:23-32.
47. Li H, Zuo J, Tang W. Phosphodiesterase-4 Inhibitors for the Treatment of Inflammatory Diseases. Front Pharmacol. 2018;9:1048.
48. Sheldon A. FDA Approves Arcutis' ZORYVE® (roflumilast) Cream 0.3% for Treatment of Psoriasis in Children Ages 6 to 11. Westlake Village: Arcutis Biotherapeutics; 2023.
49. Hashim PW, Chima M, Kim HJ, Bares J, Yao CJ, Singer G, et al. Crisaborole 2% ointment for the treatment of intertriginous, anogenital, and facial psoriasis: A double-blind, randomized, vehicle-controlled trial. J Am Acad Dermatol. 2020;82(2):360-5.
50. Bissonnette R, Stein Gold L, Rubenstein DS, Tallman AM, Armstrong A. Tapinarof in the treatment of psoriasis: A review of the unique mechanism of action of a novel therapeutic aryl hydrocarbon receptor-modulating agent. J Am Acad Dermatol. 2021;84:1059-67.
51. Carmona-Rocha E, Rusiñol L, Puig L. New and Emerging Oral/Topical Small-Molecule Treatments for Psoriasis. Pharmaceutics. 2024;16(2):239.

9

Phototherapy in the Management of Psoriasis

Chinmoy Raj, Debasmita Behera, CR Srinivas

■ INTRODUCTION

Psoriasis is a chronic inflammatory multisystem disorder affecting 3.2% population of the world. The pathogenesis involves abnormal interactions among innate immunity, T cells, keratinocytes, etc., that clinically manifest as scaly erythematous indurated plaques. Immune cells in the patients with psoriasis produce excessive proinflammatory factors, resulting in the overactivation of both innate and adaptive immune systems and differentiation of T helper (Th) cells toward Th1 and/or Th17 subtypes.[1]

Therapeutic options for psoriasis have evolved considerably over the past 100 years and broadly can be divided into two aspects: Systemic and topical treatment. Although many patients may be capable of adequately controlling their disease with the use of topical treatments alone, often these interventions are insufficient and disease severity dictates the need for alternative options. While systemic and biologic treatments are heavily relied on for severe and widespread skin disease, these medications do come with risks of systemic side effects and immunosuppression. Phototherapy, recognized as the second-line therapy for treating psoriasis involves repeated exposure of the skin to ultraviolet (UV) light. This treatment modality is one of the oldest treatment modalities in dermatology and continues to be a highly preferred one particularly, for psoriasis due to its effectiveness and relative safety.

In the recent past, there has been a resurgence of interest in the role of phototherapy in the treatment of psoriasis. This has occurred in parallel with an improved understanding of the mechanism of the action of phototherapy involving selective apoptosis and depletion of epidermal T cells, accompanied by a shift from a Th1 to a Th2 response in lesional skin.[2]

The key types of phototherapy used for treating psoriasis include narrowband UVB (NB-UVB), broadband UVB (BB-UVB), and psoralen plus UVA (PUVA). Each of these methods has unique applications and benefits. NB-UVB is often preferred due to its superior safety profile and efficacy for plaque psoriasis, making it suitable for a wide range of patients, including children, pregnant women, and those with weakened immune systems. PUVA, which involves taking a photosensitizing agent [e.g., 8-methoxypsoralen (8-MOP)] followed by UVA exposure, is effective but can have more side effects, which limits its use to more severe cases. Understanding the principles and applications of phototherapy is instrumental for dermatologists to effectively integrate this treatment into patient care, ensuring safe and cost-effective management of psoriasis.[3,4]

CHAPTER 9: Phototherapy in the Management of Psoriasis

SOURCES OF LIGHT

Sunlight

The range of terrestrial solar radiation spans from 290 to 4,000 nm including ultraviolet spectrum (UVR: 100–400 nm), visible light, and infrared rays (IR). Approximately 95% of ultraviolet radiation (UVR) is UVA, while around 5% is UVB. UVC radiation is entirely absorbed by the ozone layer and does not reach the earth's surface, making it unsuitable for use in treating skin conditions.[5,6] Different UVR wavelengths penetrate the skin to different depths with longer wavelengths reaching deeper into the skin and therefore possess distinct photochemical and photobiological characteristics.[7]

Ultraviolet radiation is divided into the following from shortest to longest wavelengths:
- *Ultraviolet C*: 100–290 nm
- *UVB*: (290–320 nm), further categorized into:
  - Broadband UVB (BB-UVB): 290–320 nm
  - Narrowband UVB (NB-UVB): 311–313 nm
  - Targeted UVB therapy: 308 nm (e.g., Excimer)

Short-wavelength UVB radiation is absorbed primarily by the proteins and nucleic acids in keratinocytes and does not penetrate deeper than the epidermis. In contrast, long-wavelength UVB radiation can reach the mid-dermis.
- *UVA*: (320–400 nm), further categorized into:
  - UVA1 (340–400 nm): Reaches the epidermis, the middle, and deep dermal components, especially blood vessels.
  - UVA2 (320–340 nm): Resembles UVB, with more superficial penetration.

Since UVB radiation interacts almost exclusively with the epidermis, it is used more for superficial dermatoses affecting the epidermis, while UVA radiation is used for deep dermatoses affecting the dermis.

Artificial Sources of Ultraviolet Radiation

Commonly employed sources in dermatotherapeutics include specialized fluorescent tubes (e.g., sunlamps such as Philips TL 01 and black-light lamps), or high-pressure mercury lamps, which are equipped with optical filters to restrict emissions to the targeted UVA or UVB spectrum. Additionally, LED technology can be used to produce spectral emissions in the UVA, UVB, or UVC ranges.[8-10]

Home phototherapy units are becoming increasingly popular, ranging from handheld devices for spot treatment of small areas (e.g., UVB comb therapy for scalp psoriasis) to walk-in units for full-body therapy. These devices offer a convenient option for patients who live far from phototherapy centers or wish to avoid frequent clinic visits. Proper training is essential for patients to safely and accurately perform this therapy at home, ensuring effective treatment and minimizing risks.

List of phototherapeutics available for psoriasis is provided in **Table 1**.[11]

MECHANISMS OF ACTION OF PHOTOTHERAPY

The mechanism of action differs with UVA and UVB, depending on their biophysical properties. So, UVA as long-wave, low-energy radiation penetrates into the dermis and acts on fibroblasts, mastocytes, endothelial cells, dendritic cells, and dermal T cells.

Ultraviolet B

It induces apoptosis of pathogenic T cells and keratinocytes, inducing local and systemic immunosuppression via the production of photoproducts [formation of cyclobutane pyrimidine dimers (CPD), pyrimidine-(6-4-)pyrimidone photoproducts (6-4PP), and Dewar valence isomers] and DNA damage.[12,13] Strong evidence suggested that Th1/Th17 and T regulatory (Treg) cells play critical roles in the pathogenesis of psoriasis. Phototherapy

CHAPTER 9: Phototherapy in the Management of Psoriasis

TABLE 1: Summary of phototherapeutics for psoriasis[11]

Classification of light source	Sublight source	Wavelengths	Indications
First line therapy UVB	NB-UVB	311 nm	• Stable plaque psoriasis, > 10% body surface
	Excimer Laser/lamp	308 nm	• Excimer: Topical plaque psoriasis, non-pustular palmoplantar psoriasis
Second line therapy PUVA PDL	Bath PUVA	320–400 nm	Refractory psoriatic plaques, palmoplantar pustular psoriasis, stable plaque psoriasis
	Oral PUVA	320–400 nm	
		585–595 nm	Nail psoriasis
Third-line therapy PDL PDT		585–595 nm	Topical plaque psoriasis chronic plaque psoriasis, nail psoriasis
	LED		
	He-Ne	632.8 nm	
	IPL	555–950 nm	
Red light		620–770 nm	Plaque psoriasis
Blue light		400–480 nm	Plaque psoriasis
NIR		830 nm, 810 nm	Plaque psoriasis
Excimer		308 nm	Nail psoriasis
IPL		550–950 nm	Plaque psoriasis
PUVB		290–320 nm	Stable plaque psoriasis
BB-UVB		290–320 nm	Stable plaque psoriasis
Sunbath		400–760 nm	Chronic plaque psoriasis

can alter this cytokine balance by shifting the immune response from the Th1/Th17 axis toward a Th2-dominant, counterregulatory axis, leading to decreased levels of interleukin-12 (IL-12), IL-18, IL-20, IL-22, IL-23, TNF-α, and (the proinflammatory) IFN-γ, as well as upregulation of anti-inflammatory cytokines such as IL-4 and IL-10.[14,15]

Ultraviolet A

It affects gene expression through the oxidation of membrane lipids via the generation of reactive oxygen species. Psoralen acts by intercalation of cellular DNA and forms monoadducts that induce apoptosis upon exposure to UVA.

Both UVA (PUVA) and UVB induce:[3,16-22]
- Reduced expression of adhesion molecules, especially intercellular adhesion molecule-1 (ICAM-1) on keratinocytes and Langerhans cells
- Apoptosis of keratinocytes, Langerhans cells, dendritic cells, macrophages, and T cells
- Isomerization of urocanic acid from trans to cis form that binds to 5-OH tryptamine receptors on mastocytes, dendritic cells, and Langerhans cells, leading to their functional immunosuppression, blocking

CHAPTER 9: Phototherapy in the Management of Psoriasis

deliberation of histamine, and causing trafficking of mastocytes to lymph nodes
- Increase Treg cells and restore Treg function via the upregulation of FOXP3 in Treg cells, alleviating psoriasis

Narrowband ultraviolet B (NBUVB) especially acts by:[15,16,19-21,23,24]
- Reducing Th1 cells and their proinflammatory cytokines (IL-2, IFN-γ and TNF-α), and downregulates the Th17 population via the IL-23 axis
- Promotes differentiation of regulatory T cells via the RANK/RANKL signaling pathway in keratinocytes and Langerhans cells, a key mechanism for maintaining self-tolerance and controlling excessive immune responses
- Increase in anti-inflammatory cytokines, including IL-10 (produced by keratinocytes, regulatory T cells and macrophages with phagocytosed apoptotic cells), alpha-MSH (by keratinocytes) and PGE2 (by keratinocytes and Langerhans cells) and others such as TGF-β, IL-4, and calcitonin gene-related peptide (CGRP).

There are four salient effects of phototherapy in psoriasis:[25]
1. Proapoptotic effects (induction of apoptosis and release of photoproducts)
2. Immunomodulatory effects (release of immunomodulatory molecules, regulation of cell migration, and induction of immunosuppression)
3. Antipruritic effects (downregulation of Th2 cytokines, degranulation of mast cells, and increase of β-endorphins)
4. Pro- and prebiotic effects (redistribution of the skin microbiome by selection of UV-resistant microbial species, decrease of *Staphylococcus aureus*, and increase of immunostimulatory microbial products)

Ultraviolet B

Broadband ultraviolet B was the first to be developed, in the 1940s, and emits wavelengths of light of between 290 and 313 nm.

Narrowband ultraviolet B now is the first-line treatment for the management for psoriasis as the wavelengths that most efficiently clear psoriasis are approximately around 313 nm.[26] The normal epidermis allows 2.4% of incident UVB to enter the dermis, while 44% passes through the stratum corneum. In psoriasis, the thicker corneal layer with air-tissue interfaces reflects much of the UVB.[27] To enhance absorption and reduce UV-induced erythema, psoriatic plaques should be treated with a thin layer of emollient or petrolatum before undergoing phototherapy.[28]

Narrowband ultraviolet B (311 ± 2 nm) has been found to be superior to conventional BB-UVB (300–320 nm), with longer remissions, lower incidence of burning, and perhaps less carcinogenicity. They have largely supplanted BB-UVB and UVA radiation sources for phototherapy.

The advantages of NBUVB over PUVA are:
- No gastrointestinal upset associated with psoralen
- No need for eye protection during the post-treatment period
- Safe to use for children and pregnant women
- Easier and less expensive to administer

Indications of NB-UVB in psoriasis are:[29]
- Stable or guttate types of psoriasis with >20% body area affected
- Failure to respond to adequate trials of topical therapies
- In cases where systemic drugs are contraindicated, poorly tolerated, or not sufficiently effective

Narrowband ultraviolet B is considered to be the first choice of phototherapy methods in moderate to severe plaque psoriasis because of safety reasons in comparison to PUVA.[30]

Treatment Methodology of Narrowband Ultraviolet B

The initial starting dose of NBUVB can be based on skin phototype or minimal erythema dose (MED). The US protocols tend to focus on individualized treatment plans based on patient skin type. **Table 2** summarizes the dosing scheme given by the American Academy of Dermatology and the National Psoriasis Foundation.[31-33]

Alternatively, the German Dermatologic Society (Deutsche Dermatologische Gesellschaft, DDG) recommends initial UVB irradiation dose determination prior to the start of phototherapy, either by assessing the MED **(Table 3)**[34] or based on Fitzpatrick skin type **(Table 4)**[34] and UVB treatment administered according to a standardized dosing schedule **(Table 5)**.[34-36]

The goal of therapy is to retain a mild perceptible erythema throughout treatment. While practitioners prefer regimens based on the patient's skin type for the convenience of both the patient and themselves, using MED-based therapy is considered the safest approach for patients.[37] Although both twice- and thrice-weekly regimens are effective, the patient gets exposed to a higher cumulative UVB dose and increased risk

---

TABLE 2: Determination of MED, subsequent visits, maintenance therapy, and maximum dose for NB-UVB phototherapy[3,31-33]

Dose category

Estimation of initial NB-UVB dose by skin type needs to be performed by skin type, as assessed by the prescribing physician and/or the phototherapist, as follows:
- Skin types I and II: 300 mJ/cm^2
- Skin types III and IV: 500 mJ/cm^2
- Skin types V and VI: 800 mJ/cm^2

Determination of MED

- MED should be tested in a sun-shielded region on the hip or buttock. All other areas of the skin should be covered. The patient should wear eye protection during the delivery of the UV doses
- The tested areas should be uniform in size, approximately 2 × 2 cm, and marked with a skin pen to identify that tested area
- The following dosage schedule should be used varying on skin types:

Skin types I–II (mJ/cm^2)	Skin types I–II (mJ/cm^2)
250	350
400	500
550	650
700	800
850	950
1,000	1,100
1,150	1,250
1,300	1,400

- Initiate the therapeutic intervention with all measurement regions exposed, then occlude following administration of the prescribed photonic dose
- Advise subjects to maintain occlusion of the treated area for a 24-hour postintervention period, ensuring avoidance of both natural and artificial ultraviolet radiation exposure
- The subject is to return for follow-up evaluation 24 hours postexposure. The minimal erythema dose (MED) is defined as the lowest administered dose that elicits any perceptible erythematous response within the designated test site

Note: MED testing should not be performed in patients with skin types V and VI. These patients should be started at an initial dose of 800 mJ/cm^2 and increased as tolerated according to the protocol below.

Continued

CHAPTER 9: Phototherapy in the Management of Psoriasis

Continued

Subsequent visits

During follow-up consultations, the therapeutic efficacy of phototherapy is evaluated through quantitative assessment of cutaneous erythema intensity and persistence, complemented by qualitative analysis of patient-reported adverse sensations, including pruritus, cutaneous dysesthesia, and nociceptive experiences.

The effect of skin erythema on UVB dosing will be as follows:
- *Minimal erythema lasting <24 hours following treatment*: Increase dose by 20%
- *Erythema persistent for > 24 hours but <48 hours*: Dose held at the previous level until erythema lasting <24 hours
- *Erythema lasting > 48 hours*: No treatment on that day followed by return of dose to the last lower dose that did not cause persistent erythema

If the patient missed a treatment, the following schedule should be used:

Duration of missed days	Dose
1 week	Hold the previous dose constant
1–2 weeks	Decrease the previous dose by 25%
2–4 weeks	Decrease the previous dose by 50%
>4 weeks	Return to the starting dose

Maintenance therapy

Upon achieving clinical resolution of psoriatic lesions, the subject may elect to pursue a continuation therapeutic regimen, either in the form of a gradual dose reduction protocol or as an indefinite maintenance intervention
- The maintenance dose should be the last dose given prior to clearing
- The standardized maintenance therapy tapering protocol comprises bi-weekly administrations for an initial 4-week period, followed by weekly administrations for a subsequent 4-week interval. Throughout this regimen, the therapeutic dose should remain constant
- For extended maintenance therapy, the subject should undergo phototherapeutic interventions at intervals of 7–14 days
- The maintenance dose should be established at 75% of the final therapeutic dose and maintained at this constant level throughout the prolonged treatment course

Maximum dose

Upon attaining the prescribed dose, consultation with the attending physician is warranted for further clinical direction.

In the absence of complete cutaneous clearance, dose escalation may be implemented, typically involving incremental increases of 5–10% per therapeutic session, contingent upon patient tolerability.

The following outlines the recommended upper limits for phototherapeutic dosage:

Note: Irrespective of the subject's Fitzpatrick phototype classification, the upper threshold for phototherapeutic intervention in facial regions should not surpass 1 J/cm².

Administration of doses exceeding this limit necessitates explicit authorization from the attending physician, predicated on individual patient-specific clinical considerations.

Skin type	Dose (mJ/cm^2)
I and II	2,000
III and VI	3,000
V and VI	5,000

(MED: minimal erythema dose; NB: narrowband; UVB: ultraviolet B) of UV-induced erythema with the latter.[38] The twice-weekly regimen generally takes approximately 1.5 times longer to clear the skin disease compared to the thrice-weekly approach.[39] Several increment strategies can be utilized for treatment. Some clinicians suggest increasing the MED by 10-20% for each session, while others favor larger increments of 15-25%.[40,41] There is no general consensus on the effectiveness of long-term maintenance with NB-UVB; however, some clinicians have observed longer remission durations in patients with plaque-type psoriasis.[33]

Psoralen Plus Ultraviolet A

Photochemotherapy (PUVA) involves the use of psoralen, an exogenous photosensitizer followed by UVA irradiation. Both components are essential for clinical improvement as either of them used singly is not beneficial. Psoralen acts by inducing intercalation

TABLE 3: Recommended UVB doses to determine the mean erythema dose (MED)[34]						
Broadband UVB (J/cm²)	0.02	0.04	0.06	0.08	0.1	0.12
UVB 311 nm (J/cm²)	0.2	0.4	0.6	0.8	1	1.2

TABLE 4: Recommendations for the initial dose for UVB phototherapy according to skin type[34]		
Skin types according to Fitzpatrick (phototype)	Broadband UVB (J/cm²)	UVB 311 nm (J/cm²)
I	0.02	0.2
II	0.03	0.3
III	0.05	0.5
IV	0.06	0.6

TABLE 5: Dose scheme for UVB phototherapy (UV broadband and UVB 311 nm)[34-36]			
Steps			
Step 1 (optional)	Determination of the MED	Reading after 24 hours	
Step 2	Start of therapy	Standard dosage according to skin type (Fitzpatrick) or 70% of MED	
Step 3	Follow treatment 3-5 times a week	No erythema	Increase by 30%
		Minimal Erythema	Maintain dose or, depending on tolerance, increase cautiously by approximately 10-15%
		Persistent Asymptomatic Erythema	No increase
		Painful erythema with or without edema or blistering	Pause irradiation until symptoms resolve, resume with a reduced dose of 30-50%, then increase by approximately 10%
Step 4	Resumption of therapy	After the symptoms have subsided	Reduction of the last dose by 50%, further increases by 10%

of cellular DNA base pairs and forming crosslinks. The DNA crosslinks result in antiproliferative, antiangiogenic, apoptotic, and immunosuppressive effects. The most frequently used psoralens for oral use are 8-MOP and 5-MOP and that for topical therapy include 8-MOP and trimethylpsoralen (TMP). Psoralen can be applied topically in a variety of ways: A bath solution for whole body treatment and soak, paint, cream, or gel for hands and feet, scalp, and other localized areas. Topical therapy is preferred over oral therapy in patients with liver dysfunction, gastrointestinal issues, cataracts, poor adherence to eye protection, or a risk of drug interactions (such as with warfarin). It is also favored to reduce irradiation time, particularly for children, the elderly, or individuals with claustrophobia.

Indications for PUVA in psoriasis are:[42]
- Psoriasis involving >20% of body surface area (BSA)
- Unresponsiveness to topical therapy/TL-O1 therapy
- Palmoplantar pustular psoriasis which is characterized by repeated eruptions of sterile pustules on the palms and soles
- Localized disease not responding to other modalities of therapy

Exclusion criteria are as follows:
- Children aged <10 years
- Pregnancy and lactation
- People suffering from photosensitivity disorders

Treatment Methodology of Psoralen Plus Ultraviolet A

There are two protocols that are followed in psoriasis:
1. *US protocol*: The initial treatment dose is determined by the patient's skin type, and therapy is administered two to three times a week. Doses are increased by 0.5–1.5 J/cm^2, depending on the development of erythema and the patient's therapeutic response. Dosing of 8-methoxypsoralen and UVA radiation for PUVA are mentioned in **Tables 6 and 7** respectively:

2. *European protocol*: The starting dose is based on MPD determination which is similar to MED except that the UVA geometric doses series is undertaken in psoralen-sensitized skin, 2 hours after oral ingestion of a standard dose of 8-MOP (or 2.5 hours for 5-MOP). MPD is defined as the minimal dose of UVA radiation that produces uniform erythema when small template test areas are exposed to increasing doses of UVA ranging from 0.5 to 5 J/cm^2. The erythema readings are performed 72–96 hours after testing when the phototoxicity has reached a peak.[43] Dose recommendations for the determination of the minimum phototoxic dose (MPD) and the initial dose for photochemotherapy depending on skin type as indicated in **Tables 8 and 9**, respectively.

TABLE 6: Dosing of 8-methoxypsoralen for oral psoralen plus ultraviolet A[3]

Patient weight		Drug dose (mg)
lbs	kgs	
<66	<30	10
66–143	30–65	20
144–200	66–91	30
>200	>91	40

TABLE 7: Dosing of ultraviolet A radiation for oral psoralen plus ultraviolet A[3]

Skin type	Initial dose, (J/cm^2)	Increments, (J/cm^2)	Maximum dose, (J/cm^2)
I	0.5	0.5	8
II	1.0	0.5	8
III	1.5	1.0	12
IV	2.0	1.0	12
V	2.5	1.5	20
VI	3.0	1.5	20

CHAPTER 9: Phototherapy in the Management of Psoriasis

TABLE 8: Dose recommendations for the determination of the minimum phototoxic dose (MPD)[34]

Method	Dose*	Skin type	UVA dose (J/cm²)					
PUVA oral (8-MOP)	0.6 mg/kg bw	I–IV	0.5	1	2	3	4	5
PUVA oral (5-MOP)	1.2 mg/kg bw	I–IV	1	2	4	6	8	10
PUVA-Bath (1 mg/L 8-MOP)	0.5–1.0 mg/L (0.00005–0.0001%)	I, II	0.25	0.5	1	1.5	2	2.5
		III, IV	0.5	1	2	3	4	5

*There is no general international consensus on this.

(bw: bodyweight; MOP: methoxypsoralen; PUVA: psoralen with UVA)

TABLE 9: Recommendations for the initial dose for photochemotherapy depending on skin type[34]

Skin type according to Fitzpatrick (phototype)[32]	Oral PUVA (8-MOP) (J/cm²)	Oral PUVA (5-MOP) (J/cm²)	Bath PUVA and Cream PUVA (J/cm²)
I	0.3	0.4	0.2
II	0.5	1.0	0.3
III	0.8	1.5	0.4
IV	1.0	2.0	0.6

(MOP: methoxypsoralen; PUVA: psoralen with UVA)

The IADVL therapeutic guidelines committee recommends a modified US regime suited to Indian patients, in which the initial treatment dose is 2–3 J/cm² and is subsequently increased by 0.5 J/cm² provided the patient has not developed erythema or burning sensation over the apparently normal skin.[42]

Minimum phototoxic dose testing helps establish the ideal starting dose for treatment, detects cases of underdosage resulting from inadequate psoralen absorption and can also identify individuals with abnormal photosensitivity.

Initial Treatment (Clearance Phase)

Usually initiated at a dose that corresponds to either the skin phototype or 50–70% of the MPD, given 2–3 times a week with at least 48-hour intervals between treatments. If mild erythema appears, the dose may be maintained or slightly reduced; however, if moderate to severe erythema occurs, treatment is deferred. On average, around 15–25 treatment sessions are needed for clearance with a final clearance dose of UVA ranging between 5 and 20 J/cm², depending on the patient's skin type.[42] Once >95% of the initial psoriatic area has cleared, the patient is transitioned to a maintenance schedule.[44]

Maintenance Treatment

The final clearance dose is maintained, while the treatment frequency is gradually decreased to as low as once a month.[44] A number of guidelines discourage the use of maintenance PUVA for patients with psoriasis, while some advocate maintenance PUVA as an option for patients with particularly aggressive disease.[45-47]

Treatment of Relapses

If there is a significant relapse after treatment cessation or during the maintenance phase, resuming the clearance regimen is advisable. For minor flare-ups during maintenance, the treatment frequency can be increased to regain disease control. Recent studies have shown that administering PUVA twice weekly reduces cumulative PUVA exposure while still maintaining remission time compared to the conventional thrice-weekly regimen. This could enhance patient compliance and improve the risk-benefit ratio.[48-51]

PUVASOL refers to the intake of psoralen followed by sunlight exposure as a rich source of UVA and has been used successfully for treating psoriasis. It can be administered at home making it a cost-effective option for patients living in tropical countries such as India.[52] Major drawbacks include lack of privacy and inability to monitor and quantify UV light, which may give rise to untoward effects. The ideal time for sun exposure is 9.15–11.15 AM or 2.30–3.30 PM, when UVB and infrared radiation are minimum.[53] Exposure to sun is advised for 10 minutes after 1.5–2 hours of 8-MOP intake (at a dose of 0.6 mg/kg body weight after breakfast). Patients are advised two to three sessions weekly, with the exposure time increased by 5 minutes each week until reaching a maximum of 30–45 minutes. To prevent eye toxicity and darkening of normal skin, it is essential to wear protective eyewear and avoid additional sun exposure for the next 8 hours.[42] Two Indian studies reported that 55 and 63% of patients experienced good to excellent improvement with PUVASOL in psoriasis.[54,55]

■ TARGETED PHOTOTHERAPY

Targeted UV therapy became more widely accepted after the development of the 308-nm monochromatic xenon-chloride laser for psoriasis (in 1997), as it reduces cumulative UV exposure, toxicity, and number of treatments required compared to full-body phototherapy.[56,57]

The exciter light utilizes a noble gas (xenon) that reacts with chloride, a reactive gas, to produce UV radiation at a wavelength of 308 nm. When electrically stimulated, this gas mixture emits a monochromatic 308 nm laser beam, allowing for precise and localized alterations to the irradiated tissue.[58]

There are two forms of excimer light therapy:
1. The excimer laser which delivers targeted phototherapy to lesions through a tip with a spot size ranging from 14 to 30 nm in diameter, leaving healthy skin unaffected.
2. The excimer lamp emits inconsistent light and requires a longer duration to achieve the same fluence, making it suitable for treating larger areas.

The use of excimer light is most appropriate in adult and pediatric patients with mild, moderate, or severe psoriasis with <10% BSA involvement and in difficult-to-treat psoriasis subtypes such as palmoplantar pustular psoriasis, scalp, nail psoriasis, flexures, and genitals.[59,60]

Treatment begins with a dose of 1 to 3 times the MED, with gradual dose increments based on clinical outcomes and patient tolerance. Excimer laser sessions are generally scheduled 2–3 times per week, with at least 48 hours between sessions, over a period of 3–6 weeks. Clearance is typically achieved after 8–10 sessions, demonstrating effectiveness comparable to PUVA in treating nonpustular palmoplantar psoriasis.[11,60]

More recently, dosing is guided by the patients' skin type and the thickness of the plaque and subsequent dosages are adjusted based on the response to therapy or the development of side effects **(Table 10)**.[61]

It is an effective treatment option for psoriasis refractory to systemic treatment and may be used as monotherapy or combined with topical steroids, calcipotriol, dithranol, tacrolimus, and 8-MOP, enhancing their effectiveness.[60]

Newer, specialized light treatments such as the monochromatic excimer light (MEL) laser have emerged, offering the benefit of covering larger areas with potentially lower operating costs compared to the excimer laser. MEL has

TABLE 10: Dosing guidelines for targeted therapy[61]

Initial dose for psoriasis

Plaque thickness	Induction score	Fitzpatrick skin type I–III (dose in mJ/cm^2)	Fitzpatrick skin type IV–VI (dose in mJ/cm^2)
None	1		
Mild	2	300	400
Moderate	3	500	600
Severe	4	700	900

	No effect	Minimal effect	Good effect	Considerable improvement	Moderate/severe erythema (with or without blistering)
Dose for subsequent treatments	No erythema at 12–24 hours and no plaque improvement	Slight erythema at 12–24 hours but no significant improvement	Mild-to-moderate erythema at 12–24 hours	Significant improvement with plaque thinning or reduced scaliness or pigmentation occurred	
Typical dosing change from prior treatment dose	Increase dose by 25%	Increase dose by 15%	Maintain dose	Maintain dose or reduce dose by 15%	Reduce dose by 25% (treat around blistered area, do not treat blistered area until it heals or crust disappears)

proven effective in treating mild-to-moderate psoriasis vulgaris, particularly palmoplantar psoriasis.[62-64]

Table 11 summarizes the dosing schedule, possible adverse effects, and contraindications of various modalities discussed before.[65]

■ COMBINATION THERAPY

Historically, Goeckermann pioneered the combination of BBUVB with coal tar in 1925, followed by Ingram, who later incorporated anthralin (dithranol). Combination therapy involves using UVB or PUVA alongside topical or systemic treatments in order to enhance the clinical response for psoriasis while reducing the frequency of phototherapy sessions and the total cumulative dose. There is strong evidence that a combination of oral retinoids with PUVA or UVB (known as Re-PUVA or Re-UVB) is superior to monotherapy. Re-PUVA is instituted at a standard dose of 0.75–1 mg/kg isotretinoin or, 0.5–0.75 mg/kg for acitretin for 5–10 days before PUVA is started. It helps accelerate the desquamation of psoriatic plaques leading to increased UVA penetration.[66-69]

Additionally, retinoids offer protective benefits against the development of non-melanoma skin cancers (NMSC) with no immunosuppressive properties.[70]

There are a myriad of other agents, topical as well as systemic that can be combined with UV therapy; however, concomitant systemic immunosuppressive agents such as cyclosporine, azathioprine, tacrolimus, and mycophenolate mofetil should be avoided as it increases the risk for developing NMSC.[71]

Table 12 list drugs that can be combined with UV therapy, either with or without additional topical or systemic treatments.

TABLE 11: Various phototherapeutics in psoriasis[65]

	Narrowband UVB (NB-UVB; 310–331 nm)	Broadband UVB (BB-UVB)	Psolaren and UVA light (PUVA)	Excimer laser (308 nm)
Dosing	• Dosage based on either the Fitzpatrick skin type or MED; determine MED; initial treatment at 50–70% of MED followed by two to five treatments weekly; apply emollient prior to treatment. • *Maintenance therapy after >95% clearance*: Once a week for 4 weeks; keep the dose the same once every 2 weeks for 4 weeks; decrease dose by 25% once every 4 weeks, 50% of highest dose	The dosage may be administered according to the Fitzpatrick skin type; initial treatment at 50% of MED followed by three to five treatments weekly	• A dose based on MPD is recommended; if MPD testing is impractical, a regimen based on skin type may be used • Initial dose: 0.5–2.0 J/cm^2, depending on skin type (or MPD) • Treat twice weekly, increments of 40% per week until erythema, and then a maximum 20% per week • No further increments when 15 J/cm^2 is reached	The dose of energy delivered is guided by the patient's skin type and thickness of plaque; further doses are adjusted based on response to treatment or development of side effects; treatment is usually given twice weekly
Indications other than psoriasis	Atopic dermatitis, vitiligo, polymorphous light eruption (PLE), nodular prurigo, parapsoriasis en plaques, mycosis fungoides, pityriasis lichenoides, lymphomatoid papulosis, and seborrheic dermatitis	Atopic dermatitis, PLE, nodular prurigo, mycosis fungoides, pityriasis lichenoides, lymphomatoid papulosis, seborrheic dermatitis, and HIV-associated pruritic eruptions	Atopic dermatitis, vitiligo, mycosis fungoides—graft-versus-host disease, pityriasis rubra pilaris, systemic sclerosis/morphea, and dyshidrotic eczema	Atopic dermatitis, vitiligo, mycosis fungoides, pityriasis lichenoides, urticaria pigmentosa, morphea, scleroderma, granuloma annulare, lichen planus, lichen simplex chronicus, and alopecia areata
Possible adverse effects	Photodamage, polymorphic light eruption, increased risk of skin aging, and skin cancers but lower than that for PUVA	Photodamage, polymorphic light eruption, and increased risk of skin aging and skin cancers	Photodamage, premature skin aging, increased risk of melanoma and nonmelanoma skin cancers, ocular damage (cataract)	Erythema, blisters, hyperpigmentation, and erosions; long-term side effects not yet clear but likely similar to NB-UVB
Contraindications	• *Absolute*: Photosensitivity disorders • *Relative*: Photosensitizing medications, melanoma, and nonmelanoma skin cancers (NMSC)	• *Absolute*: Photosensitivity disorders • *Relative*: Photosensitizing medications, melanoma, and NMSC	• *Absolute*: Photosensitivity disorders • *Relative*: Age <10 years, pregnancy, photosensitizing medications, melanoma, NMSC, and severe organ dysfunction	• *Absolute*: Photosensitivity disorders • *Relative*: Photosensitizing medications, melanoma, and NMSC

TABLE 12: Combination of UV with or without topical or systemic therapy

Combinations recommended	Not recommended
• Topical steroids • Calcipotriene) • Topical retinoids (especially tazarotene) • Anthralin • Coal tar • Methotrexate (effective in clearing psoriasis with UVB but not recommended with PUVA due to increased risk of phototoxicity and skin cancer) • Cyclosporine • Biologic agents such as alefacept, etanercept, adalimumab, and ustekinumab • Fumaric acid esters (FAEs) • Apremilast	• Cyclosporine • Azathioprine • Tacrolimus • Mycophenolate mofetil

Controlled use of UV phototherapy during pregnancy is considered safe. UV therapy holds no FDA pregnancy category but has been successfully used during gestation.[79,80] Due to possible photodegeneration of folic acid in the course of UV therapy, various authors recommend that pregnant patients receiving UVB therapy should use folic acid supplements at the standard dose of 0.8 mg/day despite lack of apparent folic acid deficiency.[81,82]

Psoralen plus ultraviolet A is listed as FDA pregnancy category C therefore should be avoided during pregnancy since psoralen has a theoretical risk of teratogenic and mutagenic effects, due to DNA synthesis and cell division inhibition.[80,83]

A consensus statement published by the American Academy of Dermatology in 2010 concluded that for moderate to severe psoriasis in HIV-positive patients, phototherapy and antiretrovirals are the recommended first-line therapeutic agents.[84,85]

■ PHOTOTHERAPY FOR PSORIASIS IN SPECIAL POPULATIONS

Phototherapy in childhood psoriasis has been observed to be effective and well tolerated despite its potential association with the risk of retinal toxicity, accelerated or premature skin aging, and induction of skin malignancy. Oral PUVA is not recommended for pediatric patients due to concerns related to long-term toxicity, photocarcinogenesis, and limited recent data on its use. However, topical psoralen may be combined with UVA therapy for children >10 years old.[72-75]

Indications:[76-78]
- Debilitating palmoplantar psoriasis
- Chronic plaque psoriasis involving 5–10% of BSA
- Guttate psoriasis
- Refractory psoriasis
- Children in whom systemic drugs are contraindicated

Patient Selection and Assessment[21,86,87]

Prior to starting phototherapy, it is wise to assess the individual for both safety and quality considerations. The following steps should be ideally taken and documented:
- Indication and proper patient selection—motivated, compliant patient
- Exclusion of contraindications—history and clinical examination of whole body
- Assessment of skin (to assess for solar damage, premalignant skin lesions, and skin cancers) and disease reactivity to sun, tanning beds, or previous phototherapy
- Previous topical/systemic immuno-suppressive drug therapy/use of photo-active drugs (e.g., thiazide and quinine)
- Assessment of severity—Psoriasis Area and Severity Index (PASI) or BSA as needed
- Verbal and written education and/or informed consent, benefits, side effects, and possible risks of phototherapy

CHAPTER 9: Phototherapy in the Management of Psoriasis

- Determination of skin type or MED or MPD, choice of phototherapy protocol, and treatment plan

Safety Measures During Phototherapy[43]

- Patients should be advised regarding the appropriate use of emollients.
- Eye protection with UVA-blocking glasses is required during treatment and for 12 hours after ingesting psoralen. For individuals with preexisting cataracts or those at higher risk (e.g., children and patients with atopic eczema), protection is needed for 24 hours.
- Male patients should wear appropriate clothing to protect the genitalia.
- The face (if not involved by the dermatosis being treated) should be shielded with a visor to avoid unnecessary UV exposure.
- Protect the skin by using clothing, sunscreen, and avoidance of sunlight both after treatment and on nontreatment days.

Management of Acute Side Effects[43,44]

- Nausea can be alleviated by psoralen with a light meal with 8-MOP or by lowering the dose.
- Symptomatic erythema may require either topical corticosteroids when mild or a short course of oral corticosteroids and/or nonsteroidal anti-inflammatory drugs (NSAIDs) when severe.
- Pruritus (commonly referred to as PUVA itch) and PUVA pain can be managed by low-frequency electrotherapy, topical capsaicin, and oral gabapentin. **Table 13** provides an overview of patient monitoring for those undergoing PUVA.
- Acute subacute PUVA phototoxicity can range from mild erythema to severe pain with edema, blistering, and systemic symptoms including malaise and fever. These reasons necessitate adjusting the dose or halting treatment until the issues are resolved.

TABLE 13: Monitoring for PUVA

Baseline	Follow-up
Cutaneous examination for skin cancer or premalignant lesions	Every 6–12 months
Ocular: Gross examination, slit-lamp examination, fundoscopy, and visual acuity assessment	Annually
Laboratory: • Renal and/or liver function test • Antinuclear antibody (if suggested by positive findings on history or examination)	• 3 monthly • Need not be repeated

(PUVA: psoralen with UVA)

Management of Long-term Side Effects[43]

- Chronic actinic damage of the skin (such as PUVA lentigines and keratoses) is dose-dependent and only partially reversible after discontinuing PUVA treatment.
- *Nonmelanoma skin cancer*:
  - Patients receiving over 250 treatments have a significantly increased risk of squamous cell carcinoma (SCC). Therefore, it is advised that the maximum lifetime dose should not exceed 1,000–1,500 J/cm^2 or 150–200 exposures.
  - The guidance and standards for phototherapy units recommend skin cancer screenings for patients with >500 UVB exposures. Those exceeding this threshold should undergo an annual skin examination to detect premalignant and malignant lesions. Regular monitoring by the physician during phototherapy, along with cumulative doses and skin cancer assessments, is thus advised.

■ CONCLUSION

Phototherapy is an excellent modality of treatment for psoriasis which is economical, safe, and highly effective with minimal to no adverse effects.

ACKNOWLEDGMENT

We acknowledge the invaluable contribution and effort of Dr Pranomita Sahoo, 3rd year PGT, PG Department of Dermatology, Kalinga Institute of Medical Sciences, in realizing this project.

TAKE HOME MESSAGE

Phototherapy must be considered as one of the effective options to treat psoriasis. When combined with other drugs such as retinoids or methotrexate, phototherapy adds to effectiveness and permits the use of smaller doses of drugs for a shorter duration.

REFERENCES

1. Greb JE, Goldminz AM, Elder JT, Lebwohl MG, Gladman DD, Wu JJ, et al. Psoriasis. Nat Rev Dis Primers. 2016;2:16082.
2. Gudjonsson JE, Johnston A, Sigmundsdottir H, Valdimarsson H. Immunopathogenic mechanisms in psoriasis. Clin Exp Immunol. 2004;135:1-8.
3. Menter A, Korman NJ, Elmets CA, Feldman SR, Gelfand JM, Gordon KB, et al. Guidelines of care for the management of psoriasis and psoriatic arthritis: section 5. Guidelines of care for the treatment of psoriasis with phototherapy and photochemotherapy. J Am Acad Dermatol. 2010;62:114-35.
4. Taylor DK, Anstey AV, Coleman AJ, Diffey BL, Farr PM, Ferguson J, et al. Guidelines for dosimetry and calibration in ultraviolet radiation therapy: a report of a British photodermatology group workshop. Br J Dermatol. 2002;146:755-63.
5. Battie C, Verschoore M. Cutaneous solar ultraviolet exposure and clinical aspects of photodamage. Indian J Dermatol Venereol Leprol. 2012;78:9-14.
6. Srinivas CR, Sekar CS, Jayashree R. Photodermatoses in India. Indian J Dermatol Venereol Leprol. 2012;78:1-8.
7. Everett MA, Yeargers E, Sayre RM, Olson RL. Penetration of epidermis by ultraviolet rays. Photochem Photobiol. 1966;5:533-42.
8. Arndt S, Lissner C, Unger P, Bäumler W, Berneburg M, Karrer S. Biological effects of a new ultraviolet A1 prototype based on light-emitting diodes on the treatment of localized scleroderma. Exp Dermatol. 2020;29:1199-208.
9. Bormann M, Alt M, Schipper L, Sand L van de, Otte M, Meister TL, et al. Disinfection of SARS-CoV-2 contaminated surfaces of personal items with UVC-LED disinfection boxes. Viruses. 2021;13:598.
10. Kalajian TA, Aldoukhi A, Veronikis AJ, Holick MF. Ultraviolet B light emitting diodes (LEDs) are more efficient and effective in producing vitamin D3 in human skin compared to natural sunlight. Sci Rep. 2017;7:11489.
11. Zhang P, Wu MX. A clinical review of phototherapy for psoriasis. Lasers Med Sci. 2018;33:173-80.
12. Kulms D, Poppelmann B, Yarosh D, Luger TA, Krutmann J, Schwarz T, et al. Nuclear and cell membrane effects contribute independently to the induction of apoptosis in human cells exposed to UVB radiation. Proc Natl Acad Sci U S A. 1999;96:7974-9.
13. Douki T, Sage E. Dewar valence isomers, the third type of environmentally relevant DNA photoproducts induced by solar radiation. Photochem Photobiol Sci. 2016;15:24-30.
14. Wong T, Hsu L, Liao W. Phototherapy in psoriasis: a review of mechanisms of action. J Cutan Med Surg. 2013;17:6-12.
15. Johnson-Huang LM, Suárez-Farinas M, Sullivan-Whalen M, Gilleaudeau P, Krueger JG, Lowes MA. Effective NBUVB radiation therapy suppresses the IL-23/IL-17 axis in normalized psoriatic plaques. J Invest Dermatol. 2010;130:2654-63.
16. Krutman J, Hoenigsman H, Elmets CA. Dermatological Phototherapy and Photodiagnostic Methods, 2nd edition. Berlin-Heidelberg: Springer; 2009. p. 448.
17. Pathirana D, Ormerod AD, Saiag P, et al. European S3-guidelines on the systemic treatment of psoriasis vulgaris [published correction appears in J Eur Acad Dermatol Venereol. 2010;24(1):117-8]. J Eur Acad Dermatol Venereol. 2009;23 Suppl 2:1-70.
18. Honigsman H, Schwarz T. Ultraviolet therapy. In: Bologna JL, Jorizzo JL, Rapini RP (Eds). Dermatology, 2nd edition. Boston: Elsevier Ltd.; 2008. pp. 2053-69.
19. Schwartz T. Photoimmunology. In: Rook's Textbook of Dermatology, 7th edition. London: Blackwell Science Ltd.; 2007. pp. 10.29-10.37.
20. Maverakis E, Miyamura Y, Bowen MP, Correa G, Ono Y, Goodarzi H. Light, including ultraviolet. J Autoimmun. 2010;34:247-57.
21. Sage RJ, Lim HW. UVB based therapy and vitamin D. Dermatol Ther. 2010;23:72-81.

22. Zhang D, Chen Y, Chen L, Yang R, Wang L, Liu W, et al. Ultraviolet irradiation promotes FOXP3 transcription via p53 in psoriasis. Exp Dermatol. 2016;25:513-8.
23. Loser K, Mehling A, Loeser S, Apelt J, Kuhn A, Grabbe S, et al. Epidermal RANKL controls regulatory T-cell number via activation of dendritic cells. Nat Med. 2006;12:372-9.
24. Akiyama T, Shimo Y, Quin J. RANL signalling regulates the development of the immune system and immune tolerance. Inflamm Regener. 2009;4:258-6.
25. Kurz B, Berneburg M, Bäumler W, Karrer S. Phototherapy: Theory and practice. J Dtsch Dermatol Ges. 2023;21:882-97.
26. Parrish JA, Jaenicke KF. Action spectrum for phototherapy of psoriasis. J Invest Dermatol. 1981;76: 359-62.
27. Bruls WA, Slaper H, van der Leun JC, Berrens L. Transmission of human epidermis and stratum corneum as a function of thickness in the ultraviolet and visible wavelengths. Photochem Photobiol. 1984;40(4):485-94.
28. Abdallah MA, El-Khateeb EA, Abdel-Rahman SH. The influence of psoriatic plaques pretreatment with crude coal tar vs. petrolatum on the efficacy of narrow-band ultraviolet B: a half-vs.-half intra-individual double-blinded comparative study. Photodermatol Photoimmunol Photomed. 2011;27: 226-30.
29. Saraswat A, Madke B. Psoriasis. In: S Sacchidanand, Savitha AS, Shilpa K, Shashi Kumar B M, (Eds). IADVL Textbook of Dermatology, 5th edition. Mumbai: Bhalani Publishing House; 2022. pp 1120-200.
30. Menter A, Korman NJ, Craig AE, Feldman SR, Gelfand JM, Gordon KB, et al. Guidelines for the management of psoriasis and psoriatic arthritis. Section 6. Case-based presentations and evidence-based conclusions. J Am Acad Dermatol. 2011; ahead of print, pp. 1-40.
31. Mehta NN, Shin DB, Joshi AA, Dey AK, Armstrong AW, Duffin KC, et al. Effect of 2 psoriasis treatments on vascular inflammation and novel inflammatory cardiovascular biomarkers: a randomized placebo-controlled trial. Circ Cardiovasc Imaging. 2018;11:e007394.
32. Zanolli M, Feldman SR. Phototherapy Treatment Protocols for Psoriasis and Other Photoherapy Responsive Dermatoses, 2nd edition. Milton, Abingdon, UK: Taylor & Francis; 2005.
33. Boztepe G, Karaduman A, Sahin S, Hayran M, Kolemen F. The effect of maintenance narrow-band ultraviolet B therapy on the duration of remission for psoriasis: a prospective randomized clinical trial. Int J Dermatol. 2006;45:245-50.
34. Herzinger T, Berneburg M, Ghoreschi K, Gollnick H, Hölzle E, Hönigsmann H, et al. S1-Guidelines on UV phototherapy and photochemotherapy. J Dtsch Dermatol Ges. 2016;14:853-76.
35. Stege H, Ghoreschi K, Hünefeld C. UV-Phototherapie. Der Hautarzt. 2021;72:14-26.
36. Fitzpatrick TB. The validity and practicality of sun-reactive skin types I through VI. Arch Dermatol. 1988;124:869-71.
37. Schneider LA, Hinrichs R, Scharffetter-Kochanek K. Phototherapy and photochemotherapy. Clin Dermatol 2008;26:464-76.
38. Dawe RS, Wainwright NJ, Cameron H, Ferguson J. Narrowband (TL-01) ultraviolet B phototherapy for chronic plaque psoriasis: three times or five times weekly treatment? Br J Dermatol. 1998;138:833-9.
39. Cameron H, Dawe RS, Yule S, Murphy J, Ibbotson SH, Ferguson J. A randomized, observer-blinded trial of twice vs. three times weekly narrowband ultraviolet B phototherapy for chronic plaque psoriasis. Br J Dermatol. 2002;147:973-8.
40. Honigsman H. Phototherapy for psoriasis. Clin Exp Dermatol. 2001;26:343-50.
41. Zanolli M. Phototherapy arsenal in the treatment of psoriasis. Dermatol Clin. 2004;22:397-406.
42. Shenoi SD, Prabhu S. Photochemotherapy (PUVA) in psoriasis and vitiligo. Indian J Dermatol Venereol Leprol. 2014;80:497-504.
43. Mckenna K, Ibbotson S. Principles of photo-therapy. In: Griffiths CEM, Barker J, Bleiker TO, Hussain W, Simpson RC (Eds). Rook's Textbook of Dermatology. West Sussex: Wiley-Blackwell Publishers; 2024. p.21.1-18.
44. Morison WL, Richard EG. PUVA photochemotherapy and other phototherapy modalities. In: Wolverton SE (Ed). Comprehensive Dermatologic Therapy, 3rd (Ed) Philadelphia: Elsevier Saunders; 2013. pp. 279-90.
45. Mysore V. Targeted phototherapy. Indian J Dermatol Venereol Leprol. 2009;75:119.
46. Nast A, Kopp I, Augustin M, Banditt KB, Boehncke WH, Follmann M, et al. German evidence-based guidelines for the treatment of psoriasis vulgaris (short version). Arch Dermatol Res. 2007;299: 111-38.
47. British Photodermatology Group guidelines for PUVA. Br J Dermatol. 1994;130:246-55.
48. Diette KM, Momtaz T, Stern RS, Arndt KA, Parrish JA. Psoralens and UV-A and UV-B twice weekly for the treatment of psoriasis. Arch Dermatol. 1984;120:1169-73.
49. Sakuntabhai A, Sharpe GR, Farr PM. Response of psoriasis to twice weekly PUVA. Br J Dermatol 1993;128:166-71.
50. Valbuena MC, Hernandez O, Rey M, Sanchez G, de Quintana LP. Twice- vs. thrice-weekly MPD PUVA

in psoriasis: a randomized-controlled efficacy study. Photodermatol Photoimmunol Photomed. 2007;23:126-9.
51. El-Mofty M, El Weshahy H, Youssef R, Abdel-Halim M, Mashaly H, El Hawary M. A comparative study of different treatment frequencies of psoralen and ultraviolet A in psoriatic patients with darker skin types (randomized-controlled study). Photodermatol Photoimmunol Photomed. 2008;24:38-42.
52. Aggarwal K, Khandpur S, Khanna N, Sharma VK, Pandav CS. Comparison of clinical and cost-effectiveness of psoralen + ultraviolet A versus psoralen + sunlight in the treatment of chronic plaque psoriasis in a developing economy. Int J Dermatol. 2013;52:478-85.
53. Balasaraswathy P, Kumar U, Srinivas CR, Nair S. UVA and UVB in sunlight, optimal utilization of UV rays in sunlight for phototherapy. Indian J Dermatol Venereol Leprol. 2002;68:198-201.
54. Marquis L, Rangwala GM. Photochemotherapy of psoriasis with oral 8-methoxypsoralen (8-MOP) and solar irradiation (PUVASOL therapy). Indian J Dermatol Venereol Leprol. 1980;46:297-8.
55. Anstey AV. Disorders of Skin Pigmentation. In: Burns T, Breathnach S, Cox N, Griffiths C (Eds). Rook's Textbook of dermatology. 8th edition. West Sussex: Wiley Blackwell Publishers; 2010. p. 58. 50-2.
56. Bonis B, Kemeny L, Dobozy A, Bor Z, Szabo G, Ignacz F. 308 nm UVB excimer laser for psoriasis. Lancet. 1997;350:1522.
57. Stein KR, Pearce DJ, Feldman SR. Targeted UV therapy in the treatment of psoriasis. J Dermatol Treat. 2008;19:141-5.
58. Ly K, Smith MP, Thibodeaux QG, Beck KM, Liao W, Bhutani T. Beyond the booth: excimer laser for cutaneous conditions. Dermatol Clin. 2020;38:157-63.
59. Miot HA, Ianhez M, Criado PR, Ramos PM. Targeted phototherapy for vitiligo and psoriasis: guidelines of the Brazilian Society of Dermatology. An Bras Dermatol. 2023;98:757-77.
60. Abrouk M, Levin E, Brodsky M, Gandy JR, Nakamura M, Zhu TH, et al. Excimer laser for the treatment of psoriasis: safety, efficacy, and patient acceptability. Psoriasis (Auckl). 2016;6:165-73.
61. Menter A, Korman NJ, Elmets CA, et al. Guidelines of care for the management of psoriasis and psoriatic arthritis. Section 3. Guidelines of care for the management and treatment of psoriasis with topical therapies. J Am Acad Dermatol. 2009;60(4):643-59.
62. Han L, Somani AK, Huang Q, Fang X, Jin Y, Xiang LH, et al. Evaluation of 308-nm monochromatic excimer light in the treatment of psoriasis vulgaris and palmoplantar psoriasis. Photodermatol Photoimmunol Photomed. 2008;24:231-6.
63. Neumann NJ, Mahnke N, Korpusik D, Stege H, Ruzicka T. Treatment of palmoplantar psoriasis with monochromatic excimer light (308-nm) versus cream PUVA. Acta Derm Venereol. 2006;86:22-4.
64. Aubin F, Vigan M, Puzenat E, Blanc D, Drobacheff C, Deprez P, et al. Evaluation of a novel 308-nm monochromatic excimer light delivery system in dermatology: a pilot study in different chronic localized dermatoses. Br J Dermatol. 2005;152:99-103.
65. Richards HL, Fortune DG, O'Sullivan TM, Main CJ, Griffiths CE. Patients with psoriasis and their compliance with medication. J Am Acad Dermatol. 1999;41(4):581-3.
66. Lauharanta J, Geiger JM. A double-blind comparison of acitretin and etretinate in combination with bath PUVA in the treatment of extensive psoriasis. Br J Dermatol. 1989;121:107-12.
67. Saurat JH, Geiger JM, Amblard P, Beani JC, Boulanger A, Claudy A, et al. Randomized double-blind multicenter study comparing acitretin-PUVA, etretinate-PUVA and placebo PUVA in the treatment of severe psoriasis. Dermatologica. 1988;177:218-24.
68. Tanew A, Guggenbichler A, Honigsmann H, Geiger JM, Fritsch P. Photochemotherapy for severe psoriasis without or in combination with acitretin: a randomized, double-blind comparison study. J Am Acad Dermatol. 1991;25:682-4.
69. Lebwohl M. Acitretin in combination with UVB or PUVA. J Am Acad Dermatol. 1999;41:S22-4.
70. Bavinck JN, Tieben LM, Van der Woude FJ, Tegzess AM, Hermans J, ter Schegget J, et al. Prevention of skin cancer and reduction of keratotic skin lesions during acitretin therapy in renal transplant recipients: a double-blind, placebo-controlled study. J Clin Oncol. 1995;13:1933-8.
71. Marcil I, Stern RS. Squamous-cell cancer of the skin in patients given PUVA and cyclosporine: nested cohort crossover study. Lancet 2001;358:1042-5.
72. Guerrier CJ, Porter DI. An open assessment of 0.1% dithranol in a 17% urea base ('Psoradrate' 0.1%) in the treatment of psoriasis of children. Curr Med Res Opin. 1983;8:446-50.
73. Menter MA, Whiting DA, McWilliams J. Resistant childhood psoriasis: an analysis of patients seen in a day-care center. Pediatr Dermatol. 1984;2:8-12.
74. Kortuem KR, Davis MD, Witman PM, McEvoy MT, Farmer SA. Results of Goeckerman treatment for psoriasis in children: a 21-year retrospective review. Pediatr Dermatol. 2010;27:518-24.
75. Oostveen AM, Beulens CA, van de Kerkhof PC, de Jong EM, Seyger MM. The effectiveness and safety of short-contact dithranol therapy in paediatric psoriasis: a prospective comparison of regular day care and day care with telemedicine. Br J Dermatol. 2014;170:454-7.

76. Walters IB, Burack LH, Coven TR, Gilleaudeau P, Krueger JG. Suberythemogenic narrow-band UVB is markedly more effective than conventional UVB in treatment of psoriasis vulgaris. J Am Acad Dermatol. 1999;40:893-900.
77. Ersoy-Evans S, Altaykan A, Sahin S, Kolemen F. Phototherapy in childhood. Pediatr Dermatol. 2008;25:599-605.
78. Pavlovsky M, Baum S, Shpiro D, Pavlovsky L, Pavlotsky F. Narrow band UVB: is it effective and safe for paediatric psoriasis and atopic dermatitis? J Eur Acad Dermatol Venereol. 2011;25:727-9.
79. Nast A, Amelunxen L, Augustin M, Boehncke WH, Dressler C, Gaskins M, et al. S3 Guideline for the treatment of psoriasis vulgaris, update - Short version part 2 - Special patient populations and treatment situations. J Dtsch Dermatol Ges. 2018;16:806-13.
80. Bangsgaard N, Rørbye C, Skov L. Treating psoriasis during pregnancy: safety and efficacy of treatments. Am J Clin Dermatol. 2015;16:389-98.
81. Rose RF, Batchelor RJ, Turner D, Goulden V. Narrowband ultraviolet B phototherapy does not influence serum and red cell folate levels in patients with psoriasis. J Am Acad Dermatol. 2009;61:259-62.
82. Zhang M, Goyert G, Lim HW. Folate and phototherapy: What should we inform our patients? J Am Acad Dermatol. 2017;77:958-64.
83. Horn EJ, Chambers CD, Menter A, Kimball AB. Pregnancy outcomes in psoriasis: why do we know so little? J Am Acad Dermatol. 2009;61:e5-8.
84. Akaraphanth R, Lim HW. HIV, UV and immuno-suppression. Photodermatol Photoimmunol Photomed. 1999;15:28-31.
85. Menon K, Van Voorhees AS, Bebo BF Jr, Gladman DD, Hsu S, Kalb RE, et al. Psoriasis in patients with HIV infection: from the medical board of the National Psoriasis Foundation. J Am Acad Dermatol. 2010;62:291-9.
86. Schlaeger M, Boehncke WH, Weberschock T. Phototherapie. In: Nast A, Boehncke WH, Mrowietz U, Ockenfels HM, Philipp S, Reich K, et al. (Eds). S-3 Leitlinie zur Therapie der Psoriasis vulgaris. Update 2011. AWMF On line; Das Portal der wissenschaftlichen Medizin. AWMF Nr. 013/001.
87. Benáková N. Phototherapy of psoriasis in the era of biologics: still in? University Department of Dermatovenereology, 1st Medical Faculty, Charles University, Prague, Czech Republic. 2011;197.

10

Conventional Systemic Therapies in Psoriasis

Konakanchi Venkata Chalam, Kavya Baddireddy

■ INTRODUCTION

Conventional systemic treatments for psoriasis are essential for managing moderate-to-severe cases of this chronic skin condition. These treatments include methotrexate (MTX), acitretin, cyclosporine, and fumaric acid esters (FAEs), each with distinct mechanisms of action. MTX, an immunosuppressant, inhibits the rapid proliferation of skin cells by targeting the folate pathway. Acitretin, a retinoid, modulates skin cell growth and differentiation. Cyclosporine, an immunomodulator, reduces inflammation by inhibiting T-cell activity. FAEs, primarily used in Europe, exert anti-inflammatory and immunomodulatory effects. These treatments offer significant relief for many patients, although they require careful monitoring due to potential side effects.[1]

■ METHOTREXATE

Methotrexate, approved by the Food and Drug Administration (FDA) in 1972 for psoriasis treatment, inhibits enzymes like dihydrofolate reductase and thymidylate synthase crucial for nucleic acid synthesis.[2] Its derivatives also block 5-aminoimidazole-4-carboxamide ribonucleotide transformylase, increasing endogenous adenosine known for anti-inflammatory effects. Originally thought to affect keratinocytes, MTX primarily suppresses lymphoid cell proliferation (especially at doses <25 mg/week), suggesting an immunosuppressive role in psoriasis. MTX additionally inhibits T and B lymphocytes, suppresses proinflammatory cytokines, and affects neutrophil and monocyte chemotaxis. It reduces DNA synthesis, induces keratinocyte apoptosis, and lowers interleukin-22 (IL-22) levels, impacting psoriasis pathogenesis.[3] MTX's anti-inflammatory effects involve adenosine release, which mitigates oxygen-free radical production and modulates immune responses. However, MTX's action on adenosine receptors (A1, A2A, A2B) may contribute to adverse effects such as hepatotoxicity and fatigue.[4]

Methotrexate is indicated for treating moderate-to-severe plaque psoriasis, psoriatic erythroderma, palmoplantar pustulosis, generalized pustular psoriasis, nail psoriasis, and psoriatic arthritis. It is recommended when topical therapies, phototherapy, or acitretin fail to improve the condition or are not feasible. MTX is also used in combination with other immunosuppressive drugs, especially biologics, to enhance their efficacy by preventing the formation of antibodies against them.[5]

Dosage

In the management of psoriasis, MTX is commonly administered orally once weekly, with doses ranging from 7.5 to 25 mg, either as a single dose or divided into three administrations over a 24-hour period. Comparative studies indicate that while a 10-mg weekly regimen has a slower onset compared to 25 mg, it also correlates with a reduced incidence of severe adverse effects. Daily dosing (2.5 mg daily for 6 days) shows lower efficacy than weekly dosing (15 mg divided into three doses every 8 hours) and carries a higher risk of liver enzyme elevation.

For specific patients, the Weinstein–Frost regimen—a tripartite dosing strategy every 12 hours—has demonstrated effectiveness in alleviating gastrointestinal side effects. This approach aims to disrupt the prolonged S phase of the psoriatic keratinocyte cell cycle, which spans 7 days.[6]

Methotrexate can be administered via various routes, including oral, intramuscular, intravenous, subcutaneous, or intrathecal. While oral administration is most common, weekly subcutaneous or intramuscular injections are viable alternatives. Treatment initiation may involve a test dose of 2.5–5 mg, followed by hematological evaluation within 5–7 days. Alternatively, an initial therapeutic dose such as 15 mg weekly may be started, with adjustments based on improvements in skin condition and tolerance over at least 1 month.

Subcutaneous MTX may be preferred for patients requiring higher doses due to its ability to reduce gastrointestinal disturbances. Clinical studies underscore its efficacy and tolerability compared to placebo.

Parenteral MTX solution, administered orally, provides cost-effectiveness. Although differences in bioavailability profiles exist between subcutaneous and oral routes, consensus suggests that oral parenteral solutions approximate oral formulations in efficacy.[7]

Efficacy

Methotrexate received FDA approval in 1972 without the need for randomized clinical trials, resulting in limited high-quality studies on its safety and efficacy. Despite this, several studies have highlighted its benefits in treating psoriasis.[8]

In one study, 868 MTX-naïve patients were randomized to receive either infliximab or MTX. After 16 weeks, 42% of those treated with MTX achieved Psoriasis Area and Severity Index (PASI) 75, indicating significant improvement. However, this study did not include a placebo group, which may lead to an overestimation of MTX's effectiveness.[9] In another large trial comparing MTX to adalimumab and placebo, MTX was more effective than placebo but less effective than adalimumab.[10] Various studies have consistently shown that biologic therapies such as infliximab, adalimumab, etanercept, ustekinumab, and narrowband ultraviolet B (NB-UVB) are more effective than MTX.[11-13]

Methotrexate is not FDA-approved for psoriatic arthritis but is used as a disease-modifying drug. Its effectiveness in managing disease activity and preventing radiographic progression needs further investigation. A recent randomized controlled trial found no evidence that MTX improves synovitis in psoriatic arthritis and showed no significant treatment effects on various endpoints. However, another study reported significant improvements in reducing dactylitis and enthesitis, as well as American College of Rheumatology outcomes.

Combining MTX with tumor necrosis factor inhibitors improves treatment efficacy for psoriasis. One study of 239 patients found that adding MTX to etanercept resulted in a better clinical response compared to etanercept alone. Additionally, MTX has been used with NB-UVB phototherapy, leading to increased efficacy and faster skin clearing. However, the long-term effects of this combination on photocarcinogenesis require further study.[14]

Adverse Effects

Methotrexate therapy can lead to various side effects, particularly soon after initiation.

Common side effects include fatigue, nausea, vomiting, anorexia, stomatitis, glossitis, and headaches. Adjusting the dosage, route, or frequency can often manage these issues. Less common adverse effects include pharyngitis, diarrhea, enteritis, tiredness, chills, fever, dizziness, leukopenia, and skin-related reactions such as pruritus, pain, urticaria, mild reversible alopecia, bruising, psoriatic lesion ulcerations, phototoxic responses, and rarely, toxic epidermal necrolysis.

Methotrexate can also trigger an acute sunburn reaction known as ultraviolet radiation recall (UV recall) when administered near UV irradiation. Other potential effects include pneumonitis, myelosuppression, and hepatotoxicity. Although myelosuppression is rare in psoriasis patients, it can occur, especially in elderly patients, those with renal issues, folate deficiency, or those on interacting medications, necessitating vigilant monitoring.

Additionally, the immunosuppressive nature of MTX raises the risk of infections and can reactivate conditions such as tuberculosis, hepatitis, and lymphoma, requiring regular monitoring. Less common adverse effects like hair loss and photosensitivity have been reported, though their exact mechanisms remain unclear.

Hematologic and Hepatotoxic Risks of Methotrexate

Patients initiating MTX therapy should be aware of potential hematologic and hepatotoxic risks. Hematologic toxicity, which includes conditions such as myelosuppression, is more prevalent among individuals with renal insufficiency, advanced age, dosing errors, drug interactions, hypoalbuminemia, and excessive alcohol intake. While extensively studied in conditions like rheumatoid arthritis, psoriasis patients generally face a low risk of MTX-induced myelosuppression when appropriately monitored and without additional risk factors.

Conversely, hepatotoxicity poses a more significant concern for psoriasis patients, particularly those with obesity, diabetes mellitus, or hyperlipidemia. Risk factors contributing to MTX-associated hepatotoxicity include a history of excessive alcohol consumption, persistent abnormal liver function tests (LFTs), preexisting liver diseases such as chronic hepatitis B or C, familial liver conditions, and exposure to hepatotoxic substances. Regular monitoring of LFTs and noninvasive fibrosis assessments are critical for early detection and management of hepatotoxicity during MTX therapy across various medical conditions.

Methotrexate toxicities are classified into four types, A to D.
- Type A toxicities encompass gastrointestinal and bone marrow issues, which are dose-dependent and linked to folate antagonism in rapidly replicating tissues. An increase in mean corpuscular volume can predict hematological toxicity.
- Type B reactions are idiosyncratic, such as pneumonitis.
- Type C toxicity involves long-term antifolate effects, including hepatotoxicity and hyperhomocysteinemia.
- Type D effects are delayed, occurring after stopping the drug, and include pregnancy-related issues and teratogenesis.[1]

Folic Acid Supplementation

Folic acid (FA) supplementation, at 1–5 mg/day, may reduce MTX side effects like nausea and megaloblastic anemia without affecting its efficacy. However, recent analyses show FA does not significantly lower mucocutaneous or gastrointestinal side effects but does reduce hepatic side effects. MTX raises homocysteine levels, increasing atherosclerosis risk, which FA can mitigate. Conflicting studies suggest high folate might reduce MTX efficacy in rheumatoid arthritis and psoriasis. Rheumatologists recommend varying FA protocols, commonly 5 mg/week after MTX, with some suggesting 5 mg/day for 1–3 days starting 48 hours post-MTX.[15]

Pregnancy and Lactation

Methotrexate, designated as pregnancy category X due to its teratogenic effects, carries a significant risk of causing fetal abnormalities throughout pregnancy. Thus, women of reproductive age are advised to use contraception while receiving MTX treatment. For those intending to conceive after therapy, it is recommended to wait a minimum of 3 months postdiscontinuation to ensure complete elimination of the drug from the body.

Methotrexate has been detected in human breast milk and poses a risk of serious adverse reactions in breastfed infants. Thus, it is contraindicated in nursing mothers.[16]

Male Fertility

While MTX is not mutagenic, its impact on spermatogenesis remains inconclusive. Some studies indicate reversible oligospermia in men taking MTX, while others show no changes in sperm count. Data on the teratogenicity of MTX when used by fathers are limited. Considering the mixed findings, men should wait at least 3 months after discontinuing MTX before attempting to conceive, allowing for the theoretical clearance of the drug's effects on sperm within the average cycle of spermatogenesis lasting 74 days.[17,18]

Contraindications

Methotrexate is contraindicated in patients who are pregnant, have moderate-to-severe hepatic or renal impairment, blood dyscrasias, active peptic ulcer disease, cirrhosis, significant thrombocytopenia, leukopenia, or anemia due to its potential for severe hematologic and hepatic side effects. Relative contraindications include chronic alcoholism, recent or severe hepatitis, concurrent use of hepatotoxic drugs, active infections, immunosuppression, recent vaccinations, obesity, diabetes mellitus, and unreliable patient adherence to treatment protocols.[19] The concurrent use of sulfa drugs and acitretin is also relatively contraindicated but may be acceptable with careful hepatic monitoring, particularly for palmar–plantar psoriasis. MTX should be used with caution in patients with human immunodeficiency virus (HIV) due to the heightened risk of adverse effects.[20]

Monitoring

Patients taking MTX require comprehensive monitoring to ensure safety and efficacy. Initially, complete blood count (CBC), serum creatinine, and transaminase levels should be checked weekly for the first 4 weeks, then at least every 2 months. Regular LFTs, including serum aspartate aminotransferase (AST), alanine aminotransferase (ALT), and serum albumin levels, are essential. If hepatotoxicity is suspected, a liver biopsy may be necessary. MTX should not be prescribed if creatinine clearance is below 50 mL/min due to nephrotoxicity risks. Pulmonary toxicity monitoring is also crucial, as patients may present with dry cough, fever, or dyspnea, necessitating baseline chest radiographs to identify interstitial and alveolar infiltrates, hilar adenopathy, pleural effusions, and pulmonary fibrosis. In regions where tuberculosis is endemic, screening for tuberculosis is required to prevent reactivation. Bone marrow toxicity should be monitored due to the risk of myelosuppression from folate deficiency, indicated by a sudden drop in blood counts. **Table 1** summarizes the initial diagnostic tests and follow-up monitoring necessary for MTX therapy.

Monitoring for hepatotoxicity involves both invasive and noninvasive methods. According to the American Academy of Dermatology (AAD) guidelines, liver biopsies are recommended for patients with risk

TABLE 1: Baseline and follow-up monitoring for methotrexate

Monitoring	AAD guidelines	European guidelines
Baseline	• Complete blood count • Liver function test • Renal function test • HIV test • Pregnancy test 2 weeks before starting treatment and on day 2 or 3 of a normal menstrual cycle • Tuberculin skin test (PPD)	• Complete blood count • Liver function test • Renal function test • HBV/HCV • Pregnancy test 2 weeks before starting treatment and on day 2 or 3 of a normal menstrual cycle • PIIINP • Serum albumin • Urinary sediment
Follow-up	• Complete blood cell counts weekly for the first 2 weeks, biweekly for the following months, and every 1–3 months after that • Liver function tests every 4–12 weeks • Renal function tests every 2–3 months	• Repeat the complete blood cell count after the first week, then biweekly for the next 2 months, and subsequently every 2–3 months • Conduct liver function tests every 4–12 weeks • Perform renal function tests every 2–3 months • Monitor liver and renal function along with urine analysis biweekly for 2 months, and then every 2–3 months. Measure PIIINP levels every 3 months

(AAD: American Academy of Dermatology; HBV: hepatitis B virus; HCV: hepatitis C virus; HIV: human immunodeficiency virus; PIIINP: amino-terminal type III procollagen peptide; PPD: purified protein derivative)

factors such as chronic alcoholism, liver disease, diabetes, obesity, hyperlipidemia, and concurrent use of hepatotoxic drugs. For patients without these risk factors, a liver biopsy is recommended after a cumulative MTX dose of 3.5–4.0 g, and for those with risk factors, it should be done at the start of treatment or within 2–6 months, and then after every 1–1.5 g of cumulative dose.[21] European guidelines suggest increased hepatotoxicity risk after a cumulative dose of >3 g of MTX or >100 g/week of alcohol consumption, recommending the use of the amino-terminal type III procollagen peptide (PIIINP) as a noninvasive tool.[22] PIIINP levels should be measured before starting MTX and every 3 months thereafter. Vibration-controlled transient elastography (Fibroscan) and the Controlled Attenuation Parameter (CAP) technique are other noninvasive methods to assess liver stiffness, early fibrosis, cirrhosis, and early steatosis. Combining transient elastography with PIIINP measurements can reduce the need for liver biopsies, especially in patients with a body mass index (BMI) below 30 kg/m². Additionally, a combination of Fibrotests, Fibroscans, and PIIINP measurements is considered ideal for monitoring liver toxicity in patients on MTX.[23,24] **Table 2** outlines the various invasive and noninvasive tests used to monitor MTX hepatotoxicity.

ACITRETIN

Acitretin, an oral retinoid derived from vitamin A, was introduced for psoriasis therapy in the early 1980s alongside its active form, etretinate. FDA approved acitretin specifically for psoriasis

CHAPTER 10: Conventional Systemic Therapies in Psoriasis

TABLE 2: Different invasive and noninvasive techniques for monitoring methotrexate (MTX) hepatotoxicity

Test	Interpretation	Comments
Liver biopsy	• *Grade I*: Normal, mild fatty changes, or slight portal inflammation • *Grade II*: Moderate-to-severe alterations • *Grade III*: Fibrosis (mild in stage IIIa and moderate-to-severe in stage IIIb) • *Grade IV*: Cirrhosis	• MTX is safe for grade II changes; for grade IIIa, continue MTX and repeat biopsy every 6 months • It is contraindicated for grades IIIb and IV
Ultrasonography	The most common and easiest way to identify nonalcoholic fatty liver disease	Limited by low inter-rater and intra-operator consistency and low sensitivity
Transient elastography	A noninvasive, ultrasonography-based scan that measures liver stiffness. It exhibits low interoperator variability and is highly effective in distinguishing cirrhosis from normal liver conditions	Most studies have involved patients with chronic liver diseases. This method requires validation in individuals with psoriasis
PIIINP	Perform a liver biopsy if pretreatment PIIINP exceeds 8.0 µg/L, or if it is above the normal range of 1.7–4.2 µg/L in at least three samples within a year, or if it is over 8.0 µg/L in two consecutive samples. Discontinue MTX if PIIINP is greater than 10.0 µg/L in at least three samples over the course of a year	Monitoring PIIINP is cost-effective, convenient for patients, and results in a seven-fold reduction in the number of liver biopsies, thereby minimizing complications associated with liver biopsy. However, PIIINP is not exclusive to liver fibrosis and can be elevated in healthy children and adolescents, as well as in individuals with inflammatory arthritis or scleroderma
MRI	Currently, there is inadequate data	Early studies using a low field-strength MRI machine did not match the histological results obtained from liver biopsies
DHS	High predictive value in early fibrosis, low predictive value in advanced fibrosis	DHS offers potential for identifying early hepatic damage caused by MTX

Other serum markers:
Direct markers: ALT, AST, C-glutamyltranspeptidase, hyaluronic acid, apolipoprotein A1, bilirubin, haptoglobin, cholesterol, platelets, and prothrombin time
Indirect markers: Collagen IV, collagen VI, human cartilage gp39, laminin, MMP-2, tenascin, TIMP-1, and undulin

(ALT: alanine aminotransferase; AST: aspartate aminotransferase; DHS: dynamic hepatic scintigraphy; gp: glycoprotein; MRI: magnetic resonance imaging; PIIINP: amino-terminal type III procollagen peptide; MMP: matrix metalloproteinase; TIMP: tissue inhibitor of metalloproteinase)

in 1997. Its mechanisms of action include influencing epidermal differentiation and proliferation, along with anti-inflammatory and immunomodulatory properties. Unlike many psoriasis treatments, acitretin does not suppress the immune system. It is FDA-approved for severe plaque-type psoriasis and generalized and localized pustular psoriasis. It is also used in combination with UVB, psoralen plus ultraviolet A (PUVA), cyclosporine, or biologics. Acitretin is the sole systemic retinoid FDA-approved for psoriasis and effective as monotherapy. It normalizes keratinocyte differentiation, reduces proinflammatory cytokines (IL-6, MRP-8, interferon gamma), and activates all nuclear retinoid X-receptors and retinoic acid receptors, enhancing its psoriasis management efficacy.

Dosage

Acitretin, available in hard gelatin capsules of 10 mg, 17.5 mg, and 25 mg strengths, is initially prescribed at 25–50 mg orally once daily for adults, preferably taken with a main meal. Following an initial response, the maintenance dose, also within the 25–50 mg daily range, is adjusted based on clinical response and tolerability. In treating psoriasis, improvement is noticeable within 4-6 weeks, with optimal benefits seen after 3-4 months. The starting dose is typically 25 mg orally daily, potentially reducing to 10 mg daily or 25 mg every other day once symptoms stabilize, primarily targeting plaque thickness, scaling, and itching. However, reductions in body surface area (BSA) may vary. When combined with phototherapy, acitretin is generally initiated at 25 mg orally daily for 2 weeks before phototherapy begins, requiring a decrease in the initial UV light dose. If acitretin is added to ongoing stable UV light therapy, the UV dose is typically reduced by 30–50% about 7 days after starting acitretin. Overall, achieving the optimal balance between effectiveness and patient tolerance is crucial, as acitretin's therapeutic benefits unfold gradually over 3–6 months.[25]

Efficacy

Acitretin, while comparably effective to other systemic psoriasis treatments, lacks head-to-head studies for direct comparison. Its efficacy correlates with dosage, and diverse dosing protocols exist. Clinical trials report varied PASI improvements, including notable responses at 50 and 40 mg/day for specified durations. Long-term therapy sustains efficacy, with significant PASI improvements observed at 6 and 12 months.[26,27] Acitretin's nonimmunosuppressive profile makes it suitable for psoriasis patients undergoing highly active antiretroviral therapy for HIV.[28] Notably, it exhibits promising outcomes in severe psoriasis variants such as erythrodermic and pustular forms, as well as hyperkeratotic palmoplantar psoriasis, either as monotherapy or in combination with phototherapy or systemic/biologic agents.[25]

Combining acitretin with phototherapy enhances treatment effectiveness compared to using either treatment alone. This approach reduces prolonged side effects and lowers overall phototherapy doses, frequency, and duration. Clinical trials demonstrate that acitretin–UVB combination therapy improves safety and efficacy, allowing for reduced acitretin doses and decreased UVB exposure. Integrating acitretin into phototherapy, whether UVB or PUVA, enhances treatment response, requiring fewer sessions and reducing cumulative phototherapy doses for clinical improvement. Additionally, adjunctive acitretin therapy reduces the risk of cutaneous squamous cell carcinoma associated with PUVA treatment alone, in contrast to the increased risk with cyclosporine therapy. Optimal treatment starts with acitretin before phototherapy begins.[28,29]

Adverse Effects

The foremost concern associated with acitretin therapy pertains to its teratogenic potential when utilized by women of childbearing age, necessitating stringent contraindications during pregnancy. Administration during gestational weeks 3-6 poses a significant risk of multiple malformations across various organ systems. Patients are advised against acitretin use prior to or during lactation due to potential adverse effects on offspring. Despite its relatively short half-life of 49 hours, acitretin may spontaneously convert to etretinate, which persists significantly longer. The precise alcohol threshold for this conversion remains unknown, posing potential risks with inadvertent exposure to alcohol-containing items. Consequently, the use of acitretin is discouraged in women of childbearing potential, with contraception being imperative for those contemplating pregnancy. However, there appears to be no evidence of fertility or teratogenic effects in men taking acitretin, although based on limited data.[30]

Virtually all patients experience mucocutaneous adverse effects, ranging from mild-to-severe, including xerosis, dry eyes, nasal/oral dryness, epistaxis, cheilitis, pruritus, burning skin, and brittle nails. Hair loss, particularly in women, is more prevalent with doses exceeding 17.5 mg/day. "Retinoid dermatitis", characterized by scaly, erythematous plaques with superficial fissuring, is a less common yet noteworthy adverse effect. Long-term acitretin therapy has been associated with pyogenic granulomas, predominantly in periungual regions.

Hyperlipidemia is the most common laboratory abnormality, affecting 25–50% of patients, with a higher risk in individuals with obesity, diabetes, or excessive alcohol consumption. Severe hypertriglyceridemia may precipitate pancreatitis, potentially fatal in some cases, and elevate the risk of atherosclerosis. Elevated transaminases occur in 13–16% of patients, with significant increases potentially indicating acitretin-induced toxic hepatitis, necessitating prompt discontinuation. Other less common adverse effects include pseudotumor cerebri-like symptoms, mood changes, altered vision, and minor myalgia/arthralgia. Diffuse idiopathic hyperostosis, characterized by skeletal changes, is a rare adverse effect of systemic retinoids, while acitretin's impact on osteoporosis remains a subject of debate. Nevertheless, there is a potential risk of premature epiphyseal growth plate closure in young patients undergoing long-term, high-dose retinoid therapy.[31]

Drug Interactions

Substances affecting cytochrome P450, like cyclosporine, alter acitretin metabolism. Medications competing for plasma proteins, such as phenytoin, impact plasma levels. Concurrent oral retinoid and vitamin A use raises hypervitaminosis A risk. Acitretin may affect glyburide's glucose-lowering effects, requiring caution in combined use.[32]

Pregnancy and Lactation

Acitretin is categorized as pregnancy category X due to its severe risks to fetal development, causing abnormalities such as meningoencephalocele, meningomyelocele, multiple synostoses, absence of terminal phalanges, facial dysmorphia, syndactyly, malformations of the hip, ankle, and forearm, low-set ear, high palate, cardiovascular malformation, decreased cranial volume, and alterations of the skull and cervical vertebrae. It should not be prescribed to pregnant women, those planning pregnancy during treatment, or within 3 years after stopping therapy. Strict monitoring programs like the Take to Prevent Pregnancy Program (TAPP) ensure safe usage due to acitretin's known teratogenic potential. Lactating women are also advised against using acitretin due to potential adverse effects on offspring. Despite its short half-life of 49 hours, acitretin can convert to etretinate, which persists longer in the body. The exact alcohol threshold that triggers this conversion is unclear, necessitating caution regarding alcohol consumption. While acitretin may not affect male fertility or cause teratogenic effects based on current evidence, contraception is still recommended for men considering fathering children during treatment.[33]

Monitoring

Monitoring during acitretin therapy should include baseline evaluations such as medical history, physical examination, LFTs, lipid profile assessment, and pregnancy testing for women of childbearing age. Initially, liver enzymes (AST, ALT) should be checked monthly for 3 months, followed by every 3 months thereafter. Lipid profiles should be assessed initially and then every 3 months. Due to acitretin's teratogenic effects, monthly pregnancy tests are necessary and should continue for 3 years after treatment ends. Regular clinical assessments are essential to evaluate treatment response, manage potential side effects like dry skin and mucosal dryness, and monitor for psychiatric symptoms. Monitoring cumulative doses is crucial for long-term safety. Scheduled follow-up visits every 3 months help ensure treatment effectiveness and patient well-being. If lipid levels are elevated, consideration should be given to administering triglyceride-lowering medications such as fibrates. Given the heightened cardiovascular risk in psoriasis patients, lifestyle modifications to manage hyperlipidemia should be recommended alongside acitretin therapy.

Contraindications

Acitretin carries significant warnings and contraindications. It is absolutely contraindicated in pregnant or potentially pregnant women due to its severe teratogenic effects. Noncompliance with effective contraception during and for at least 3 years after treatment discontinuation is also prohibited. Nursing mothers should avoid acitretin due to potential harm to infants. Absolute contraindications also include hypersensitivity to acitretin or its components, severe hepatic or renal dysfunction, chronic high blood lipid levels, and concurrent use with MTX or tetracyclines. Ethanol consumption is strongly discouraged during acitretin therapy and for at least 2 months afterward to prevent conversion to the highly teratogenic etretinate. Caution is advised when combining acitretin with MTX, cyclosporine, or other vitamin A compounds due to increased risks of adverse effects. Additionally, individuals prescribed acitretin should refrain from donating blood for at least 3 years to avoid potential transmission of its effects, including genetic defects.[34]

■ CYCLOSPORINE

Cyclosporine, approved by the FDA for psoriasis treatment in 1997, functions as a potent immunomodulator. It operates by binding to cyclophilin, inhibiting calcineurin activity, which disrupts inflammatory signaling pathways. This mechanism reduces cytokines like interferon-gamma and IL-2, thereby dampening T-cell activation. Due to its extensive range of potential side effects, cyclosporine is reserved for short-term management of severe, persistent, or acute psoriasis, such as erythroderma. It serves as a crucial bridge therapy, facilitating the transition to safer, long-term treatments.[35]

Dosage

In managing psoriasis with cyclosporine, dosage strategies can vary. One common method is the "step-up" approach, which begins with a moderate dose of 2.5–3.0 mg/kg/day, administered in two daily doses. This dose is gradually increased by 0.5 mg/kg/day until the desired control of symptoms is achieved, allowing for close monitoring of side effects. This strategy is particularly useful for moderate cases. For more severe cases, a "step-down" strategy may be utilized, where treatment starts with a higher dose of up to 5 mg/kg/day to quickly manage symptoms. Once control is established, the dose is gradually reduced. Modified formulations of cyclosporine ensure steady absorption, especially at lower doses such as 2–3 mg/kg/day or 1–2 mg/kg/day. For obese patients, dosing based on actual body weight can enhance effectiveness, and weight loss may further improve outcomes. While some studies support dosing adjustments based on weight, others suggest that fixed doses can be equally effective. Cyclosporine oral suspension, available in a concentration of 100 mg/mL, is primarily used in pediatric patients and allows for precise dosing adjustments based on the specific needs and weight of the child.[36]

Efficacy

Cyclosporine is highly effective for treating severe plaque psoriasis, with doses of 2.5–5 mg/kg/day providing rapid and substantial

CHAPTER 10: Conventional Systemic Therapies in Psoriasis

symptom relief in 80–90% of patients. Even at 3 mg/kg/day, 50–70% achieve a PASI 75 response. Lower maintenance doses, like 1.25 mg/kg/day, can sustain these improvements, though relapses often occur upon discontinuation, requiring alternative or adjunctive therapies for long-term control. While combining cyclosporine with NB-UVB phototherapy is not recommended due to the risk of photocarcinogenesis, sequential usage can enhance efficacy, particularly in reducing pruritus and treatment duration.[37]

Adverse Effects

Nephrotoxicity and hypertension are common adverse effects associated with cyclosporine use. Despite close monitoring, reversible nephrotoxicity occurs in 19–24% of patients during short-term treatment, while long-term use beyond 2 years significantly increases the risk of irreversible kidney damage. Elevated serum creatinine levels often persist even after reducing the cyclosporine dose. Hypertension, especially common among elderly patients, typically resolves upon discontinuation of the drug. Regular blood pressure monitoring is crucial to prevent chronic hypertension and kidney injury. If hypertension persists despite dose adjustments, discontinuation of cyclosporine is recommended. Calcium channel blockers are preferred for managing hypertension due to cyclosporine-induced renal arteriole vasoconstriction. Less severe adverse effects include headache, paresthesia, musculoskeletal pain, and hypertrichosis. Neurologic effects, such as fatigue, tremor, asthenia, and rare seizures, have been reported. Gastrointestinal effects are generally mild and transient, including abdominal pain, diarrhea, nausea, and vomiting. Respiratory effects, such as dyspnea, cough, and rhinitis, affect approximately 5% of patients. Additionally, hyperuricemia and hypomagnesemia may occur.

Pregnancy and Lactation

Research on cyclosporine use during pregnancy primarily draws from studies involving organ transplant recipients, where it is commonly co-administered with other medications, making it challenging to isolate its specific effects. Animal studies indicate no fertility issues but suggest lower fetal weight and increased mortality rates. Human studies suggest a higher incidence of premature births. Cyclosporine, categorized as pregnancy category C, contains ethanol and is excreted into breast milk, potentially posing risks to nursing infants. Therefore, decisions about continuing cyclosporine therapy or breastfeeding require careful evaluation of the associated benefits and risks.[38]

Drug Interactions

Cyclosporine is primarily metabolized by the cytochrome P450 3A4 subtype (CYP3A4), influencing the levels of drugs metabolized by this enzyme such as statins, calcium channel blockers, and warfarin. Concurrent use of statins can increase the risk of severe rhabdomyolysis. Combining cyclosporine with aminoglycosides, nonsteroidal anti-inflammatory drugs, or potassium-sparing diuretics can increase the likelihood of nephrotoxicity and hyperkalemia. Alcohol consumption may elevate cyclosporine levels, with limited impact from moderate intake. The immunosuppressive effects of cyclosporine may weaken vaccine effectiveness, notably affecting transplant patients' responses to influenza vaccines. Despite these concerns, vaccinations are strongly recommended due to the increased infection susceptibility while on cyclosporine, with caution warranted for live attenuated vaccines.[39]

Monitoring

Comprehensive assessments should include medical history, physical examination, and baseline evaluations for blood pressure, hepatitis, tuberculosis, and family history of renal disease. A detailed medication history is crucial due to potential interactions with cyclosporine. Factors increasing the risk of nephrotoxicity, like obesity, age, diabetes, and nephrotoxic agents, should be considered. Initial tests include urinalysis, serum creatinine, blood urea nitrogen, CBC, electrolytes, lipid profile, bilirubin, and liver enzymes.

Regular monitoring of renal function is vital to prevent permanent kidney damage. For the first 3 months, biweekly checks of blood urea nitrogen and creatinine are recommended, switching to monthly thereafter. Adjustments to cyclosporine doses should be made if creatinine levels rise persistently, with possible discontinuation if needed. Monthly monitoring includes blood pressure, creatinine, and blood urea nitrogen. Women should be informed about pregnancy risks.

Routine blood pressure checks are essential to prevent hypertension and kidney damage. Calcium channel blockers are preferred; beta blockers can also be used. Thiazide and potassium-sparing diuretics should be avoided. Although routine monitoring of cyclosporine levels is unnecessary, closer attention may be required in specific cases, such as concurrent medication use or liver disease.[40]

Contraindications

Careful consideration is warranted when contemplating the use of cyclosporine in elderly or expectant patients, as well as those with immunodeficiency disorders. Contraindications to cyclosporine therapy encompass a history of systemic malignancy (except non-melanoma skin cancer), renal insufficiency, hypertension, previous treatment with PUVA, uncontrolled infections, and hypersensitivity to cyclosporine. Caution should be exercised when prescribing cyclosporine to patients taking other medications that may interact with CYP3A4. Administration of live vaccinations is not recommended for patients using cyclosporine.[39]

■ FUMARIC ACID ESTERS

Fumaric acid esters, which include compounds such as dimethyl fumarate and monoethyl fumarate salts, are widely used in Europe for the treatment of moderate-to-severe psoriasis. In the United States, however, the FDA has not approved these esters for this specific indication, although they are approved for conditions such as psoriatic arthritis. Initially, it was believed that the primary mechanism of FAEs involved modulation of the immune system. Recent research, however, has demonstrated that FAEs also have significant antiangiogenic and antioxidant properties.[41]

Dosage

The dosing regimen for FAEs starts with one daily pill of lower strength (105 mg of FAE mixtures) and gradually increases over 8 weeks to six pills of regular strength (215 mg of FAE mixtures).

Efficacy

The 2015 Cochrane review, encompassing six studies and 544 participants, demonstrated a notable decrease in PASI scores with the administration of FAEs at varying doses for psoriasis treatment. Additionally, a meta-analysis of two additional studies underscored the efficacy of FAEs, surpassing placebo in achieving PASI 50. FAE therapy also significantly improved participants' quality of life and increased the proportion achieving PASI 75. However, when comparing the combination of MTX and FAEs with MTX alone, no significant difference in efficacy emerged, even after adjusting for baseline disease severity.[42]

Adverse Effects

Adverse reactions to FAEs, like gastrointestinal discomfort and flushing, were more common in users than in placebo recipients (76% vs. 16%). Other effects include anaphylaxis/angioedema, malaise, hematological issues, hepatotoxicity, elevated lipids, increased creatinine, potassium, proteinuria, and potential renal problems. Gastrointestinal symptoms affect about two-thirds of patients, often with mild lymphopenia. Regular monitoring of liver function, lipids, and creatinine is crucial. Rare renal disease and leukoencephalopathy cases were not seen in trials, suggesting FAEs may not be the direct cause. Starting with low doses and gradually increasing may ease gastrointestinal effects.

Pregnancy and Lactation

Pregnancy and breastfeeding are absolute contraindications for FAEs due to insufficient safety data for these populations.

Drug Interactions

Potential drug interactions include other fumaric acid derivatives, MTX, cyclosporine, as well as immunosuppressive and cytostatic medications, which could enhance toxicity. Additionally, caution is warranted with drugs known to cause renal dysfunction.[43]

Monitoring

Before initiating FAE therapy, it is imperative to conduct a thorough medical history and physical examination. Initial assessments should include a CBC with platelet counts and a urinalysis. Continuous monitoring throughout treatment is vital, with CBC and platelet count evaluations planned biweekly for the initial 2 months, monthly for up to 6 months, and bimonthly thereafter.

Contraindications

Contraindications to FAEs include severe liver, gastrointestinal, or kidney disease, malignancy or a history of it, leukopenia, and other hematologic abnormalities, pregnancy, and breastfeeding.[44]

■ CONCLUSION

While advancements in small molecules and biologics have significantly expanded the arsenal of treatments for psoriasis, conventional systemic therapies—such as MTX, acitretin, cyclosporine, and FAEs—remain foundational in managing moderate-to-severe cases of this chronic skin condition. These traditional treatments, each with its unique mechanism of action, continue to offer substantial benefits for many patients, particularly where newer therapies may not be available or suitable. Despite the promise of novel therapies, the importance of these conventional options cannot be overstated, as they provide reliable and effective management strategies. However, their use requires diligent monitoring due to potential side effects. As the field evolves, integrating these traditional treatments with emerging therapies will be crucial in achieving optimal patient outcomes and advancing the comprehensive management of psoriasis.

TAKE HOME MESSAGE

- *Core treatments*: MTX, acitretin, cyclosporine, and FAEs are crucial for severe psoriasis.
- *Distinct actions*: Each therapy offers unique benefits with specific mechanisms.
- *Ongoing relevance*: Conventional treatments remain vital despite new advancements.
- *Reliable management*: These therapies provide effective and dependable control of psoriasis.
- *Monitoring required*: Regular monitoring is essential due to potential side effects.
- *Integrated strategy*: Combining traditional and new therapies enhances treatment outcomes.

REFERENCES

1. Menter A, Strober BE, Kaplan DH, Kivelevitch D, Prater EF, Stoff B, et al. Joint AAD-NPF guidelines of care for the management and treatment of psoriasis with biologics. J Am Acad Dermatol. 2019;80:1029-72.
2. Matthews DA, Alden RA, Bolin JT, Freer ST, Hamlin R, Xuong N, et al. Dihydrofolate reductase: x-ray structure of the binary complex with methotrexate. Science. 1977;197:452-5.
3. Rajitha P, Biswas R, Sabitha M, Jayakumar R. Methotrexate in the Treatment of Psoriasis and Rheumatoid Arthritis: Mechanistic Insights, Current Issues and Novel Delivery Approaches. Curr Pharm Des. 2017;23:3550-66.
4. Montesinos MC, Desai A, Delano D, Chen JF, Fink JS, Jacobson MA, et al. Adenosine A2A or A3 receptors are required for inhibition of inflammation by methotrexate and its analog MX-68. Arthritis Rheum. 2003;48:240-7.
5. Kalb RE, Strober B, Weinstein G, Lebwohl M. Methotrexate and psoriasis: consensus conference. J Am Acad Dermatol. 2011;64:1179.
6. van Huizen AM, Sikkel R, Caron AGM, Menting SP, Spuls PI. Methotrexate dosing regimen for plaque-type psoriasis: an update of a systematic review. J Dermatolog Treat. 2022;33:3104-18.
7. Bedoui Y, Guillot X, Sélambarom J, Guiraud P, Giry C, Jaffar-Bandjee MC, et al. Methotrexate an Old Drug with New Tricks. Int J Mol Sci. 2019;20:5023.
8. West J, Ogston S, Foerster J. Safety and efficacy of methotrexate in psoriasis: a meta-analysis of published trials. PLoS One. 2016;11:e0153740.
9. Sbidian E, Chaimani A, Garcia-Doval I, Do G, Hua C, Mazaud C, et al. Systemic pharmacological treatments for chronic plaque psoriasis: a network meta-analysis. Cochrane Database Syst Rev. 2017;12:CD011535.
10. Barker J, Hoffmann M, Wozel G, Ortonne JP, Zheng H, van Hoogstraten H, et al. Efficacy and safety of infliximab vs. methotrexate in patients with moderate-to-severe plaque psoriasis: results of an open-label, active-controlled, randomized trial (RESTORE1). Br J Dermatol. 2011;165:1109-17.
11. Saurat JH, Stingl G, Dubertret L, Papp K, Langley RG, Ortonne JP, et al.; CHAMPION Study Investigators. Efficacy and safety results from the randomized controlled comparative study of adalimumab vs. methotrexate vs. placebo in patients with psoriasis (CHAMPION). Br J Dermatol. 2008;158:558-66.
12. Gelfand JM, Wan J, Callis Duffin K, Krueger GG, Kalb RE, Weisman JD, et al. Comparative effectiveness of commonly used systemic treatments or phototherapy for moderate to severe plaque psoriasis in the clinical practice setting. Arch Dermatol. 2012;148:487-94.
13. Coates LC, Helliwell PS. Methotrexate efficacy in the tight control in psoriatic arthritis study. J Rheumatol. 2016;43: 356-61.
14. Busard C, Zweegers J, Limpens J, Langendam M, Spuls PI. Combined use of systemic agents for psoriasis: a systematic review. JAMA Dermatol. 2014;150:1213-20.
15. Brownell I, Strober BE. Folate with methotrexate: big benefit, questionable cost. Br J Dermatol. 2007;157:213.
16. El-Beheiry A, El-Mansy E, Kamel N, Salama N. Methotrexate and fertility in men. Arch Androl. 1979;3:177-9.
17. Estop AM, Cieply K, Van Kirk V, Levison F, Buckingham R. Sperm chromosome studies in patients taking low dose methotrexate. Am J Hum Genet. 1992;51:A314.
18. Sussman A, Leonard JM. Psoriasis, methotrexate, and oligospermia. Arch Dermatol. 1980;116:215-7.
19. Barker J, Horn EJ, Lebwohl M, Warren RB, Nast A, Rosenberg W, et al.; International Psoriasis Council. Assessment and management of methotrexate hepatotoxicity in psoriasis patients: report from a consensus conference to evaluate current practice and identify key questions toward optimizing methotrexate use in the clinic. J Eur Acad Dermatol Venereol. 2011;25:758-64.
20. Dalla Pria A, Bendle M, Ramaswami R, Boffito M, Bower M. The pharmacokinetics of high-dose methotrexate in people living with HIV on antiretroviral therapy. Cancer Chemother Pharmacol. 2016;77:653-7.
21. Kalb RE, Strober B, Weinstein G, Lebwohl M. Methotrexate and psoriasis: 2009 National Psoriasis Foundation Consensus Conference. J Am Acad Dermatol. 2009;60:824-37.
22. Pathirana D, Ormerod AD, Saiag P, Smith C, Spuls PI, Nast A, et al. European S3-Guidelines on the systemic treatment of psoriasis vulgaris. J Eur Acad Dermatol Venereol. 2009;23:S1-70.
23. Patel NP. Comment on: 'Monitoring for methotrexate-induced liver fibrosis in many UK dermatology centres is out of date and needs reform'. Clin Exp Dermatol. 2022;47:1724-5.
24. Hamed KM, Dighriri IM, Baomar AF, Alharthy BT, Alenazi FE, Alali GH, et al. Overview of Methotrexate Toxicity: A Comprehensive Literature Review. Cureus. 2022;14:e29518.
25. Dogra S, Yadav S. Acitretin in psoriasis: an evolving scenario. Int J Dermatol. 2014;53:525-38.
26. Murray HE, Anhalt AW, Lessard R, Schacter RK, Ross JB, Stewart WD, et al. A 12-month treatment of severe psoriasis with acitretin: results of a Canadian open multicenter study. J Am Acad Dermatol. 1991;24:598-602.

27. Wang CY, Wang CW, Chen CB, Chen WT, Chang YC, Hui RC, et al. Pharmacogenomics on the Treatment Response in Patients with Psoriasis: An Updated Review. Int J Mol Sci. 2023;24:7329.
28. Chaiyabutr C, Jiamton S, Silpa-Archa N, Wongpraparut C, Wongdama S, Chularojanamontri L. Retrospective study of psoriasis in people living with HIV: Thailand's experience. J Dermatol. 2022;49:607-14.
29. Yentzer BA, Yelverton CB, Pearce DJ, Camacho FT, Makhzoumi Z, Clark A, et al. Adherence to acitretin and home narrowband ultraviolet B phototherapy in patients with psoriasis. J Am Acad Dermatol. 2008;59:577-81.
30. Katz HI, Waalen J, Leach EE. Acitretin in psoriasis: an overview of adverse effects. J Am Acad Dermatol. 1999;41:S7-S12.
31. Pearce DJ, Klinger S, Ziel KK, Murad EJ, Rowell R, Feldman SR. Low-dose acitretin is associated with fewer adverse events than high-dose acitretin in the treatment of psoriasis. Arch Dermatol. 2006;142:1000-4.
32. Lambert WE, Meyer E, De Leenheer AP, De Bersaques J, Kint AH. Pharmacokinetics and drug interactions of etretinate and acitretin. J Am Acad Dermatol. 1992;27:S19-22.
33. Bangsgaard N, Rørbye C, Skov L. Treating Psoriasis During Pregnancy: Safety and Efficacy of Treatments. Am J Clin Dermatol. 2015;16:389-98.
34. Lee CS, Li K. A review of acitretin for the treatment of psoriasis. Expert Opin Drug Saf. 2009;8:769-79.
35. Rosmarin DM, Lebwohl M, Elewski BE, Gottlieb AB; National Psoriasis Foundation. Cyclosporine and psoriasis: 2008 National Psoriasis Foundation Consensus Conference. J Am Acad Dermatol. 2010;62:838-53.
36. Colombo MD, Cassano N, Bellia G, Vena GA. Cyclosporine regimens in plaque psoriasis: an overview with special emphasis on dose, duration, and old and new treatment approaches. Sci World J. 2013;2013:805705.
37. Spencer RK, Jin JQ, Elhage KG, Davis MS, Hakimi M, Bhutani T, et al. Comparative efficacy of biologics and oral agents in palmoplantar psoriasis and palmoplantar pustulosis: A systematic review and network meta-analysis of randomized clinical trials. J Am Acad Dermatol. 2023;89:423-5.
38. Markham T, Watson A, Rogers S. Adverse effects with long-term cyclosporin for severe psoriasis. Clin Exp Dermatol. 2002;27:111-4.
39. Ryan C, Amor KT, Menter A. The use of cyclosporine in dermatology: part II. J Am Acad Dermatol. 2010;63:949-72; quiz 973-4.
40. Soleymani T, Vassantachart JM, Wu JJ. Comparison of Guidelines for the Use of Cyclosporine for Psoriasis: A Critical Appraisal and Comprehensive Review. J Drugs Dermatol. 2016;15:293-301.
41. Balak DM. Fumaric acid esters in the management of psoriasis. Psoriasis (Auckl). 2015;5:9-23.
42. Atwan A, Ingram JR, Abbott R, Kelson MJ, Pickles T, Bauer A, et al. Oral fumaric acid esters for psoriasis. Cochrane Database Syst Rev. 2015;2015:CD010497.
43. Balak DM, Fallah Arani S, Hajdarbegovic E, Hagemans CA, Bramer WM, Thio HB, et al. Efficacy, effectiveness and safety of fumaric acid esters in the treatment of psoriasis: a systematic review of randomized and observational studies. Br J Dermatol. 2016;175:250-62.
44. Atwan A, Ingram JR, Abbott R, Kelson MJ, Pickles T, Bauer A, et al. Oral fumaric acid esters for psoriasis: abridged Cochrane systematic review including GRADE assessments. Br J Dermatol. 2016;175:873-81.

Small Molecules in Psoriasis

Farhat Fatima, SK Shahriar Ahmed, Sudip Das

INTRODUCTION

Small molecules are nonbiologic pharmaceuticals, which have a molecular weight of <1 kDa. They can enter cells and specifically alter the production of different proinflammatory cytokines and inhibit inflammatory cytokines by altering signaling pathways in immune cells. Unlike biologics, which neutralize cytokines and different receptors, small compounds lead to transcription or many intracellular enzymes by inhibiting factors. Additionally, unlike biologics, there are no immunogenicity reactions, which is an extra benefit.

JANUS KINASE INHIBITOR IN PSORIASIS

Janus kinase (JAK) inhibitors target the JAK pathways, which are crucial in the immunopathogenesis of psoriasis. The JAK family includes four members: JAK1, JAK2, JAK3, and tyrosine kinase 2 (TYK2). These kinases are involved in intracellular signaling affecting various cytokines, which then cause downstream effects. These inhibitors work by blocking the upstream components of the proinflammatory signaling pathways. This action alters the immune response and suppresses the abnormal activation of the inflammatory cascade in psoriasis. By targeting these pathways, JAK inhibitors can reduce the severity of psoriasis and improve the patient's quality of life.

According to standardized measures like the Psoriasis Area and Severity Index (PASI), clinical trials have shown that JAK inhibitors are effective in reducing psoriasis symptoms.[1] Oral versions of JAK inhibitors provide a possible benefit over injectable biologics. Although promising, more research is needed to determine their long-term safety and effectiveness in comparison to current biologics. JAK inhibitors can be divided into two categories: First-generation inhibitors, which target many JAKs, and second-generation inhibitors, which are more specific and may have better safety profiles. All things considered, JAK inhibitors offer a fresh strategy for treating psoriasis, which merits more study and clinical testing.

Deucravacitinib, a TYK2 inhibitor, is the only Food and Drug Administration (FDA)-approved (in the year 2022) JAK inhibitor for the treatment of psoriasis while the pan JAK inhibitor, tofacitinib and the JAK1 inhibitor, upadacitinib are approved for psoriatic arthritis (PsA). No topical JAK inhibitor has been approved for psoriasis till now.

Systemic Janus Kinase Inhibitors

Deucravacitinib

Deucravacitinib disrupts interleukin 23 (IL-23), IL-12, and type I interferon signaling—all important cytokines in the pathophysiology of psoriasis—by specifically targeting TYK2.

Clinical trials demonstrated significant improvements in PASI scores, with 67–75% of patients achieving PASI 75 at week 12 for higher doses, compared to 7% for placebo.[2] Real-world data from Japan reported PASI 75 achievement rates of 78.3% at week 16.[3] Deucravacitinib also improved quality of life measures, including the Dermatology Life Quality Index (DLQI).[2] The drug's onset of action is rapid, with improvements observed as early as week 2. While adverse events (AEs) were more common than with placebo, they were generally mild and manageable.[3]

Tofacitinib

Tofacitinib is a first-generation JAK1 and JAK3 inhibitor implicated in the T helper 1 (Th1) and Th2 signaling pathways. Despite not being approved for the treatment of psoriasis, tofacitinib's effectiveness and safety have been examined in a number of randomized controlled trials (RCTs) that have enrolled patients with moderate-to-severe plaque psoriasis. In terms of tofacitinib's safety, it has demonstrated a satisfactory profile with, for the most part, mild-to-severe AEs, primarily headache, upper respiratory tract infection, nasopharyngitis, and gastrointestinal symptoms (constipation, nausea, vomiting, and diarrhea). Studies conducted over an extended period of time have demonstrated sustained efficacy for up to 24 months, with 10 mg twice day demonstrating higher efficacy than 5 mg.[4] Over a 52-week period, both 5-mg and 10-mg doses showed effectiveness in treating psoriasis and PsA in Japanese patients.[5]

Upadacitinib

Upadacitinib, a JAK inhibitor, has shown efficacy in treating PsA in phase 3 clinical trials. In patients with PsA and inadequate response to biologic disease-modifying antirheumatic drugs (DMARDs), upadacitinib 15 mg and 30 mg once daily demonstrated superior efficacy compared to placebo in improving signs and symptoms over 24 weeks.[6] The efficacy was maintained through 56 weeks, with improvements in American College of Rheumatology (ACR) and PASI responses. While upadacitinib demonstrated a generally comparable safety profile to adalimumab, higher rates of certain AEs, such as serious infections and herpes zoster, were observed with upadacitinib, particularly at the 30 mg.

Janus Kinase Inhibitors under Investigation for Psoriasis[1]

Baricitinib: It is a JAK1/2 inhibitor, which has showed promise in the treatment of psoriasis. In a mouse model of psoriasis, topical administration of baricitinib markedly decreased inflammatory indicators, ear edema, leukocyte infiltration, and epidermal cell proliferation. Its effectiveness in treating moderate-to-severe psoriasis was shown in a randomized phase 2b experiment. Notably, a case of paradoxical psoriasis brought on by baricitinib has been documented, underscoring the necessity of more studies on the long-term consequences.

Abrocitinib: In a phase 2 clinical research, up to 60% of patients exhibited PASI 75 responses after using abrocitinib. However, the enrollment period was not finished as scheduled, and the sponsor stopped funding the study. The medication is currently authorized to treat atopic dermatitis.

Peficitinib: A JAK inhibitor with JAK3 selectivity has demonstrated favorable results in a phase II RCT.

Filgotinib: Filgotinib, JAK1 inhibitor, significantly improved patient-reported outcomes, peripheral arthritis, psoriasis, enthesitis, and ACR response in patients with active PsA, in a phase 2 study.

Itacitinib: It is a JAK inhibitor, which has only produced noticeable improvements at a dose of 600 mg/day in a phase 2 study for plaque psoriasis.

Brepocitinib and *ropsacitinib* are two of the investigational TYK2 inhibitors that show promise in terms of articular (ACR20 response rate) and cutaneous outcomes [PASI 50/75/90/100 and Physician Global Assessment (PGA) 0/1 response; up to 52 weeks each].

Topical Janus Kinase Inhibitors

Brepocitinib

In a phase 2b double-blind experiment, topical formulations with varying doses of brepocitinib applied once or twice daily were compared to the vehicle.[7] The study's initial 12-week phase involved the randomization and treatment of 344 individuals. However, as compared to a placebo, brepocitinib did not result in statistically significant improvements. In general, the treatment was favorably received. One trial participant experienced herpes zoster and herpes simplex lesions in nonpsoriasis plaque-affected locations a few days apart.

Ruxolitinib

Ruxolitinib was evaluated in an unblinded study after showing similar efficacy to calcipotriol and betamethasone formulations in a small, double-blinded trial.[8] Ruxolitinib-improved lesion area and severity compared to nontreated sites, and it also improved calculated PGA scores. The formulations were generally well-tolerated, with two patients reporting local reactions, stinging, and hypoesthesia, one patient developing mild leukopenia, and another patient developing mild reticulocytosis.

Tofacitinib

In a phase 2a trial, two topical formulations of tofacitinib 2% ointment were compared to a vehicle in individuals with mild-to-moderate psoriasis.[9] In comparison to the vehicle, one of the ointments showed a statistically significant decrease in Target Plaque Severity Score (TPSS) at week 4. In general, the treatment was favorably received. A few individuals complained of burning or stinging sensations along with localized erythema. In 430 individuals with mild-to-moderate psoriasis, a phase 2b research comparing two concentrations of tofacitinib ointment (1% or 2%) to a placebo revealed that the 2% formulation significantly improved versus the vehicle, but by week 12, there were no discernible changes from the vehicle.[10]

PHOSPHODIESTERASE 4 INHIBITOR IN PSORIASIS[11]

Phosphodiesterase 4 (PDE-4) inhibitors work by blocking the degradation of cyclic adenosine monophosphate (cAMP), which leads to a reduction in inflammation. PDE-4 is an enzyme that degrades cAMP to adenosine monophosphate (AMP), which subsequently leads to the production of proinflammatory mediators. By inhibiting PDE-4, cAMP levels increase, which in turn suppresses proinflammatory cytokines, such as tumor necrosis factor alpha (TNF-α), IL-2, IL-12, and IL-23, and increases anti-inflammatory cytokines, like IL-10. This occurs through the activation of protein kinase A (PKA), which then activates cAMP response element-binding protein (CREB). CREB is a response element found in genes involved in the pathophysiology of psoriasis, thus reducing inflammation. This mechanism of action makes PDE-4 inhibitors a promising target for psoriasis treatment.

Apremilast

Apremilast is an oral PDE-4 inhibitor approved for the treatment of moderate-to-severe plaque psoriasis. It works by inhibiting the degradation of cAMP, which leads to a reduction in inflammation.

Efficacy: Clinical trials, such as ESTEEM 1 and ESTEEM 2, have demonstrated that apremilast is significantly more effective than placebo in achieving a 75% reduction in the PASI (PASI 75) score in patients with moderate-to-severe plaque psoriasis.[12,13] Apremilast has shown efficacy in difficult-to-treat areas, such as the scalp and nails. In the LIBERATE trial, apremilast was compared to placebo and etanercept, and showed a significantly greater proportion of patients achieved PASI 75 compared to placebo.[14] Apremilast has also shown significant improvements in the DLQI scores, indicating an improvement in the quality of life for patients with psoriasis. Apremilast has also shown improvement in scalp itch and whole-body itch.

Dosage: The typical dosage of apremilast is 30 mg twice a day (BID).

Adverse events: The most common AEs associated with apremilast are diarrhea, nausea, headache, and upper respiratory tract infections. These AEs are generally mild to moderate in severity, transient, and tend to decrease over time. Although rare, some patients have reported depression, and one patient reported suicidal ideation, in the LIBERATE trial.

Other uses: In addition to psoriasis, apremilast is also approved for the treatment of PsA.

Roflumilast

Topical roflumilast is being investigated for psoriasis. It has been shown that roflumilast is 25–300 times more potent than either crisaborole or apremilast. Using roflumilast cream increased the TPSS × target plaque area (TPA) considerably in a phase 1/2a research.[15] The 0.3% and 0.15% roflumilast groups at 6 weeks had mean changes from baseline PASI scores of −50.0% and −49.0%, respectively, compared to −17.8% in the vehicle group, indicating a significant improvement in the Investigator Global Assessment (IGA) score of clear or almost clear. Mild application-site responses are the most common side effects. In contrast to oral PDE-4 inhibitors, topical roflumilast has few adverse effects on the gastrointestinal tract.

Crisaborole

Topical crisaborole has been investigated for plaque psoriasis in sensitive areas. According to a recent pilot trial, 2% crisaborole was more effective than the vehicle.[16] Even though several trials have demonstrated effectiveness in treating psoriasis, the majority have not been published, and it is doubtful that more research will be conducted. Topical crisaborole works best for thin, nonscaly plaques because the thickness of the stratum corneum is inversely correlated with topical drug absorption. The pilot research of patients with plaque psoriasis did not reveal any adverse skin reactions, despite reports of local burning and stinging after crisaborole injection in atopic dermatitis. This is probably because psoriatic skin does not have the same innate barrier failure as eczematous skin.

■ OTHER MOLECULES

Tapinarof:[17] This topical aryl hydrocarbon receptor-modulating drug (agonist) improves psoriasis by lowering IL-17. Moreover, it possesses antioxidant properties and strengthens the skin's barrier. The FDA-approved 1% topical cream is used once a day. Local side effects such as contact dermatitis and folliculitis were observed.

Esters of fumaric acid: Efficacy comparable to methotrexate was reported in an RCT.[18] One side effect that is occasionally observed is lymphopenia.

PICLIDENOSON

Piclidenoson is an oral agonist of the A3 adenosine receptor (A3AR) linked to the Gi protein. Piclidenoson may have anti-inflammatory properties through inhibiting TNF-α through downregulating the nuclear factor kappa B (NF-κB) signaling pathway. According to a phase 3 trial,[19] 35.3% of patients in the group that received a 2-mg dose of piclidenoson twice a day experienced improvement when compared to a placebo. AEs occurred in the 1-, 2-, and 4-mg dosing arms at rates of 58.3%, 17.6%, and 13.3%, respectively, while the placebo arm saw a rate of 21.1%.

PONESIMOD

Ponesimod is an oral sphingosine-1-phosphate receptor 1 (S1PR1) selective modulator. Lymphocytes leave secondary lymphoid tissues and enter the bloodstream through this receptor. Ponesimod inhibits the egress of lymphocytes caused by sphingosine-1-phosphate (S1P) by causing the internalization of S1PR1. In a phase II study, 20–40 mg significantly improved PASI 75 in patients with moderate–to-severe psoriasis.[20] It can result in increased liver enzymes, dizziness, and dyspnea in addition to bradycardia.

RETINOIC ACID RECEPTOR-RELATED ORPHAN RECEPTOR GAMMA T INHIBITORS

Vimirogant is an oral, selective RORγt (retinoic acid receptor-related orphan receptor gamma t) inverse agonist, which was reported to reduce the PASI score by 30% in a phase II experiment. It was generally well tolerated, with only minor side effects like headache and nausea, and four patients experienced reversible transaminitis. Phase III trials were not conducted, however, because of liver damage. Recent trials have demonstrated the effectiveness of topical preparations of RORγt inverse agonists, which are currently being studied.[21]

RHO-ASSOCIATED COILED-COIL CONTAINING PROTEIN KINASE 2 INHIBITOR

Phase II trials of the targeted oral ROCK2 (Rho-associated coiled-coil containing protein kinase 2) inhibitor belumosudil (KD025) revealed that it was well tolerated but not as effective.[22] It dramatically lowers T-cell infiltration as well as IL-17 and IL-23 levels.

CONCLUSION

Small molecule immunomodulators offer diverse approaches to treating psoriasis by targeting various inflammatory pathways. JAK inhibitors, such as Deucravacitinib, block pro-inflammatory signaling and improve psoriasis symptoms, with significant clinical trial results. Other JAK inhibitors like Tofacitinib and Upadacitinib are effective for psoriatic arthritis and are being studied for psoriasis. Investigational JAK inhibitors, such as Baricitinib and Abrocitinib, show promise but require further research. PDE-4 inhibitors like Apremilast work by increasing cAMP levels, reducing inflammation, and are approved for moderate-to-severe plaque psoriasis. Topical JAK inhibitors, including Brepocitinib and Tofacitinib, have shown mixed results in trials. Other investigational treatments, such as Tapinarof, Piclidenoson, and Ponesimod, also target various inflammatory pathways and are under study. These small molecules provide new, potentially safer, alternatives to biologics for psoriasis treatment.

CHAPTER 11: Small Molecules in Psoriasis

> **TAKE HOME MESSAGE**
> - Small molecule immunomodulators are promising treatment options in psoriasis, offering oral alternatives to biologics.
> - Deucravacitinib is the only FDA-approved JAK inhibitor for psoriasis, while Tofacitinib and Upadacitinib approved for psoriatic arthritis are under investigation for psoriasis treatment.
> - PDE-4 inhibitors like Apremilast are effective in reducing inflammation and improving PASI scores, with demonstrated efficacy in challenging psoriasis areas like the scalp and nails.
> - Topical JAK inhibitors (e.g., Brepocitinib, Tofacitinib), PDE-4 inhibitors (e.g., Roflumilast, Crisaborole) and other investigational treatments (e.g., Tapinarof, Piclidenoson) show promise but require additional clinical studies to establish their full potential.

REFERENCES

1. Megna M, Potestio L, Ruggiero A, Cacciapuoti S, Maione F, Tasso M, et al. JAK Inhibitors in Psoriatic Disease. Clin Cosmet Investig Dermatol. 2023;16:3129-45.
2. Thaçi D, Strober B, Gordon KB, Foley P, Gooderham M, Morita A, et al. Deucravacitinib in Moderate to Severe Psoriasis: Clinical and Quality-of-Life Outcomes in a Phase 2 Trial. Dermatol Ther (Heidelb). 2022;12(2):495-510.
3. Hagino T, Saeki H, Fujimoto E, Kanda N. Effectiveness and safety of deucravacitinib treatment for moderate-to-severe psoriasis in real-world clinical practice in Japan. J Dermatolog Treat. 2024;35(1):2307489.
4. Papp KA, Krueger JG, Feldman SR, Langley RG, Thaci D, Torii H, et al. Tofacitinib, an oral Janus kinase inhibitor, for the treatment of chronic plaque psoriasis: Long-term efficacy and safety results from 2 randomized phase-III studies and 1 open-label long-term extension study. J Am Acad Dermatol. 2016;74(5):841-50.
5. Asahina A, Etoh T, Igarashi A, Imafuku S, Saeki H, Shibasaki Y, et al.; study investigators. Oral tofacitinib efficacy, safety and tolerability in Japanese patients with moderate to severe plaque psoriasis and psoriatic arthritis: A randomized, double-blind, phase 3 study. J Dermatol. 2016;43(8):869-80.
6. Mease PJ, Lertratanakul A, Anderson JK, Papp K, Van den Bosch F, Tsuji S, et al. Upadacitinib for psoriatic arthritis refractory to biologics: SELECT-PsA 2. Ann Rheum Dis. 2021;80(3):312-20.
7. Landis MN, Smith SR, Berstein G, Fetterly G, Ghosh P, Feng G, et al. Efficacy and safety of topical brepocitinib cream for mild-to-moderate chronic plaque psoriasis: a phase IIb randomized double-blind vehicle-controlled parallel-group study. Br J Dermatol. 2023;189(1):33-41.
8. Punwani N, Scherle P, Flores R, Shi J, Liang J, Yeleswaram S, et al. Preliminary clinical activity of a topical JAK1/2 inhibitor in the treatment of psoriasis. J Am Acad Dermatol. 2012;67(4):658-64.
9. Ports WC, Khan S, Lan S, Lamba M, Bolduc C, Bissonnette R, et al. A randomized phase 2a efficacy and safety trial of the topical Janus kinase inhibitor tofacitinib in the treatment of chronic plaque psoriasis. Br J Dermatol. 2013;169(1):137-45.
10. Papp KA, Bissonnette R, Gooderham M, Feldman SR, Iversen L, Soung J, et al. Treatment of plaque psoriasis with an ointment formulation of the Janus kinase inhibitor, tofacitinib: a Phase 2b randomized clinical trial. BMC Dermatol. 2016;16(1):15.
11. Wittmann M, Helliwell PS. Phosphodiesterase 4 inhibition in the treatment of psoriasis, psoriatic arthritis and other chronic inflammatory diseases. Dermatol Ther (Heidelb). 2013;3(1):1-15.
12. Papp K, Reich K, Leonardi CL, Kircik L, Chimenti S, Langley RG, et al. Apremilast, an oral phosphodiesterase 4 (PDE4) inhibitor, in patients with moderate to severe plaque psoriasis: Results of a phase III, randomized, controlled trial (Efficacy and Safety Trial Evaluating the Effects of Apremilast in Psoriasis [ESTEEM] 1). J Am Acad Dermatol. 2015;73(1):37-49.
13. Paul C, Cather J, Gooderham M, Poulin Y, Mrowietz U, Ferrandiz C, et al. Efficacy and safety of apremilast, an oral phosphodiesterase 4 inhibitor, in patients with moderate-to-severe plaque psoriasis over 52 weeks: a phase III, randomized controlled trial (ESTEEM 2). Br J Dermatol. 2015;173(6):1387-99.
14. Reich K, Gooderham M, Green L, Bewley A, Zhang Z, Khanskaya I, et al. The efficacy and safety of apremilast, etanercept and placebo in patients with moderate-to-severe plaque psoriasis: 52-week results from a phase IIIb, randomized, placebo-controlled trial (LIBERATE). J Eur Acad Dermatol Venereol. 2017;31(3):507-17.

15. Papp KA, Gooderham M, Droege M, Merritt C, Osborne DW, Berk DR, et al. Roflumilast Cream Improves Signs and Symptoms of Plaque Psoriasis: Results from a Phase 1/2a Randomized, Controlled Study. J Drugs Dermatol. 2020;19(8):734-40.
16. Hashim PW, Chima M, Kim HJ, Bares J, Yao CJ, Singer G, et al. Crisaborole 2% ointment for the treatment of intertriginous, anogenital, and facial psoriasis: A double-blind, randomized, vehicle-controlled trial. J Am Acad Dermatol. 2020;82(2):360-5.
17. Nogueira S, Rodrigues MA, Vender R, Torres T. Tapinarof for the treatment of psoriasis. Dermatol Ther. 2022;35(12):e15931.
18. Fallah Arani S, Neumann H, Hop WC, Thio HB. Fumarates vs. methotrexate in moderate to severe chronic plaque psoriasis: a multicentre prospective randomized controlled clinical trial. Br J Dermatol. 2011;164(4):855-61.
19. Papp KA, Beyska-Rizova S, Gantcheva ML, Slavcheva Simeonova E, Brezoev P, Celic M, et al.; COMFORT-1 Study Investigators. Efficacy and safety of piclidenoson in plaque psoriasis: Results from a randomized phase 3 clinical trial (COMFORT-1). J Eur Acad Dermatol Venereol. 2024;38(6):1112-20.
20. Vaclavkova A, Chimenti S, Arenberger P, Holló P, Sator PG, Burcklen M, et al. Oral ponesimod in patients with chronic plaque psoriasis: a randomised, double-blind, placebo-controlled phase 2 trial. Lancet. 2014;384(9959):2036-45.
21. Tang L, Yang X, Liang Y, Xie H, Dai Z, Zheng G. Transcription Factor Retinoid-Related Orphan Receptor γt: A Promising Target for the Treatment of Psoriasis. Front Immunol. 2018;9:1210.
22. Carmona-Rocha E, Rusiñol L, Puig L. New and Emerging Oral/Topical Small-Molecule Treatments for Psoriasis. Pharmaceutics. 2024;16(2):239.

12

Use of Biologics in Psoriasis

Abhishek De, Disha Chakraborty

■ INTRODUCTION

The introduction of biological agents over the past two decades has revolutionized the treatment landscape for both psoriasis and psoriatic arthritis (PsA). Before their development, systemic treatments for moderate-to-severe psoriasis were limited to oral medications like methotrexate. While methotrexate was relatively effective, its safety profile raised significant concerns. Most traditional systemic treatments such as oral retinoids and cyclosporine carry serious black box warnings. In contrast, biological agents offer a highly effective alternative with none of the black box warnings seen in their predecessors. Furthermore, some newer biologics require as few as four injections annually during the maintenance phase, adding convenience to their benefits.[1]

The advancements in biological therapy have marked significant progress in terms of both efficacy and safety. This shift in treatment is largely due to the evolving understanding of psoriasis pathophysiology. 30 years ago, psoriasis was predominantly viewed as a disorder of epidermal hyperproliferation. However, recent discoveries have emphasized the role of the immune system in driving the disease.[2]

■ KEY CYTOKINES INVOLVED IN PSORIASIS

Scientists now have a detailed understanding of the molecular mechanisms involved, including the specific cytokines that play a key role in psoriatic disease. The early stages of psoriasis pathogenesis involve multiple cell types such as keratinocytes, natural killer T cells, plasmacytoid dendritic cells, and macrophages, which secrete cytokines that activate myeloid dendritic cells. These activated dendritic cells then release interleukin 12 (IL-12) and IL-23, both of which are crucial to the cellular cascade of psoriasis. IL-12 promotes the differentiation of naïve T cells into T helper 1 (Th1) cells, which in turn produce interferon gamma (IFN-γ) and tumor necrosis factor alpha (TNF-α), while IL-23 is vital for the expansion of Th17 and Th22 cells. Th17 cells release IL-17, IL-22, and TNF-α, all of which are central to the inflammatory process in psoriasis.[3]

The prominence of the IL-23/Th17 pathway in psoriasis pathogenesis suggests that this particular pathway may be the primary driver of inflammation in many patients. The superior efficacy of IL-17 and IL-23-targeting biologics likely reflects the crucial role of this pathway in the disease, highlighting a more targeted approach to treatment that aligns with the underlying immunological mechanisms.[4] With the approval of 11 biologic agents for psoriasis by the Food and Drug Administration (FDA), and additional treatments in development, the therapeutic landscape has significantly expanded. However, the sheer number of available options has introduced a level of complexity, leading to uncertainty among healthcare providers. This has sometimes resulted in the random selection of biologic treatments. To address this issue, this chapter is designed to highlight the most clinically relevant information about each FDA-approved biologic agent, including those in the pipeline. It specifically focuses on the distinctive benefits and drawbacks of each option, aiming to simplify the decision-making process for providers in selecting the most suitable treatment for individual patients. As is often the case in medical practice, the use of biologic agents for psoriasis requires both scientific precision and an artistic approach tailored to each patient's unique needs.

TREATMENT TARGETS EVOLVED IN PSORIASIS MANAGEMENT

Moderate-to-severe psoriasis is associated with substantial psychosocial challenges, which significantly diminish a patient's health-related quality of life (HRQoL) and elevate the risk for psychiatric conditions such as depression and anxiety. Systemic treatments are recommended for individuals with moderate-to-severe psoriasis, and this includes both traditional systemic therapies and biologics. Clinical trials have reported that many patients achieve either a 90% or complete reduction in their Psoriasis Area and Severity Index (PASI) scores. These outcomes, coupled with the recognition of diverse manifestations of psoriasis, have prompted ambitious treatment goals, including achieving PASI 90 or PASI 100 or reaching a Physician's Global Assessment (PGA) score of 0-1 (indicating clear or nearly clear skin). Such targets are increasingly seen as achievable for those undergoing treatment for moderate-to-severe plaque psoriasis.[5,6]

Concurrently, there has been growing interest among dermatologists in adopting a treat-to-target (T2T) approach for psoriasis management. Multiple treatment targets have been proposed, with guidelines on systemic therapy for moderate-to-severe plaque psoriasis emphasizing that clear or almost clear skin should be the primary goal, with PASI 90 being the most important outcome. Additionally, achieving an absolute PASI score of 1-2 is considered meaningful within these guidelines.

However, despite these advancements, the T2T strategy is inconsistently applied in clinical practice. Research shows that a significant number of patients with moderate-to-severe psoriasis either remain untreated or are managed solely with topical treatments, reflecting suboptimal care.

The concept of T2T in psoriasis management continues to evolve and requires clear, standardized guidelines that address both skin and systemic symptoms of the disease. Importantly, these strategies must be patient-centered, not solely focused on achieving clear skin. It should consider HRQoL, comorbid conditions, treatment side effects, and patient preferences.[5-7]

CLASSIFICATION OF BIOLOGICS USED IN PSORIASIS[8]

Classification of biologics used in psoriasis is given in **Table 1**.

CHAPTER 12: Use of Biologics in Psoriasis

TABLE 1: Classification of biologics used in psoriasis[8]

Biologic	Structure	Target	Standard dosing	Average half-life	Efficacy (primary trial endpoint) at standard dose
Adalimumab[8]	Human IgG1κ	TNF-α	80 mg loading dose; 40 mg every 2 weeks	14 days	71% PASI 75 at week 16
Certolizumab pegol[8]	PEGylated Fab fragment of humanized IgG1	TNF-α	400 mg at weeks 0, 2, and 4; then 200 mg every 2 weeks	14 days	76.7% PASI 75 at week 16
Etanercept[8]	TNFR and IgG Fc fusion protein	TNF-α	50 mg weekly	3 days	34% PASI 75 at week 12
Infliximab[8]	Human-murine chimeric IgG1	TNF-α	5 mg/kg at weeks 0, 2, and 6; then every 8 weeks	8–9.5 days	89% PASI 75 at week 10
Secukinumab[8]	Human IgG1κ	IL-17A	300 mg at weeks 1–5; then 300 mg monthly	27 days	81.6% PASI 75 at week 12
Ixekizumab[8]	Humanized IgG4	IL-17A	160 mg at week 0; 80 mg at weeks 2, 4, 6, 8, 10, 12; then 80 mg every 4 weeks	13 days	82.6% PASI 75 at week 12
Brodalumab[8]	Human IgG2	IL-17RA	210 mg at weeks 0, 1, and 2; then every 2 weeks	11 days	86% PASI 75 at week 12
Bimekizumab[8]	Humanized IgG1	IL-17A, IL-17F, IL-17AF	320 mg at weeks 0, 4, 8, 12, 16; then every 8 weeks	23 days	91% PASI 90 at week 16
Ustekinumab[8]	Human IgG1κ	p40 subunit of IL-12 and IL-23	45 mg at weeks 0 and 4; then every 12 weeks	21 days	67% PASI 75 at week 12
Guselkumab[8]	Human IgG1λ	p19 subunit of IL-23	100 mg at weeks 0 and 4; then every 8 weeks	15–18 days	70% PASI 90 at week 16
Risankizumab[8]	Humanized IgG1	p19 subunit of IL-23	150 mg at weeks 0 and 4; then every 12 weeks	28–29 days	75% PASI 90 at week 16
Tildrakizumab[8]	Humanized IgG1κ	p19 subunit of IL-23	100 mg at weeks 0 and 4; then every 12 weeks	23.4 days	64% PASI 75 at week 12

(IgG1: immunoglobulin G1; IL-17A: interleukin-17A; TNF-α: tumor necrosis factor alpha; TNFR: tumor necrosis factor receptor)

ELIGIBILITY OF BIOLOGICS IN PSORIASIS

When prescribing biologic treatments, it is critical to consider both absolute and relative contraindications. Absolute contraindications include known hypersensitivity reactions, active infections like sepsis or tuberculosis (TB) (which can be managed under supervision after 2 months of TB treatment), and conditions like Crohn's disease when using brodalumab or moderate-to-severe heart failure [New York Heart Association (NYHA) class III/IV] when using anti-TNFs. Relative contraindications encompass a history of depression (specific to brodalumab), demyelinating diseases (such as multiple sclerosis or optic neuritis, particularly with anti-TNFs), and a history of malignancy, excluding basal cell carcinoma (BCC) and squamous cell carcinoma (SCC). Other relative concerns include pregnancy, planned surgeries, and viral infections like hepatitis B or C and HIV.

Vaccination is a crucial step before initiating biologic therapy, with live attenuated vaccines such as measles, mumps, and rubella (MMR), varicella, and oral polio recommended 2–4 weeks prior to starting treatment. Inactivated vaccines, such as those for hepatitis A and B, varicella (if not immune), herpes zoster (for patients over 50), and human papillomavirus (HPV), may be given both before and during therapy. Monitoring includes TB screening through chest X-ray and skin or blood tests (e.g., purified protein derivative (PPD)/tuberculin skin test (TST) or QuantiFERON), along with serology for hepatitis and human immunodeficiency virus (HIV). Liver function tests (LFTs) are specifically important for infliximab (IFX) users. Comorbidities to be checked include PsA, metabolic syndrome, inflammatory bowel disease (IBD), uveitis, and depression. Patients at high risk for infections should be counseled on infection control measures, including caution with pets, food, and travel.[8]

■ INTERLEUKIN 12/23 BLOCKERS IN PSORIASIS

Ustekinumab is a human immunoglobulin G1 (IgG1) kappa monoclonal antibody that binds to the shared p40 subunit of IL-12 and IL-23, both of which are heterodimers—IL-12 consists of p40 and p35, and IL-23 consists of p40 and p19. By binding to the p40 subunit, ustekinumab prevents these cytokines from interacting with the IL-12 receptor β1 subunit on T-cells, inhibiting the signaling pathways involved in immune cell activation and inflammatory responses.

Interleukin 12 is secreted by activated dendritic cells and macrophages, leading to the differentiation of naïve T-cells into Th1 cells, which produce IFN-γ and TNF-α. IL-23 promotes the expansion of Th17 and Th22 cells, which release proinflammatory cytokines like IL-17, IL-22, and TNF-α. These cytokines drive keratinocyte proliferation, vascular dilation, and immune cell infiltration, contributing to the development of psoriatic skin lesions.[9]

By blocking IL-12 and IL-23, ustekinumab disrupts this inflammatory cycle, making it effective in treating conditions like psoriasis and PsA, among others. It is FDA-approved for moderate-to-severe plaque psoriasis (since 2009), PsA (since 2015), Crohn's disease, and ulcerative colitis. Clinical trials, such as PHOENIX 1 and 2, PEARL, ACCEPT, PSUMMIT I and II, have demonstrated its efficacy and safety in these conditions.[10]

In terms of administration, ustekinumab is available for subcutaneous and intravenous use, with dosing based on weight. Side effects are generally mild, with headaches and nasopharyngitis being the most common. However, serious infections like cellulitis and pneumonia are less frequent compared to other biologics. There are reports of paradoxical pustular psoriasis flares and adverse reactions like fatigue, hypersensitivity, and reversible posterior leukoencephalopathy syndrome.

Ustekinumab is contraindicated in patients with hypersensitivity and active infections. The presence of anti-ustekinumab antibodies (AUA), which occur in a small percentage of patients, can reduce the treatment's efficacy. Methotrexate co-medication does not significantly affect serum ustekinumab levels or AUA formation.[11]

For patients on ustekinumab, live vaccines should be avoided during treatment, and precautions are necessary for household contacts receiving live vaccines. Ustekinumab is classified as category B in pregnancy, with recommendations to discontinue treatment

CHAPTER 12: Use of Biologics in Psoriasis

due to potential risks, although no adverse maternal or neonatal outcomes were found in a series of pregnant patients. In lactation, the secretion of ustekinumab in breast milk is minimal, so breastfeeding may not need to be discontinued, though caution is advised.[12,13]

■ TUMOR NECROSIS FACTOR ALPHA BLOCKERS IN PSORIASIS[14,15]

The TNF-α blockers in psoriasis are given in **Table 2**.

TABLE 2: Tumor necrosis factor alpha (TNF-α) blockers in psoriasis[14,15]

Name of the drug	Type of monoclonal antibody	Indication (FDA-approved)	Dose	Adverse effects	Special populations
Infliximab[14]	Chimeric (25% mouse and 75% human) IgG1 monoclonal antibody specific for TNF-α only	Psoriasis, psoriatic arthritis, ankylosing spondylitis, rheumatoid arthritis, ulcerative colitis, Crohn's disease	• Available as lyophilized concentrate of 100 mg in 1 vial • Each 100 reconstituted with 10 mL of sterile water and diluted with 250 mL of normal saline and infused over at least 2 hours	Infusion reactions, hepatotoxicity	• Category B safe during lactation • Live vaccines should be administered 6–12 months after birth for infants exposed in utero to infliximab
Etanercept[14,15]	Dimeric fully human fusion protein; it consists of two ligand-binding domains of TNF receptor 2 fused to Fc portion of IgG1	• It is the only TNF-α blocker, which is approved by the FDA for pediatric psoriasis (above 6 years of age). • Plaque psoriasis, psoriatic arthritis	• *Starting dose*: 50 mg twice weekly for 3 months • *Maintenance dose*: 50 mg once weekly after 3 months • *138 lb or more*: 50 mg once weekly • *<138 lb*: 0.8 mg/kg once weekly	• Injection site reactions are the most common side effect • Management includes warm compresses, topical corticosteroids, and antihistamines	Pregnancy category B, detected at low levels in breast milk
Certolizumab[14,15]	Recombinant, humanized fragment of Fab antibody conjugated with polyethylene glycol	• Psoriasis • Psoriatic arthritis	• Lyophilized powder reconstituted with 1 mL water and administered by a healthcare provider • Single-dose 1 mL prefilled syringe containing 200 mg of drug (self-administered)	Upper respiratory tract infections, abscesses, pneumonia, antidrug antibodies	Safe in pregnancy and lactation

Continued

CHAPTER 12: Use of Biologics in Psoriasis

Continued

Name of the drug	Type of monoclonal antibody	Indication (FDA-approved)	Dose	Adverse effects	Special populations
Adalimumab[14,15]	Fully human IgG1 recombinant antibody to TNF-α only and prevents its binding to both p55 and p75 receptors	Psoriasis, psoriatic arthritis, hidradenitis suppurativa	80-mg loading dose (week 0) followed by 40 mg every alternate week starting at week 1 after the initial dose	*Injection site reactions (3.2%)*: Erythema, swelling, and itching	Safe in pregnancy
Golimumab[14,15]	Fully human anti-TNF-α monoclonal antibody created in specific transgenic mice (mice with human genes inserted into their genome)	Psoriatic arthritis	Prefilled syringe or autoinjector for subcutaneous injection of 50 mg 50 mg/4 mL (12.5 mg/mL) solution supplied in a single-dose vial for intravenous infusion	Antidrug antibodies, injection site reactions, upper respiratory tract infections, and deranged LFTs	Not recommended

(FDA: Food and Drug Administration; IgG1: immunoglobulin G1; LFTs: liver function tests)

■ INTERLEUKIN-17 INHIBITORS IN PSORIASIS

There are four IL-17 inhibitors currently in use: Ixekizumab, brodalumab, secukinumab, and bimekizumab.

The FDA-approved indications are for moderate-to-severe plaque psoriasis in adults who are candidates for systemic therapy, PsA, ankylosing spondylitis (AS), rheumatoid arthritis, nail psoriasis, and palmoplantar psoriasis. The off-label indications are pustular psoriasis and chronic noninfectious uveitis **(Table 3)**.[16-18]

■ INTERLEUKIN-23 BLOCKERS IN PSORIASIS

For the treatment of moderate-to-severe psoriasis, three inhibitors specifically targeting IL-23 p19 are available, guselkumab, tildrakizumab, and risankizumab **(Table 4)**.

The adverse events (AEs) observed in clinical trials for IL-23 inhibitors—tildrakizumab, guselkumab, and risankizumab—were reported as follows:

- *Tildrakizumab (reSURFACE 1 and reSURFACE 2 trials)*:
  - In the reSURFACE 1 trial (100-mg dose), <1 AE was seen in 47% of patients. Serious AEs were reported in 25 patients, but no deaths occurred. The most common AEs were nasopharyngitis (8%), upper respiratory infection (3%), and psoriasis (1%). Severe infections occurred in fewer than 15 patients, with no reports of malignancy, nonmelanoma skin cancer (NMSC), major adverse cardiac events (MACE), or drug-related hypersensitivity reactions.
  - In the reSURFACE 2 trial, two cases of injection site erythema were observed, and one death was reported.[21]

CHAPTER 12: Use of Biologics in Psoriasis

TABLE 3: Interleukin 17 (IL-17) blockers in psoriasis[17,18]

Name of the drug	Year of FDA approval	Type of monoclonal antibody	Dose	Adverse effects	Considerations in special populations
Ixekizumab[17,18]	March 22, 2016	Humanized	• 160 mg (two 80-mg injections) at week 0; 80 mg every 2 weeks at weeks 2, 4, 6, 8, 10, and 12 • Thereafter, 80 mg every 4 weeks SC	Neutropenia, injection site reactions, hypersensitivity reactions, fungal infections, nausea, thrombocytopenia	No data on pregnancy and lactation Can be used in children 6 years or older
Brodalumab[17,18]	February 15, 2017	Human	• 210 mg at weeks 0, 1 and 2 • Thereafter 210 mg every 2 weeks SC	Headache, arthralgia, diarrhea, nausea, myalgia, oropharyngeal pain, injection site reactions	No data available
Secukinumab[17,18]	January 2015	Human	• 300 mg at weeks 0, 1, 2, 3, and 4 • Thereafter, 300 mg every 4 weeks SC	Injection site reactions, upper respiratory tract infections, candidiasis, oral herpes, diarrhea, neutropenia	• Pregnancy category B • Exercise caution during lactation • Can be used in children >6 years • Live vaccines not to be used concurrently
Bimekizumab[17,18]	October 18, 2023	Humanized	320 mg (given as 2 SC injections of 160 mg each) at weeks 0, 4, 8, 12, and 16, then every 8 weeks thereafter; for patients weighing ≥120 kg, consider a dosage of 320 mg every 4 weeks after week 16	Upper respiratory tract infections, hypertension, oral candidiasis, diarrhea	No data available yet

(FDA: Food and Drug Administration; IgG1: immunoglobulin G1; LFTs: liver function tests; SC: subcutaneous)

CHAPTER 12: Use of Biologics in Psoriasis

TABLE 4: Interleukin 23 (IL-23) blockers in psoriasis[19,20]

Name of the drug	Type of monoclonal antibody	Year of FDA (Food and Drug Administration) approval	Dose
Tildrakizumab[19,20]	Humanized	May, 2018	It is given in the dose of 100 mg subcutaneously on day 0 and week 4 followed by one injection every 12 weeks
Guselkumab[19,20]	Human	June, 2017	The recommended dose of guselkumab is 100 mg on day 0 and week 4, followed by 100 mg every 8 weeks, given subcutaneously
Risankizumab[19,20]	Humanized	April, 2019	It is given in the dose of 150 mg (75 mg 2 injections) subcutaneously on day 0, week 4 and every 12 weeks thereafter

- *Guselkumab (VOYAGE 1 trial)*:
  - At least one AE was reported in 74.5% of patients during the 0–48 week period. Common AEs included nasopharyngitis (25.2%), upper respiratory infection (14.3%), injection site erythema (2.4%), headache (5.5%), arthralgia (5.5%), pruritus (2.4%), and back pain (3.6%). About 2.7% of cases discontinued the study due to AEs, and 4.9% of patients experienced at least one serious AE.
  - Infections were seen in 52.3% of patients, with 16.4% requiring treatment. Serious infections were reported in 0.6% of patients, malignancy in 0.6%, NMSC in 0.6%, and MACE in 0.3%.[22]
- *Risankizumab (phase 2 trials)*:
  - The rate of any AE over the 0–48 week period was around 80%, with severe AEs in 10% of patients. Discontinuation of the study occurred in 2% of cases due to AEs, and serious AEs were reported in 15% of patients. Common AEs included nasopharyngitis (34%), headache (5%), gastroenteritis (10%), and back pain (10%).
  - Serious AEs included neoplasms (benign/malignant) (5%), BCC (2%), salivary gland neoplasm (2%), central nervous system accidents (2%), and cardiac disorders such as myocardial infarction (2%) and coronary artery occlusion (2%).[23]

They are FDA category B drugs for pregnancy and lactation, and their safety and efficacy in pediatric populations (under 18 years) have not been established.[21-23]

We have summarized the treatment guidelines and key trial results for biologic therapies used in the management of PsA from various global organizations.

Guidelines: GRAPPA (Group for Research and Assessment of Psoriasis and Psoriatic Arthritis) (2015, updated 2021), ACR/NPF (American College of Rheumatology/National Psoriasis Foundation) (2018), and EULAR (European Alliance of Associations for Rheumatology) (2019) have established guidelines for the treatment of PsA.

The ACR/NPF defines severe PsA as having erosive disease, elevated inflammatory markers, significant functional impairment, or rapidly progressing PsA with involvement at multiple sites (e.g., dactylitis, enthesitis).[24]

- *TNF inhibitors (TNFi)*:
  - IFX: Approved for PsA at 5 mg/kg intravenously; the IMPACT (Infliximab Multinational Psoriatic Arthritis Controlled Trial) and IMPACT 2 trials demonstrated significant improvement in ACR20 and PASI responses, with notable reductions in dactylitis, enthesitis, and radiographic progression.[25]
  - Adalimumab (ADA): Effective in the ADEPT trial, achieving significant

ACR20 and PASI 75 responses; the trial also noted sustained improvements in radiographic progression and quality of life (QoL).[26]
- Certolizumab pegol (CZP): RAPID-PsA trial demonstrated significant improvement in ACR20 and other outcomes (e.g., dactylitis, radiographic progression) up to 96 weeks.[27]
- Golimumab (GOL): GO-REVEAL trial showed significant ACR20 responses, with sustained benefits in skin, enthesitis, and radiographic progression up to 5 years.[28]
- Etanercept (ETN): Effective in reducing disease progression and improving ACR20 and PASI scores, with benefits sustained for up to 2 years.[29]
- IL-17 inhibitors:
  - Secukinumab: Proven efficacy in the FUTURE trials with significant improvements in ACR20 responses, patient-reported outcomes, and inhibition of radiographic progression[30]
  - Ixekizumab: The SPIRIT trials demonstrated robust ACR20 responses, skin improvement, and inhibition of structural damage.[31]
- IL-12/23 and IL-23 inhibitors:
  - Ustekinumab: The PSUMMIT trials confirmed its efficacy in both TNF-naïve and TNF nonresponder patients, with minimal radiographic progression.[32]
  - Guselkumab: DISCOVER trials showed efficacy in both biologic-naïve and TNF-experienced PsA patients, with a good safety profile.[33]
  - Tildrakizumab and risankizumab: Both have shown promise in phase II and III trials with substantial ACR20 responses and skin improvements.[34]

Each biologic offers varying degrees of efficacy across joint, skin, and other PsA manifestations, with data supporting long-term benefits and safety.

BIOLOGICS IN SPECIAL SITUATIONS

Vaccination

Patients should stop biologic therapy for 6–12 months before administering live vaccines, such as the varicella and herpes zoster (shingles) vaccines, to minimize potential risks. It is preferable to vaccinate the patient with any necessary live vaccines before starting biologic therapy. It typically takes about 2 weeks for vaccines to be effective, after which biologic therapy can be initiated. Patients on biologic therapy should avoid live vaccines to reduce the risk of complications associated with live attenuated viruses, which may be more dangerous in immunocompromised individuals.[35]

Pregnancy

Tumor necrosis factor alpha inhibitors are considered safe during pregnancy and lactation. However, their use in the third trimester may carry a theoretical risk due to transplacental transfer of medication. All IL-17 inhibitors are likely acceptable for men attempting conception with their partner, suggesting they do not pose a significant risk to fertility or pregnancy outcomes from the paternal side.[36]

Lactation

There is limited data on the use of biologics during lactation, but available reports have not identified significant adverse effects in breastfed infants or negative impacts on lactation. Due to their high molecular weight, biologics are unlikely to transfer into breast milk in significant amounts. It is recommended to avoid biologics in the first few weeks post delivery because large alveolar gaps might increase the potential for transfer. If biologics do appear in breast milk, they are unlikely to be absorbed by the infant, as they are likely destroyed in the infant's gastrointestinal tract, further minimizing risk.[37]

Hepatitis

In hepatitis B surface antigen (HBsAg)-positive patients, TNFi and IL-12/23 inhibitors carry a risk of hepatitis B virus (HBV) reactivation, while IL-17 inhibitors are considered safe when used after antiviral prophylaxis with close monitoring of LFTs and viral titers. There is no data on the safety of apremilast and IL-23 inhibitors in these patients. For anti-HBc-positive patients, TNFi, ustekinumab, and IL-17 inhibitors are usable but require careful monitoring, and again, no data exists for apremilast or IL-23 inhibitors. In chronic hepatitis C virus (HCV) patients, TNFi can be administered with antiviral therapy and close LFT and viral titer monitoring, while IL-12/23 inhibitors have a controversial safety profile. IL-17 inhibitors and apremilast show favorable safety, though data is limited, and there is little data on IL-23 inhibitors in HCV cases.[38]

Tuberculosis

Interleukin 17 inhibitors are considered safe for use in patients with latent tuberculosis infection (LTBI). However, TNFi and ustekinumab should only be used after initiating TB prophylaxis for at least 1 month to minimize the risk of reactivation.[39]

Elective Surgery

For elective surgery, it is recommended to stop biologic therapy 3–5 times the drug's half-life before surgery. Biologics can be restarted postoperatively if there are no signs of infection and wound healing is satisfactory. Typically, biologics should be discontinued about 3–4 half-lives prior to surgery and resumed 1–2 weeks after surgery, provided there are no postoperative complications.[40]

Malignancy

In a large safety analysis involving approximately 15,000 patients treated with secukinumab, the risk of malignancy was found to be low over up to 5 years of treatment. Among these patients, 1.7% (242 individuals) had a medical history of malignancy, including 168 with psoriasis, 60 with PsA, and 14 with AS. In contrast, TNFi carry a black box warning from the FDA regarding an increased risk of non-Hodgkin lymphoma and leukemia.[41]

■ BIOLOGICS AND COMORBIDITIES

Psoriasis significantly impacts mental health, with higher rates of depression, anxiety, and suicidal behaviors compared to the general population. A meta-analysis involving over 1.7 million participants found psoriasis patients to be at greater risk for suicidal ideation, attempts, and completions. Studies on biologic therapies, such as ustekinumab and ADA, have shown a reduction in depressive symptoms in psoriasis patients compared to those on conventional therapies. However, phototherapy did not exhibit the same benefit. The Psoriasis Longitudinal Assessment and Registry (PSOLAR) study confirmed biologics' positive impact on mental health by lowering the risk of depressive symptoms.[42,43]

Psoriasis is also associated with comorbid conditions like IBD and cardiovascular disease. Research revealed psoriasis patients have a higher risk of Crohn's disease and ulcerative colitis, with IL-17 inhibitors exacerbating these conditions. On the other hand, TNF-α and IL-23 inhibitors demonstrated improvements in IBD. The "psoriatic march" concept links systemic inflammation from psoriasis to cardiovascular risk through insulin resistance, leading to atherosclerosis. A study reported that biologic therapies, particularly IL-17 inhibitors, were effective in reducing coronary plaque burden, showing favorable cardiovascular outcomes in severe psoriasis patients.[44]

Metabolic syndrome, obesity, and hyperglycemia are commonly associated with psoriasis, further contributing to cardiovascular risk. Anti-IL-17 therapies have been shown to reduce blood glucose levels in psoriasis patients, and TNF-α inhibitors improved endothelial function and reduced major cardiovascular events. Studies have emphasized the importance of choosing biologic therapies based on patient comorbidities, with TNF-α inhibitors reducing cardiovascular event risk compared to methotrexate, further supporting personalized treatment approaches for psoriasis patients.[45]

■ SWITCHING BETWEEN BIOLOGICS

The efficacy of switching biologic therapies for psoriasis patients who experience inadequate responses to their current treatments is discussed. The ACCEPT trial demonstrated the benefits of switching from ETN to ustekinumab, particularly for nonresponders. It was revealed that although high doses of ustekinumab showed some effectiveness, the efficacy was still inferior compared to patients who were initially assigned to ustekinumab. Similar findings were reported in other trials, where improved response rates were observed in patients who switched to different biologics like tildrakizumab or guselkumab after being unresponsive to treatments such as ADA or ETN.[46,47]

The significance of switching between different classes of biologics for patients with a history of treatment failure is emphasized. Data suggests that better outcomes are often achieved when switching to a different mode of action, rather than remaining within the same class. For instance, markedly higher response rates were recorded for patients switching from ADA to risankizumab compared to those who continued on ADA. Additionally, while intraclass switches can still be effective, the overall response tends to be poorer in patients with prior failures compared to those without such a history.[48]

A washout period between treatments is suggested to be unnecessary, and induction doses may not be required when transitioning to another agent. Evidence indicates that improvement is more likely to be seen in patients who switch compared to those who remain on ineffective therapies, with some real-world data supporting the effectiveness of switching from IL-17 inhibitors to other biologics. However, more research is needed, particularly concerning the efficacy of switching between IL-17 and IL-23 inhibitors, as this data remains limited.[49]

■ COMBINATIONS OF BIOLOGICS WITH OTHER BIOLOGICS OR IMMUNOMODULATORS

Several small controlled trials and observational studies suggest that combining phototherapy with biologics may yield higher efficacy than biologic monotherapy in patients with moderate-to-severe psoriasis. Notably, patients receiving narrowband UVB (NBUVB) phototherapy alongside biologic agents like ETN and ADA often exhibit better outcomes than those on biologic monotherapy. However, in obese patients on ETN, the addition of NBUVB for 3 months may not confer significant additional benefits. Importantly, NBUVB appears to expedite the therapeutic effects in patients treated with ustekinumab.[50]

Despite this, long-term safety data on combining biologics with NBUVB remain scarce. This combination has been explored in 75 patients who had not achieved a PASI 90 after 12 weeks of ETN monotherapy. These patients were randomized to either continue ETN alone or receive it in conjunction with thrice-weekly NBUVB. At week 24, 16% of the combination group reached a PASI 90, similar to the 16% in the monotherapy group. Notably, only 22% of the combination group adhered to at least 80% of the NBUVB sessions. Among those with high adherence, 43% achieved PASI 90 compared to just 3% in the monotherapy group by week 16.[51]

Another study assessed the combined use of ADA and NBUVB in 20 patients with psoriasis covering >10% of body surface area (BSA). ADA (80 mg initially, followed by 40 mg biweekly) was initiated at week 1, with thrice-weekly NBUVB. After 12 weeks, patients showed an impressive 95% improvement in PASI scores. Specifically, 95% achieved PASI 75, 75% reached PASI 90, and 55% achieved complete clearance (PASI 100). By week 24, without further systemic treatment, 65% of patients maintained PASI 75. The most common adverse effect reported was erythema, but the combination was generally well tolerated.[52]

A randomized intraindividual, half-body trial by Wolf et al. evaluated ustekinumab with 311-nm NBUVB phototherapy in 10 patients. Treated thrice weekly for 6 weeks, the half body exposed to NBUVB showed an 82% PASI reduction, compared to 54% in the nonirradiated half ($p < 0.05$). Thus, 311-nm NB-UVB can significantly speed up the therapeutic response in patients receiving ustekinumab.[53]

Among the biologic combinations approved by the FDA, ETN combined with methotrexate is the most extensively studied, showing superior efficacy compared to either drug alone. This combination is often recommended when monotherapy fails to provide sufficient results. Similarly, combinations of IFX or ADA with methotrexate have demonstrated enhanced efficacy, though data is limited. Methotrexate dosage varies across studies, and the optimal dose remains uncertain, likely influenced by patient factors and the biologic used.[54]

Several studies have evaluated biologics paired with methotrexate for plaque psoriasis, with two randomized trials and one retrospective review focusing on ETN and methotrexate. Studies on IFX and methotrexate have been more limited. A separate investigation examined the cellular impact of ADA combined with methotrexate in both psoriatic and nonpsoriatic skin, suggesting that the combination may help reduce antidrug antibody formation compared to biologic monotherapy.[54]

Gottlieb et al. conducted a study to compare the combination of ETN and methotrexate versus ETN alone in patients with moderate-to-severe psoriasis. A total of 478 participants were randomized, with the combination therapy group receiving methotrexate (7.5–15 mg/week) alongside ETN. By week 24, 77% of the combination group achieved PASI 75, compared to 60% in the monotherapy group ($p < .001$). AEs were reported more frequently in the combination therapy group (75%) versus monotherapy (60%).[55]

In the IMPACT 2, a subanalysis revealed that 53% of patients receiving IFX with methotrexate achieved PASI 75 at week 54, compared to 48% of those not on methotrexate. Although the study design did not clarify whether methotrexate had additive or synergistic effects, AEs were comparable between the two groups.[56]

Acitretin, a systemic therapy with antiproliferative and immunomodulatory effects, may provide additional efficacy when combined with biologics. For instance, Gisondi et al. randomized 60 patients to receive ETN plus acitretin, ETN alone, or acitretin alone. At week 24, PASI 75 was achieved in 44% of the combination group, 45% of the ETN group, and 30% of the acitretin group. Both ETN regimens outperformed acitretin alone, with similar safety profiles across all groups.[57]

Combination therapies of biologics with cyclosporine have been explored in case reports as transitional treatments. For example,

Yamauchi and Lowe demonstrated that combining ETN with cyclosporine maintained disease control during cyclosporine tapering and discontinuation. While biologic–biologic combinations are largely unexplored, they may carry theoretical risks, such as infections and malignancies, emphasizing the need for careful patient selection and monitoring.[58]

TREAT-TO-TARGET APPROACH IN PSORIASIS

The concept of T2T strategies has been increasingly applied in chronic diseases to optimize patient outcomes. In psoriasis, a comprehensive approach has been developed based on clinical experience, published data, and a survey among Italian dermatologists. The key topics identified by the expert panel included: (1) Achieving clinical remission, (2) improving QoL, (3) abrogating systemic inflammation, and (4) ensuring safety. Consensus was reached on the treatment goals for each of these areas.[5,6]

Clinical Remission

The recommended target for clinical remission is a 90% improvement from baseline in the PASI 90 or an absolute PASI score of ≤3. Achieving this level of improvement not only reflects effective disease control but also serves as an important measure in clinical trials and real-world practice. For example, the CLEAR trial compared the efficacy of secukinumab and ustekinumab, showing that secukinumab achieved PASI 90 in 79% of patients at week 16, significantly higher than the 58% with ustekinumab. Additionally, PASI 100 rates were better with secukinumab (44% vs. 28%).[7,59]

Quality of Life

Patient-reported outcomes, particularly related to QoL, are vital in psoriasis management. A Dermatology Life Quality Index (DLQI) score of ≤3, indicating very low to no impact on daily living, is recommended as the target. Studies have shown that achieving PASI 90 is often associated with marked improvements in DLQI scores, reflecting an enhanced HRQoL. If these targets—PASI 90 or DLQI ≤ 3—are not reached within 3–4 months of treatment initiation, it is advised that the treatment regimen be changed.[6,60]

Abrogation of Systemic Inflammation

Preventing or delaying the development of PsA and other inflammatory comorbidities is another central goal of the T2T strategy. Abrogating systemic inflammation can potentially reduce the burden of cardiovascular diseases, diabetes, metabolic syndrome, and IBD, all of which are commonly associated with psoriasis. The choice of treatment should therefore consider its ability to not only control skin symptoms but also mitigate underlying inflammation that may contribute to these comorbidities.[60,61]

Safety

The safety profile of psoriasis therapies, particularly biologics, plays a crucial role in long-term management. Biological treatments are generally better tolerated than traditional systemic therapies, though they are associated with specific risks, such as infections. For instance, TNF-α inhibitors increase the risk of upper respiratory infections, while IL-17 inhibitors have been linked to a higher incidence of *Candida* infections. Ongoing monitoring and careful patient selection are essential to balancing efficacy and safety in treatment plans.[61,62]

ROLE OF ABSOLUTE PSORIASIS AREA AND SEVERITY INDEX SCORES

An absolute PASI score of ≤3 has been recommended in various national guidelines, including those from France and Spain, as a more practical and reliable marker for clinical remission. Recent analyses have shown a strong correlation between absolute PASI scores and percentage improvement measures, such as PASI 75 or PASI 90. A British analysis found a 90% concordance between an absolute PASI ≤ 2 and PASI 90, underscoring its utility in clinical practice. Absolute scores are also independent of baseline disease severity, making them easier to apply across different patient populations.[59,60]

As psoriasis treatment continues to evolve with the advent of newer biologics and systemic therapies, the T2T strategy will require ongoing refinement. Current treatment targets, such as PASI 90 and DLQI ≤ 3, reflect the best available evidence but may need to be adjusted as more data emerge on the correlation between clinical outcomes and patient-reported measures. Furthermore, the integration of patient preferences and long-term safety data will be crucial in shaping future treatment targets.

Thus, the T2T approach in psoriasis management prioritizes clinical remission, QoL, and safety, with the overarching goal of preventing systemic inflammation and its associated comorbidities. Adjustments in treatment should be made promptly if established targets are not met within the recommended time frame, ensuring that patients receive the most effective and individualized care.[61]

■ FUTURE DIRECTION

As the landscape of psoriasis treatment continues to evolve, the future of biologics holds great promise for even more targeted and individualized therapies. Advances in immunology and biotechnology are expected to drive the development of new biologics and small molecules with improved efficacy, safety profiles, and mechanisms that more precisely modulate the immune pathways involved in psoriasis. One of the emerging trends is the exploration of personalized medicine, where patient-specific factors such as genetics, biomarkers, and disease phenotypes are used to tailor biologic therapy, optimizing outcomes while minimizing adverse effects.

Another area of focus is the combination of biologics with other treatment modalities, such as phototherapy or conventional systemic therapies, to enhance response rates and manage refractory cases more effectively. Clinical trials are increasingly evaluating these combinations to establish safe and effective protocols. Moreover, research into dual-action biologics—those targeting more than one cytokine pathway—could lead to more comprehensive suppression of psoriatic inflammation, potentially improving patient QoL and reducing comorbidities.

Additionally, there is a growing interest in developing biosimilars, which offer cost-effective alternatives to current biologic therapies, increasing accessibility for patients. As patent protections for many biologics expire, biosimilars are expected to play a significant role in reducing the economic burden of psoriasis treatment. Long-term real-world data from pharmacovigilance programs will also continue to shape the future of biologics, ensuring their safety and efficacy over extended periods.

■ CONCLUSION

Biologics have revolutionized the management of moderate-to-severe psoriasis by offering highly targeted and effective treatment options that significantly improve clinical outcomes and patient QoL. The T2T approach, with defined goals such as PASI 90 and DLQI ≤ 3, has become central to optimizing care and minimizing disease impact. While biologics have demonstrated superior efficacy and safety profiles to conventional systemic therapies, ongoing research into future trends, such as personalized medicine, dual-action biologics, and biosimilars, promises to refine

CHAPTER 12: Use of Biologics in Psoriasis

further and expand the treatment landscape. As therapeutic strategies evolve, continual assessment of safety, efficacy, and patient-reported outcomes will remain critical to delivering the best possible care for psoriasis patients.

> **TAKE HOME MESSAGE**
>
> The advent of biologics has transformed the management of moderate-to-severe psoriasis by offering targeted, efficacious, and safer treatment options compared to traditional therapies. Key developments include the treat-to-target approach, aiming for milestones like PASI 90 and improved quality of life metrics. These advancements are underpinned by a deeper understanding of psoriasis' immunopathology, highlighting the IL-17 and IL-23 pathways as critical targets. Personalized medicine, dual-action biologics, and biosimilars promise to refine treatment strategies further. As therapies evolve, a balance between efficacy, safety, and patient-centric care remains essential to improving clinical outcomes and addressing comorbidities.

REFERENCES

1. Lee HJ, Kim M. Challenges and Future Trends in the Treatment of Psoriasis. Int J Mol Sci. 2023;24(17):13313.
2. Billi AC, Gudjonsson JE, Voorhees JJ. Psoriasis: Past, Present, and Future. J Invest Dermatol. 2019;139(11):e133-42.
3. Fitch E, Harper E, Skorcheva I, Kurtz SE, Blauvelt A. Pathophysiology of psoriasis: recent advances on IL-23 and Th17 cytokines. Curr Rheumatol Rep. 2007;9(6):461-7.
4. Stockinger B, Veldhoen M. Differentiation and function of Th17 T cells. Curr Opin Immunol. 2007;19:281-6.
5. Armstrong A, Jarvis S, Boehncke WH, Rajagopalan M, Fernández-Peñas P, Romiti R, et al. Patient perceptions of clear/almost clear skin in moderate-to-severe plaque psoriasis: results of the clear about psoriasis worldwide survey. J Eur Acad Dermatol Venereol. 2018;32(12):2200-7.
6. Lebwohl MG, Kavanaugh A, Armstrong AW, Van Voorhees AS. US perspectives in the management of psoriasis and psoriatic arthritis: patient and physician results from the population-based multinational assessment of psoriasis and psoriatic arthritis (MAPP) survey. Am J Clin Dermatol. 2016;17(1):87-97.
7. Lynde CW, Beecker J, Dutz J, Flanagan C, Guenther LC, Gulliver W, et al. Treating to target(s) with interleukin-17 inhibitors. J Cutan Med Surg. 2019;23(2_suppl):3S-34S.
8. Al-Janabi A, Yiu ZZN. Biologics in Psoriasis: Updated Perspectives on Long-Term Safety and Risk Management. Psoriasis (Auckl). 2022;12:1-14. Erratum in: Psoriasis (Auckl). 2022;12:187-8.
9. Poelman SM, Keeling CP, Metelitsa AI. Practical Guidelines for Managing Patients With Psoriasis on Biologics: An Update. J Cutan Med Surg. 2019;23(1_suppl):3S-12S.
10. Benson JM, Peritt D, Scallon BJ, Heavner GA, Shealy DJ, Giles-Komar JM, et al. Discovery and mechanism of ustekinumab: a human monoclonal antibody targeting interleukin-12 and interleukin-23 for treatment of immune-mediated disorders. MAbs. 2011;3(6):535-45.
11. Tsai TF, Ho JC, Song M, Szapary P, Guzzo C, Shen YK, et al. Efficacy and safety of ustekinumab for the treatment of moderate-to-severe psoriasis: a phase III, randomized, placebo-controlled trial in Taiwanese and Korean patients (PEARL) J Dermatol Sci. 2011;63(3):154-63.
12. Flanagan E, Prentice R, Wright EK, Gibson PR, Ross AL, Begun J, et al. Ustekinumab levels in pregnant women with inflammatory bowel disease and infants exposed in utero. Aliment Pharmacol Ther. 2022;55(6):700-4.
13. Gisbert JP, Chaparro M. Safety of New Biologics (Vedolizumab and Ustekinumab) and Small Molecules (Tofacitinib) During Pregnancy: A Review. Drugs. 2020;80(11):1085-100.
14. Li SJ, Perez-Chada LM, Merola JF. TNF Inhibitor-Induced Psoriasis: Proposed Algorithm for Treatment and Management. J Psoriasis Psoriatic Arthritis. 2019;4(2):70-80.
15. Brown G, Wang E, Leon A, Huynh M, Wehner M, Matro R, et al. Tumor necrosis factor-α inhibitor-induced psoriasis: Systematic review of clinical features, histopathological findings, and management experience. J Am Acad Dermatol. 2017;76(2):334-41.
16. Kearns DG, Uppal S, Chat VS, Wu JJ. Comparison of Guidelines for the Use of Interleukin-17 Inhibitors for Psoriasis in the United States, Britain, and Europe: A Critical Appraisal and Comprehensive Review. J Clin Aesthet Dermatol. 2021;14(6):55-9.
17. Țiburcă L, Bembea M, Zaha DC, Jurca AD, Vesa CM, Rațiu IA, et al. The Treatment with Interleukin 17

18. Mosca M, Hong J, Hadeler E, Hakimi M, Liao W, Bhutani T. The Role of IL-17 Cytokines in Psoriasis. Immunotargets Ther. 2021;10:409-18.
19. Huang X, Shentu H, He Y, Lai H, Xu C, Chen M, et al. Efficacy and safety of IL-23 inhibitors in the treatment of psoriatic arthritis: a meta-analysis based on randomized controlled trials. Immunol Res. 2023;71(4):505-15.
20. Yang K, Oak ASW, Elewski BE. Use of IL-23 Inhibitors for the Treatment of Plaque Psoriasis and Psoriatic Arthritis: A Comprehensive Review. Am J Clin Dermatol. 2021;22(2):173-92.
21. Reich K, Warren RB, Iversen L, Puig L, Pau-Charles I, Igarashi A, et al. Long-term efficacy and safety of tildrakizumab for moderate-to-severe psoriasis: pooled analyses of two randomized phase III clinical trials (reSURFACE 1 and reSURFACE 2) through 148 weeks. Br J Dermatol. 2020;182(3):605-17.
22. Blauvelt A, Papp KA, Griffiths CE, Randazzo B, Wasfi Y, Shen YK, et al. Efficacy and safety of guselkumab, an anti-interleukin-23 monoclonal antibody, compared with adalimumab for the continuous treatment of patients with moderate to severe psoriasis: Results from the phase III, double-blinded, placebo- and active comparator-controlled VOYAGE 1 trial. J Am Acad Dermatol. 2017;76(3):405-17.
23. Gordon KB, Lebwohl M, Papp KA, Bachelez H, Wu JJ, Langley RG, et al. Long-term safety of risankizumab from 17 clinical trials in patients with moderate-to-severe plaque psoriasis. Br J Dermatol. 2022;186(3):466-75.
24. D'Angelo S, Tramontano G, Gilio M, Leccese P, Olivieri I. Review of the treatment of psoriatic arthritis with biological agents: choice of drug for initial therapy and switch therapy for non-responders. Open Access Rheumatol. 2017;9:21-8.
25. Kavanaugh A, Antoni CE, Gladman D, Wassenberg S, Zhou B, Beutler A, et al. The Infliximab Multinational Psoriatic Arthritis Controlled Trial (IMPACT): results of radiographic analyses after 1 year. Ann Rheum Dis. 2006;65(8):1038-43.
26. Mease PJ, Ory P, Sharp JT, Ritchlin CT, Van den Bosch F, Wellborne F, et al. Adalimumab for long-term treatment of psoriatic arthritis: 2-year data from the Adalimumab Effectiveness in Psoriatic Arthritis Trial (ADEPT). Ann Rheum Dis. 2009;68(5):702-9.
27. Mease P, Deodhar A, Fleischmann R, Wollenhaupt J, Gladman D, Leszczyński P, et al. Effect of certolizumab pegol over 96 weeks in patients with psoriatic arthritis with and without prior antitumour necrosis factor exposure. RMD Open. 2015;1(1):e000119.
28. Kavanaugh A, McInnes IB, Mease P, Krueger GG, Gladman D, van der Heijde D, et al. Clinical efficacy, radiographic and safety findings through 5 years of subcutaneous golimumab treatment in patients with active psoriatic arthritis: results from a long-term extension of a randomised, placebo-controlled trial (the GO-REVEAL study). Ann Rheum Dis. 2014;73(9):1689-94.
29. Kivelevitch D, Mansouri B, Menter A. Long term efficacy and safety of etanercept in the treatment of psoriasis and psoriatic arthritis. Biologics. 2014;8:169-82.
30. Mease PJ, Landewé R, Rahman P, Tahir H, Singhal A, Boettcher E, et al. Secukinumab provides sustained improvement in signs and symptoms and low radiographic progression in patients with psoriatic arthritis: 2-year (end-of-study) results from the FUTURE 5 study. RMD Open. 2021;7(2):e001600.
31. Mease PJ, van der Heijde D, Ritchlin CT, Okada M, Cuchacovich RS, Shuler CL, et al. SPIRIT-P1 Study Group. Ixekizumab, an interleukin-17A specific monoclonal antibody, for the treatment of biologic-naive patients with active psoriatic arthritis: results from the 24-week randomised, double-blind, placebo-controlled and active (adalimumab)-controlled period of the phase III trial SPIRIT-P1. Ann Rheum Dis. 2017;76(1):79-87.
32. Kavanaugh A, Ritchlin C, Rahman P, Puig L, Gottlieb AB, Li S, et al.; PSUMMIT-1 and 2 Study Groups. Ustekinumab, an anti-IL-12/23 p40 monoclonal antibody, inhibits radiographic progression in patients with active psoriatic arthritis: results of an integrated analysis of radiographic data from the phase 3, multicentre, randomised, double-blind, placebo-controlled PSUMMIT-1 and PSUMMIT-2 trials. Ann Rheum Dis. 2014;73(6):1000-6.
33. Ritchlin CT, Deodhar A, Boehncke WH, Soriano ER, Kollmeier AP, Xu XL, et al. Multidomain Efficacy and Safety of Guselkumab Through 1 Year in Patients With Active Psoriatic Arthritis With and Without Prior Tumor Necrosis Factor Inhibitor Experience: Analysis of the Phase 3, Randomized, Placebo-Controlled DISCOVER-1 Study. ACR Open Rheumatol. 2023;5(3):149-64.
34. Ruggiero A, Picone V, Martora F, Fabbrocini G, Megna M. Guselkumab, Risankizumab, and Tildrakizumab in the Management of Psoriasis: A Review of the Real-World Evidence. Clin Cosmet Investig Dermatol. 2022;15:1649-58.
35. Papp KA, Haraoui B, Kumar D, Marshall JK, Bissonnette R, Bitton A, et al. Vaccination Guidelines for Patients With Immune-Mediated Disorders on Immunosuppressive Therapies. J Cutan Med Surg. 2019;23(1):50-74.
36. Johansen CB, Jimenez-Solem E, Haerskjold A, Sand FL, Thomsen SF. The Use and Safety of TNF Inhibitors during Pregnancy in Women with Psoriasis: A Review. Int J Mol Sci. 2018;19(5):1349.
37. Beltagy A, Aghamajidi A, Trespidi L, Ossola W, Meroni PL. Biologics During Pregnancy and Breastfeeding Among Women With Rheumatic

38. Bonek K, Roszkowski L, Massalska M, Maslinski W, Ciechomska M. Biologic Drugs for Rheumatoid Arthritis in the Context of Biosimilars, Genetics, Epigenetics and COVID-19 Treatment. Cells. 2021;10(2):323.
39. Torres T, Chiricozzi A, Puig L, Lé AM, Marzano AV, Dapavo P, et al. Treatment of Psoriasis Patients with Latent Tuberculosis Using IL-17 and IL-23 Inhibitors: A Retrospective, Multinational, Multicentre Study. Am J Clin Dermatol. 2024;25(2):333-42.
40. Rezaieyazdi Z, Sahebari M, Khodashahi M. Preoperative Evaluation and Management of Patients Receiving Biologic Therapies. Arch Bone Jt Surg. 2019;7(3):220-8.
41. Lebwohl M, Deodhar A, Griffiths CEM, Menter MA, Poddubnyy D, Bao W, et al. The risk of malignancy in patients with secukinumab-treated psoriasis, psoriatic arthritis and ankylosing spondylitis: analysis of clinical trial and postmarketing surveillance data with up to five years of follow-up. Br J Dermatol. 2021;185(5):935-44.
42. Humphreys J, Hyrich K, Symmons D. What is the impact of biologic therapies on common co-morbidities in patients with rheumatoid arthritis? Arthritis Res Ther. 2016;18(1):282.
43. Wang Y, Zhang P, Lv Y, Deng Y, Yao M, Wang L, et al. Advancements in the Study of Biologic Agents in Comorbidities of Psoriasis: A Literature Review. Clin Cosmet Investig Dermatol. 2023;16:3487-95.
44. Pelaia C, Pelaia G, Busse W. Do Comorbidities Influence the Response to Biologics in Severe Asthma? Am J Respir Crit Care Med. 2024;209(3):233-5.
45. Akbar A, Orchard T, Powell N, Selinger C, Tibbatts C. Influence of comorbidities on treatment considerations for first-line biologic prescribing in patients with inflammatory bowel disease in the UK. Frontline Gastroenterol. 2022;13(6):490-6.
46. Young MS, Horn EJ, Cather JC. The ACCEPT study: ustekinumab versus etanercept in moderate-to-severe psoriasis patients. Expert Rev Clin Immunol. 2011;7(1):9-13.
47. Blauvelt A, Papp KA, Griffiths CEM, Puig L, Weisman J, Dutronc Y, et al. Efficacy and Safety of Switching to Ixekizumab in Etanercept Non-Responders: A Subanalysis from Two Phase III Randomized Clinical Trials in Moderate-to-Severe Plaque Psoriasis (UNCOVER-2 and -3). Am J Clin Dermatol. 2017;18(2):273-80.
48. Kearsley-Fleet L, Heaf E, Davies R, Baildam E, Beresford MW, Foster HE, et al.; BCRD and BSPAR-ETN study groups. Frequency of biologic switching and the outcomes of switching in children and young people with juvenile idiopathic arthritis: a national cohort study. Lancet Rheumatol. 2020;2(4):e217-26.
49. Kerdel F, Zaiac M. An evolution in switching therapy for psoriasis patients who fail to meet treatment goals. Dermatol Ther. 2015;28(6):390-403.
50. Farahnik B, Patel V, Beroukhim K, Zhu TH, Abrouk M, Nakamura M, et al. Combining biologic and phototherapy treatments for psoriasis: safety, efficacy, and patient acceptability. Psoriasis (Auckl). 2016;6:105-111.
51. Cather JC, Crowley JJ. Use of biologic agents in combination with other therapies for the treatment of psoriasis. Am J Clin Dermatol. 2014;15(6):467-78.
52. Bagel J. Adalimumab plus narrowband ultraviolet B light phototherapy for the treatment of moderate to severe psoriasis. J Drugs Dermatol. 2011;10(4):366-71.
53. Wolf P, Weger W, Legat FJ, Posch-Fabian T, Gruber-Wackernagel A, Inzinger M, et al. Treatment with 311-nm ultraviolet B enhanced response of psoriatic lesions in ustekinumab-treated patients: a randomized intraindividual trial. Br J Dermatol. 2012;166(1):147-53.
54. Mease PJ, Gladman DD, Collier DH, Ritchlin CT, Helliwell PS, Liu L, et al. Etanercept and Methotrexate as Monotherapy or in Combination for Psoriatic Arthritis: Primary Results From a Randomized, Controlled Phase III Trial. Arthritis Rheumatol. 2019;71(7):1112-4.
55. Gottlieb AB, Langley RG, Strober BE, Papp KA, Klekotka P, Creamer K, et al. A randomized, double-blind, placebo-controlled study to evaluate the addition of methotrexate to etanercept in patients with moderate to severe plaque psoriasis. Br J Dermatol. 2012;167(3):649-57.
56. Baranauskaite A, Raffayová H, Kungurov NV, Kubanova A, Venalis A, Helmle L, et al. Infliximab plus methotrexate is superior to methotrexate alone in the treatment of psoriatic arthritis in methotrexate-naive patients: the RESPOND study. Ann Rheum Dis. 2012;71(4):541-8.
57. Gisondi P, Del Giglio M, Cotena C, Girolomoni G. Combining etanercept and acitretin in the therapy of chronic plaque psoriasis: a 24-week, randomized, controlled, investigator-blinded pilot trial. Br J Dermatol. 2008;158(6):1345-9.
58. Yamauchi PS, Lowe NJ. Cessation of cyclosporine therapy by treatment with etanercept in patients with severe psoriasis. J Am Acad Dermatol. 2006;54(3 Suppl 2):S135-8.
59. Bagel J, Blauvelt A, Nia J, Hashim P, Patekar M, de Vera A, et al. Secukinumab maintains superiority over ustekinumab in clearing skin and improving quality of life in patients with moderate to severe plaque psoriasis: 52-week results from a double-blind phase 3b trial (CLARITY). J Eur Acad Dermatol Venereol. 2021;35(1):135-42.

60. Gelfand JM, Weinstein R, Porter SB, Neimann AL, Berlin JA, Margolis DJ. Prevalence and treatment of psoriasis in the United Kingdom: a population-based study. Arch Dermatol. 2005;141(12):1537-41.
61. Stern RS, Nijsten T, Feldman SR, Margolis DJ, Rolstad T. Psoriasis is common, carries a substantial burden even when not extensive, and is associated with widespread treatment dissatisfaction. J Investig Dermatol Symp Proc. 2004;9(2):136-9.
62. Gelfand JM, Neimann AL, Shin DB, Wang X, Margolis DJ, Troxel AB. Risk of myocardial infarction in patients with psoriasis. JAMA. 2006;296(14):1735-41.

13. Combination and Rotational Therapy in the Management of Psoriasis

Lydia Mathew, Dharshini Sathishkumar

■ INTRODUCTION

Psoriasis is a chronic immune-mediated disorder that significantly impacts patients' quality of life. With a better understanding of the underlying pathogenesis, numerous drugs are added to the armamentarium of drugs to treat psoriasis to control acute flare and provide long-term maintenance. Many times, the disease can be severe and difficult to treat, and more than one modality of treatment is required and the various ways of concomitantly administering drugs, include combination therapy, rotational therapy, and sequential therapy. Combination therapy is used for better control of disease and provides longer remission. While there is strong evidence for certain combinations like topical vitamin D analogs and topical corticosteroids (CS), phototherapy plus retinoids, clear-cut evidence is lacking for many other combinations. In this chapter, we shall review the various possible combinations of drugs used to treat psoriasis and their risks and benefits.

■ COMBINATION THERAPY

Combination therapy involves the concurrent use of two or more medications of a single modality with different mechanisms of action and safety profile or the use of two or more different treatment modalities such as topicals, systemic or physical therapies. It is advantageous as it provides increased therapeutic benefit due to synergistic effects, targets varied pathogenetic pathways, and minimizes adverse effects due to lower dose of individual medications. US health insurance databases on psoriasis or psoriatic arthritis (PsA) reported the practice of combination therapy with either biologicals or apremilast in up to 42.9%.[1]

Topical therapy which is important in the treatment of specific anatomical sites and localized disease is also often used in varied combinations for the above advantages. Combining topicals into a single formulation also increases patient convenience and hence compliance.

Combination therapy is intended to induce faster remission in patients with severe or recalcitrant disease, frequent relapses, involvement of anatomical sites, such as scalp, flexures, genitalia, palms and soles, or associated PsA. There can be disastrous consequences when certain systemic medications and modalities are combined, and hence an evidence-based scientific approach is recommended. The adverse effects of combining systemic therapy involve immunosuppression and thereby infections, malignancies, organ toxicities, and those of topical therapy involve irritation.

Topical Combination Therapies

There are five strategies of combination therapy with topical agents, including proactive flare prevention, rotation therapy, sequential therapy, topical jump start therapy to enhance the efficacy of slow-acting topicals, and combining less effective but safer drugs for synergistic effects.[2] Topical CS are commonly used in combination with nonsteroidal topicals in the treatment of limited lesions of psoriasis.

Dithranol–CS: There are many studies on the use of clobetasol-17-propionate ointment with short-contact dithranol[3] with benefits of reducing treatment duration and faster clearance compared to either treatments alone. Steroids enhance the antipsoriatic action and reduce the irritation potential of dithranol. However, other topicals have largely replaced dithranol due to its irritation potential.

Calcipotriol–CS: Anti-inflammatory and immunoregulatory synergy has been best proven with calcipotriol and betamethasone dipropionate (Cal/BD) combination for the scalp, trunk, and extremities, the most efficacious being the supersaturated formulation. Calcipotriol modulates keratinocyte proliferation whereas steroids reduce inflammation and irritation induced by calcipotriol.[4] The combination received United States Food and Drug Administration (US FDA) approval in 2014 for the treatment of scalp psoriasis from the age of 12 years of age.[5]

Tazarotene–CS: This combination is beneficial as the therapeutic mechanisms are complementary and synergistic. In addition, CS reduces tazarotene-induced irritation and tazarotene can reduce CS-induced atrophy by its action on collagen.[6] Observational studies and randomized trials on tazarotene with betamethasone dipropionate/valerate, mometasone furoate, clobetasol propionate 0.05% ointment, and halobetasol show therapeutic effects. Once-daily application of fixed-dose combination of halobetasol propionate (0.01%) and tazarotene (0.045%) lotion (HP/TAZ) is approved for plaque psoriasis in adults and found effective in moderate-to-severe psoriasis, palmoplantar and scalp psoriasis based on open-label reports.[7] The polymeric emulsion technology employed in HP/TAZ lotion allows uniform delivery at lower doses and has hydrating properties as well.[6]

Tacrolimus–CS: The combination of halobetasol and tacrolimus was more efficacious and cost-effective compared to calcipotriol in a case report.[8]

Keratolytic–CS: Salicylic acid is used in varying concentrations for various anatomical sites, often as fixed-dose combinations for up to 20% body surface area (BSA). It facilitates removal of scales and, thereby, penetration of the CS and has antipruritic, bacteriostatic, and bactericidal activity. In a systematic review, combination of topical corticosteroids with keratolytics showed significant clinical response compared to monotherapy with topical steroids.[9]

Dithranol–calcipotriol: The preliminary open-label study did not show any superiority of this combination. Nevertheless, an randomized controlled trial (RCT), with short-contact dithranol and calcipotriol showed greater therapeutic efficacy than plain calcipotriol alone over a 6-week treatment duration. Mild skin irritation was observed in both groups, but this did not lead to treatment withdrawal.[10]

Tacrolimus–calcipotriene: This combination was superior to monotherapy with tacrolimus and comparable to calcipotriene monotherapy.[11]

Tacrolimus–salicylic acid: This combination (0.1 and 6%, respectively) was found to improve penetration of tacrolimus and thereby, clinical efficacy in plaque psoriasis.[12]

Tazarotene–calcipotriene: This combination did not achieve the desired effects compared to clobetasol ointment in a pilot study.[13] However, animal studies using the tazarotene-calcipotriol-loaded nanolipid carrier hydrogel formulation showed therapeutic effect and holds promise for a more effective combination.[14]

Tacrolimus–calcipotriol–CS: Case reports of rare psoriatic involvement of the lip responded to this combination.[15]

Topicals with Phototherapy

Coal tar–ultraviolet B (UVB): The traditional Goeckerman regimen uses coal tar and UVB and was developed in 1925 by the Mayo Clinic. It involves the application of 2–5% crude coal tar or any other tar three times daily or as often to keep the skin continually covered. After 24 hours, excess tar is removed by gentle wiping with cottonseed oil and exposed to broad-spectrum UV light. This is followed by a bath with ordinary soap to remove the residual tar and oil before reapplication of fresh tar for the next 24 hours. It has undergone various modifications for ease of use, compliance and efficacy, utilizing narrowband ultraviolet B (NB-UVB) and crude coal tar in varying concentrations from 2 to 10% with or without salicylic acid or lactic acid with a reduced duration of application from 1 to 6 hours. Variations include wrapping the coal tar applied area with cling film, combining with anthralin (1–10%), calcipotriene, tazarotene, acitretin, and bath psoralen-UVA (PUVA) three times a week.[16,17] Goeckerman therapy is more effective compared to NB-UVB in various studies.[18]

Corticosteroid-UVB: Clobetasol propionate with UVB was found to have better clearance than placebo with UVB.[19]

Dithranol–NBUVB: UVB followed by short-contact dithranol is an effective treatment modality and showed quicker response when combined with clobetasol.[20] The traditional Ingram regime involved daily tar baths followed by UVB and then application of dithranol in hard Lassar's paste wrapped by stockinette. This paste was removed by arachis oil after 24 hours.[21]

Calcipotriene–UVB/PUVA: Phototherapy when combined with calcipotriene is more efficacious than isolated phototherapy. This combination helps to reduce the dosage and frequency and at the same time augments the action of phototherapy. However calcipotriene should be applied only after and not before phototherapy as light can degrade calcipotriene.[2]

Tazarotene–UVB: This treatment also had additive therapeutic effects without significant adverse effects.[2]

Other combinations with phototherapy: Cal/BD aerosol foam with twice weekly NB-UVB,[22] calcipotriol/tacalcitol ointment, or tazarotene gel with PUVA are combinations that are comparably effective with earlier onset of action than PUVA alone, thereby reducing the cumulative dose of phototherapy.[23]

The combination of topical tacrolimus with phototherapy (UVA1) in palmar or plantar psoriasis was not found to be effective.[24]

Topicals with Systemic Medications

Systemic therapy is almost always augmented with topical therapy to target certain recalcitrant sites, which thereby helps lower the dose of the systemic drug. Topical CS and calcipotriol have been used effectively with methotrexate (MTX), cyclosporine A (CsA), acitretin, etretinate, and biologicals.[12] Evidence exists for the safe and effective use of dithranol with CsA.[25] It has even been suggested that using Cal/BD in combination with biologicals reduced the chances of switching therapy due to augmenting clinical response.[26]

Systemic Combination Therapies

Unlike other specialties, the combined use of disease-modifying antirheumatic drugs (DMARDs) is not common in dermatological practice. Data is available on drugs like MTX, CsA, acitretin, and lesser so, for mycophenolate mofetil (MMF) and hydroxyurea. A systematic review of MTX with other DMARDs suggested that since lower doses of each DMARD were used, it provided immunomodulatory benefits rather than immunosuppressive effects and earlier onset of action. There have been studies on its combination in rheumatoid arthritis (RA) and PsA even before psoriasis.[27] Combining systemic agents with topicals, phototherapy, or biologicals seems safer than combining conventional systemic drugs.

Methotrexate–CsA: This combination helps in rapid induction of disease control, which is especially beneficial in severe forms including pustular psoriasis and with PsA.[25] A systematic review on combination therapies with MTX found that the combination of MTX–CsA enabled lower doses of individual drugs with better response than monotherapy with either drug. When used in combination, the dose of MTX ranged from 7.5 to 20 mg/week and the dose of CsA went up to a maximum of only 3.5 mg/kg/day in various studies.[27] Lowering the daily dose of CsA (≤3 mg/kg/day) as studied in uveitis patients was found to have less risk of nephrotoxicity.[28] However, MTX–CsA pharmacokinetics potentially increases blood levels of each drug and decreases drug elimination, thereby causing increased serum creatinine and liver enzymes.[29] Though pharmacokinetic studies showed that MTX could be augmented by CsA, there was no clinically relevant outcome.[30] However, till larger studies are available, low-dose MTX is safer with CsA with stringent laboratory and clinical monitoring. When given for short durations ranging from 3 months to 1 year, the adverse effects seem to be minor and reversible and mainly attributed to CsA especially when given >3 months with few reports of transaminitis.[31-33]

Acitretin: Based on small studies and reports, acitretin works best in combination with phototherapy or other systemic agents or as sequential therapy rather than monotherapy.[34]

Acitretin–CsA combination was derived from its use for skin cancer prophylaxis in transplant recipients. Lipid levels need to be monitored closely.[35] There are variable reports of the usefulness of this combination in erythrodermic and plaque psoriasis with efficacy in some case series and lack of response in other case series. Reported adverse effects include dyslipidemia and effects related to CsA as well as retinoid dermatitis. Both drugs are metabolized by cytochrome-P450-dependent system in the liver and hence a potential risk for increased CsA exists.[36]

Methotrexate–acitretin: Based on the risk of hepatitis with MTX and etretinate (not available in most countries), there were similar concerns with acitretin, which can exist with alcohol intake (which can convert acitretin to etretinate). The incidence of hepatic fibrosis was similar in MTX monotherapy as well as MTX–acitretin and was associated with diabetes obesity.[27]

Apremilast: Due to its safety profile, it has been used effectively with many systemic agents such as MTX, acitretin, CsA, though current evidence is based on retrospective studies and case series only.[37]

Fumaric acid esters (FAE)–MTX: It leads to increased risk of immunosuppression.

According to a Delphi consensus, combinations that can be used with low-dose MTX for moderate-to-severe psoriasis in order of preference include tumor necrosis factor alpha (TNF-α) inhibitor (etanercept/adalimumab/infliximab), NBUVB, acitretin, alefacept, and CsA.[38] Reported adverse effects appeared more with MTX–CsA com-

CHAPTER 13: Combination and Rotational Therapy in the Management of Psoriasis

bination such as nephrotoxicity, nausea and vomiting, leukopenia, thrombocytopenia, and transaminitis compared to other combinations.[27] Hepatic fibrosis with MTX–acitretin and nausea and vomiting with MTX–apremilast are reported though none reached statistical significance compared to MTX monotherapy. Cumulative cancerogenic risks when combining immunomodulators are yet to be ascertained though short follow-up studies show no such effects.[27]

Combination therapy with Janus kinase (JAK) inhibitors: Real-time data is lacking on combinations with tofacitinib in psoriasis, which is increasingly being used due to its cost-effectiveness and availability. Recommendations are derived from its use in PsA and other immunological conditions. While JAK inhibitors can be combined with MTX, the National Psoriasis Foundation guidelines advise against combining potent immunosuppressive drugs such as CsA, tacrolimus, azathioprine, or biologics with JAK inhibitor. In PsA, it can also be combined with sulfasalazine and leflunomide **(Table 1)**.[37]

TABLE 1: Miscellaneous systemic combination therapies

Combination	Evidence	Benefits	Notable adverse effects	Comments
MMF (maximum 3 g daily) + low dose CsA (mean dose 2.5 mg/kg/day)[39]	Single retrospective study (n = 9)	Effective in severe, recalcitrant psoriasis (plaque/erythrodermic/pustular/with PsA) who had failed CsA either as monotherapy or with MTX, retinoids, hydroxyurea combinations	None	• Established regimen in organ transplantation • Lack of response in 2/9 patients • MMF may also have a therapeutic advantage in PsA and the combination does not appear to increase the toxicity of either drug; short-term MMF–CsA therapy appears safe; however, a small lymphoproliferative risk (1.2%) was reported with MMF in combination with cyclosporin and prednisolone in a transplant study
Hydroxyurea 1 g + acitretin 25 mg[40]	Single retrospective study (n = 13)	50% response	Bicytopenia in 1 patient at 4 weeks	• Potentially safe in psoriatic HIV patients • Acitretin may have protective effects against NMSC due to hydroxyurea
Hydroxyurea 500 mg + MTX 5–10 mg/week	Single study (n = 14) in psoriasis +/− PsA	Adequate response in 13/14 patients	GI intolerance in one patient	Theoretically can cause myelosuppression

(CsA: cyclosporine A; GI: gastrointestinal; HIV: human immunodeficiency virus; MMF: mycophenolate mofetil; MTX: methotrexate; NMSC: nonmelanoma skin cancers; PsA: psoriatic arthritis)

Unconventional medications as combinations: Other unconventional combinations include *acitretin–calcitriol* and *acitretin–pioglitazone* based on single RCTs, which proved effective without significant adverse effects.[41]

Systemic Medications with Phototherapy

Acitretin–UVB/PUVA: According to a systematic review, combining acitretin with UVB/PUVA was efficacious compared to either treatment as monotherapy and reduced the cumulative PUVA dose.[41] Acitretin may prevent nonmelanoma skin cancers (NMSC) while on long-term phototherapy. In a retrospective study, the combination of NBUVB was superior to broad-band UVB.[42] Re-PUVA[43] and re-UVB refers to the combination of retinoid derivatives (acitretin/etretinate) with PUVA and UVB, respectively. Acitretin is followed by phototherapy after 2 weeks, and if acitretin is added to an existing phototherapy regimen, the UV dose should be reduced by 50%. The dose of acitretin is recommended to be 25 mg/day or less.

Methotrexate–NBUVB: Based on RCTs, this combination effectively responds quicker than NBUVB alone without safety concerns.[41] *MTX–PUVA* is, however, associated with subacute phototoxicity, potential carcinogenesis, and suboptimal response in those previously refractory to PUVA.[35]

Apremilast–NBUVB: This combination is safe and useful, though not considered a routine option, with evidence based on case reports, retrospective studies, and an open-label prospective study.[41]

Biologicals with UVB/PUVA: Combination with TNF-α inhibitors (adalimumab/etanercept) was highly effective based on RCTs and open-label studies; however, there was limited evidence on the efficacy of its combination with ustekinumab. However, there are conflicting outcomes with alefacept-NBUVB combination when compared to NBUVB.[44] There are recommendations to limit its use for not longer than 24 weeks to avoid risk of malignancies.[41] There is a report of photocarcinogenicity in a patient using etanercept.[45] Based on a retrospective study comparing patients with psoriasis and RA who received TNF inhibitor therapy, the increased incidence of NMSC in psoriatics was suggested to be due to disease-related risk factors including phototherapy.[46]

Fumaric acid esters–NBUVB combination resulted in quicker and better response compared to monotherapy with FAE without increased adverse effects.[41]

Contraindicated combinations: These include CsA with NBUVB and PUVA to avoid NMSC.[25]

Biologicals with DMARDS, Acitretin, and Small Molecules

Biologicals used in the management of psoriasis include TNF-α inhibitors (etanercept, adalimumab, infliximab, golimumab), interleukin 17A (IL-17A) inhibitors (ixekizumab, secukinumab), and IL-12/23 inhibitors (ustekinumab). As per the recommendations of the Medical Board of the National Psoriasis Foundation 2015, when combination therapy with biologicals is resorted to, the preferred order would be MTX followed by acitretin followed by phototherapy. At the same time, there was insufficient data on the combination with acitretin, cyclosporine, or another biologic.[47] Factors that need consideration when combining a systemic agent with biological agent include teratogenicity, immunosuppression, nephrotoxicity, hepatotoxicity, bone marrow suppression, and carcinogenesis and can be used as an intermittent bridging therapy during flares.

Biologicals–MTX: The cohort study from the BIOBADADERM registry had demonstrated that there was no statistically significant increase in overall adverse events or infections when MTX was combined with TNF-α/IL-23/IL-17 inhibitors compared to biologic monotherapy. However an increase in gastrointestinal adverse effects with TNF-α inhibitor–MTX combination was attributable to the oral MTX used.[48]

Tumor necrosis factor alpha inhibitors–MTX: Most existing evidence is from using MTX with etanercept in psoriasis. MTX, the most combined DMARD with biologicals, particularly TNF inhibitors, reduces the immunogenicity and improves drug survival. A meta-analysis of RCTs on monotherapy with biologicals versus combination therapy of biologics with MTX in psoriasis showed therapeutic advantages without serious adverse effects. The study, however, mentioned a higher incidence of infections and nausea when combined, without highlighting the nature of infections, which could be a limitation in certain situations.[49] Similar conclusions on efficacy were drawn from a systematic review of TNF-α inhibitors–MTX combination, which looked at infliximab and etanercept in psoriasis and golimumab in PsA. Studies on infliximab have shown that antidrug antibodies reduced the efficacy, and MTX addition improved the clinical efficacy and cleared these antibodies.[41] Similar effects were observed while adding MTX or thiopurine to infliximab or adalimumab in patients with inflammatory bowel disease, leading to improved clinical response.[50] Nevertheless, the development of antidrug antibodies with etanercept was not found to be clinically relevant. The efficacy of MTX-biologic combination therapy, however, does not sometimes extend to PsA where monotherapy with biologics was sufficient.[49,51]

Tumor necrosis factor alpha inhibitors–CsA: CsA was more effective than MTX when combined with etanercept, especially for moderate-to-severe psoriatic skin disease in patients with PsA in an RCT.[52] There are case series, case reports, and retrospective studies that also show efficacy of this combination without serious side effects.[53]

Tumor necrosis factor alpha inhibitors-acitretin: RCTs looking at the efficacy of combining etanercept with acitretin showed that it was superior to acitretin monotherapy and advantageous as the dose of etanercept could be lowered.[41]

Various other biologicals with acitretin had suboptimal responses in case reports.

Biologicals–apremilast: This is a reasonable and safe combination in psoriasis with PsA, especially when the effect of the biological agent wears off.[41] A systematic review on this combination in plaque psoriasis, palmoplantar pustulosis and pustular psoriasis found no difference in adverse effects compared to apremilast monotherapy, which were primarily gastrointestinal. Few discontinued therapy due to lack of efficacy. However, clinical trials with well-defined outcomes are necessary to make accurate conclusions.[54] Examples of biologicals used include secukinumab, TNF-α inhibitors, and ustekinumab.

Tumor necrosis factor alpha inhibitor–FAE: An RCT combining etanercept and FAE showed quicker response and tolerability compared to etanercept alone; however, there was no significant difference in overall.[41] There are concerns of immunosuppression and lymphopenia.[55]

A systematic review on the combination of conventional DMARDs with *IL-17 inhibitors* in psoriasis failed to show any benefit; however case series/reports showed some benefit on combining IL-17 inhibitors with *acitretin* or *apremilast*.[56] In those with inadequate response to secukinumab, the addition of low dose acitretin helped to achieve clearance of psoriasis (plaque, erythrodermic and pustular variants) in case series.[57]

Dual Biologic Therapy

Combination of biologicals are rare in dermatology and are used in special scenarios such as a single agent cannot address all aspects of the diseases such as, additional PsA or palmoplantar pustulosis; loss of efficacy of one biological; quick induction in severe disease; paradoxical psoriasis with TNF-α inhibitors; and other concomitant immune-mediated diseases. Examples of such combinations include ustekinumab/guselkumab/risankizumab/secukinumab with TNF-α inhibitors (etanercept/adalimumab/golimumab/certolizumab pegol or adalimumab with omalizumab or guselkumab with dupilumab.[58] However, the financial burden has to be factored in before considering dual biological therapy.

Biologics with Janus Kinase/Tyrosine Kinase 2 Inhibitors

A case series on five patients with psoriasis and one with PsA had demonstrated the efficacy and safety profile of the combination of oral JAK/TYK2 (tyrosine kinase 2) inhibitors with biologics involving combinations of upadacitinib/deucravacitinib with IL-17 inhibitors such as ixekizumab/brodalumab/guselkumab in those who had previously failed systemic monotherapies. It is postulated that combination therapy leads to a marked reduction of total cytokines. As there is a difference in the cytokine expression in the synovium and skin (higher IL-17, IL-23 signatures in the skin), agents targeting the IL-17 axis have a greater impact on the skin. Though TYK2 inhibitors do not have the potential of malignancy or cardiac events, unlike JAK1 inhibitors, follow-up studies are recommended to assess long-term adverse effects.[59]

A retrospective review of three patients with psoriasis and PsA has highlighted the efficacy of combining upadacitinib with biological agents, such as risankizumab, brodalumab, and ixekizumab. The efficacy is probably due to the independent inhibition of dual pathways STAT3/IL-6 (upadacitinib) and IL-17/IL-23 axis (biologics). The authors, however, warn to look out for infections with this combination.[60]

ROTATIONAL THERAPY

Rotational therapy refers to the periodic rotation of medications to minimize cumulative dosing and toxicities, giving long gaps for each medication. Treatment is switched abruptly to agents with unrelated target organ toxicities. In 1993, Weinstein and White first proposed rotating various therapies (UVB/PUVA, MTX, and etretinate) every 1–2 years. It seems logical to rotate immunosuppressive therapies with retinoids to decrease overall carcinogenicity. However, there are multiple reports and studies on rotating immunosuppressive therapy.

Rotational Therapy with Cyclosporine A

It is recommended to limit CsA use to 1–2 years to prevent long-term toxicities as per US and UK guidelines, respectively. However, CsA can be used intermittently as its effects persist for 2–3 months after discontinuation.[25] Rotational therapy of CsA and *MTX* can be used with caution. Intermittent short courses (12 weeks) of cyclosporine have less risk of nephrotoxicity compared to continuous therapy.[61] Giving a break from CsA in patients with uveitis has been found to help recover early changes of CsA-induced nephrotoxicity, which may take up to 6 months to 2 years. Switching over to a potent DMARD like MTX helps maintain clinical response.[62] Irreversible renal changes with CsA and the hepatic changes with MTX are related to cumulative dosage.[63]

Rotational Therapy with Biologicals

Biologicals are devoid of organ toxicities and hence can be alternated with DMARDs or preferable retinoids to prevent further immunosuppression. Switching to etanercept following induction with CsA effectively maintained clinical response in psoriasis without any significant adverse effects directly related to the drugs.[64]

Rotating between biologicals occurs more often than reported in clinical practice. A retrospective study found that 46% of patients switched between efalizumab (suspended), infliximab, etanercept, or adalimumab. Few did not respond to up to three biologicals and ultimately responded to ustekinumab. The reasons for inefficacy might be neutralizing antibodies or genetic variations.

Rotational Use of Topicals

It typically involves rotating a steroid and a nonsteroidal topical to prevent cutaneous side effects of topical steroids and at the same time avoiding a rebound of disease.

Weekly rotation between augmented betamethasone dipropionate 0.05% cream once daily and calcipotriene 0.005% ointment was found to be more effective than betamethasone dipropionate 0.05% cream once daily over 4 weeks, probably due to lower chance of tachyphylaxis.[65]

The same principle is utilized in using calcitriol ointment twice daily on weekdays and clobetasol propionate spray twice daily on weekends.[66]

■ SEQUENTIAL THERAPY

Therapy is switched intentionally in a specific sequence to induce remission, followed by maintenance. First described by Koo, the process involves (1) the clearing phase—when a potent, quick-acting agent is initiated, often at the maximum dose, (2) the transitional phase—when a safer, well-tolerable medication is added for maintenance, such as acitretin is while the initial agent is gradually tapered off, and (3) the maintenance phase—the maintenance drug is continued with additional therapy if required. It involves a strategic change in therapies, unlike rotational therapy. However, deliberate sequencing may not always be the case, and therapy may be sequentially changed due to lack of sustained efficacy. The requirement of a washout period between the two drugs is dependent on the type of drug. With acitretin and biological agents, a washout period is not required, but the period of contraception needs to be remembered; however, when two immunosuppressive agents are considered, it is wise to keep the overlap period as minimum as possible.

Cyclosporine A followed by acitretin: Based on case reports, CsA (at a maximum of 5 mg/kg) sequentially followed by acitretin while tapering off CsA and adding UVB/PUVA when necessary was suggested as a treatment strategy; the only potential adverse effect being dyslipidemia during the transition phase when both drugs are combined briefly.[67,68]

Cyclosporine A followed by phototherapy: Short-course low-dose CsA (3 mg/kg for 4 weeks) followed by sequential NBUVB phototherapy with rapid tapering of CsA showed quick response and low phototherapy dosing.[69]

Biologicals: A systematic review and meta-analysis showed that clinical efficacy can occur up to 4th line biological treatment in sequential therapy with biologicals and targeted small molecule drugs.[70] Two biologicals can be used sequentially where a biologic with a faster onset of action, such as efalizumab (not approved) or infliximab, is used for induction, and those known to provide long remissions, such as alefacept or etanercept, are used as maintenance.[45]

Topicals

A randomized open-label study showed that sequential therapy of tazarotene 0.1% and calcitriol 0.003% in either direction was comparable to calcitriol monotherapy and superior to tazarotene monotherapy in plaque psoriasis.[71]

An RCT on sequential therapy of mometasone furoate 0.1% and salicylic acid 5% for 7 days followed by mometasone furoate 0.1% for 14 days was efficacious compared to using mometasone alone.[72]

An open-label study on sequential therapy with clobetasol propionate 0.05% spray for up to 4 weeks followed by calcitriol 3 µg/g ointment for 8 weeks was effective in the management of moderate-to-severe plaque psoriasis.[73]

A summary of the salient points to remember while combining various treatment modalities in psoriasis is given in **Table 2**.

TABLE 2: Highlights of various combination therapies

Combination	Highlight
Vitamin D analog + phototherapy	Vitamin D analog must be applied after phototherapy as light can degrade it
Tazarotene + phototherapy	A low dose of UVB is required when combined with topical tazarotene
Acitretin + phototherapy	• Synergistic effect reducing the number and dose of phototherapy and retinoids • Acitretin reduces cancer incidence and is beneficial when combined with PUVA
Acitretin + cyclosporine	While cyclosporine increases the risk of cancer, acitretin has anticancer properties
Cyclosporine + phototherapy	Not recommended in view of carcinogenicity
Cyclosporine + acitretin	To be cautious of dyslipidemia
Cyclosporine + methotrexate	When combined both can be given at lower doses reducing the risk of hepatotoxicity (methotrexate) and nephrotoxicity (cyclosporine)
Acitretin + methotrexate	Liver function and risk of fibrosis are to be closely monitored
Methotrexate + apremilast	Augmentation of gastrointestinal side effects
Methotrexate + NSAIDs	NSAIDs, in particular naproxen, increase the blood level of methotrexate
Hydroxyurea + acitretin	Useful in HIV patients as these are not immunosuppressive; additional benefit of the antiviral effect of hydroxyurea
Methotrexate + hydroxyurea	High risk of bone marrow toxicity
Methotrexate + TNF-α inhibitors	Methotrexate can decrease the immunogenicity associated with TNF blockers

(HIV: human immunodeficiency virus; NSAIDs: nonsteroidal anti-inflammatory drugs; PUVA: psoralen-UVA; TNF-α: tumor necrosis factor alpha; UVB: ultraviolet B)

TAKE HOME MESSAGE

- Various drugs, topical and/or systemic medications can be used together as combination, rotational or sequential therapy.
- Combination therapy is advantageous as it provides increased therapeutic benefit due to synergistic effects, targets varied pathogenetic pathways and minimize adverse effects due to lower doses of individual medications.
- While certain combination therapies like vitamin D analogues and topical corticosteroids have good evidence, most combinations lack clear-cut evidence
- There can be untoward side effects with certain combinations (e.g., cyclosporine and phototherapy); hence, an evidence-based systematic approach needs to be followed.
- Topical corticosteroid is the most common topical agent used in combination therapy.
- Due to the safety profile, apremilast is used with various systemic agents.
- Methotrexate is the most preferred conventional systemic agent with biological agents.

CONCLUSION

Dermatologists often resort to various therapeutic combinations in difficult-to-treat psoriasis. Understanding evidence-based outcomes of combination, rotational, and sequential therapy and their potential side effects will help the clinician to manage this chronic condition optimally without fear, even while exercising caution where required.

REFERENCES

1. Feldman SR, Zhang J, Martinez DJ, Lopez-Gonzalez L, Hoit Marchlewicz E, Shrady G, et al. Real-world biologic and apremilast treatment patterns in patients with psoriasis and psoriatic arthritis. Dermatol Online J. 2021;27.
2. Koo K, Jeon C, Bhutani T. Beyond monotherapy: a systematic review on creative strategies in topical therapy of psoriasis. J Dermatolog Treat. 2017;28:702-8.
3. Swinkels OQJ, Prins M, Kucharekova M, de Boo T, Gerritsen MJP, van der Valk PGM, et al. Combining lesional short-contact dithranol therapy of psoriasis with a potent topical corticosteroid. Br J Dermatol. 2002;146:621-6.
4. Satake K, Amano T, Okamoto T. Calcipotriol and betamethasone dipropionate synergistically enhances the balance between regulatory and proinflammatory T cells in a murine psoriasis model. Sci Rep. 2019;9:16322.
5. Osier E, Gomez B, Eichenfield LF. Adolescent Scalp Psoriasis: Update on Topical Combination Therapy. J Clin Aesthet Dermatol. 2015;8:43-7.
6. Lebwohl MG, Tanghetti EA, Stein Gold L, Del Rosso JQ, Gilyadov NK, Jacobson A. Fixed-Combination Halobetasol Propionate and Tazarotene in the Treatment of Psoriasis: Narrative Review of Mechanisms of Action and Therapeutic Benefits. Dermatol Ther (Heidelb). 2021;11:1157-74.
7. Kircik L, Tanghetti EA, Friedman A, Kucera K, Jacobson A. Challenges in Psoriatic Disease Addressed by Fixed-Combination Halobetasol Propionate 0.01% and Tazarotene 0.045% Lotion. J Clin Aesthet Dermatol. 2023;16:21-6.
8. Sarwar MZ, Khan NH, Beg MiMA, Ankolvi NMJ, Osmonaliev K. The Management of Plaque Psoriasis With Halobetasol and Tacrolimus Combination Therapy Versus Calcipotriol Monotherapy: A Case Report. Cureus. 16:e52445.
9. Jacobi A, Mayer A, Augustin M. Keratolytics and Emollients and Their Role in the Therapy of Psoriasis: a Systematic Review. Dermatol Ther (Heidelb). 2015;5:1-18.
10. Monastirli A, Georgiou S, Pasmatzi E, Sakkis T, Badavanis G, Drainas D, et al. Calcipotriol plus short-contact dithranol: a novel topical combination therapy for chronic plaque psoriasis. Skin Pharmacol Appl Skin Physiol. 2002;15:246-51.
11. Tirado-Sánchez A, Ponce-Olivera RM. Preliminary study of the efficacy and tolerability of combination therapy with calcipotriene ointment 0.005% and tacrolimus ointment 0.1% in the treatment of stable plaque psoriasis. Cutis. 2012;90:140-4.
12. Chat VS, Kearns DG, Uppal SK, Han G, Wu JJ. Management of Psoriasis With Topicals: Applying the 2020 AAD-NPF Guidelines of Care to Clinical Practice. Cutis. 2022;110:8-14.

13. Bowman PH, Maloney JE, Koo JYM. Combination of calcipotriene (Dovonex) ointment and tazarotene (Tazorac) gel versus clobetasol ointment in the treatment of plaque psoriasis: a pilot study. J Am Acad Dermatol. 2002;46:907-13.
14. Thakur S, Anjum MM, Jaiswal S, Gautam AK, Rajinikanth PS. Tazarotene-calcipotriol loaded Nanostructured lipid carrier enriched hydrogel: A novel dual drug synergistic approach towards Psoriasis management. J Drug Del Sci Tech. 2023;88:104944.
15. Sehgal VN, Sehgal S, Verma P, Singh N, Rasool F. Exclusive plaque psoriasis of the lips: efficacy of combination therapy of topical tacrolimus, calcipotriol, and betamethasone dipropionate. Skinmed. 2012;10:183-4.
16. Lee E, Koo J. Modern modified "ultra" Goeckerman therapy: a PASI assessment of a very effective therapy for psoriasis resistant to both prebiologic and biologic therapies. J Dermatolog Treat. 2005;16:102-7.
17. Perry HO, Soderstrom CW, Schulze RW. The Goeckerman treatment of psoriasis. Arch Dermatol. 1968;98:178-82.
18. Çalışkan E, Tunca M, Açıkgöz G, Arca E, Yürekli A, Akar A. Narrow band ultraviolet-B versus Goeckerman therapy for psoriasis with and without acitretin: A retrospective study. Indian J Dermatol Venereol Leprol. 2015;81:584-7.
19. Larkö O, Swanbeck G, Svartholm H. The effect on psoriasis of clobetasol propionate used alone or in combination with UVB. Acta Derm Venereol. 1984;64:151-4.
20. Lidbrink P, Johannesson A, Hammar H. Psoriasis treatment: faster clearance when UVB-dithranol is combined with topical clobetasol propionate. Dermatologica. 1986;172:164-8.
21. Statham BN, Ryatt KS, Rowell NR. Short-contact dithranol therapy--a comparison with the Ingram regime. Br J Dermatol. 1984;110:703-8.
22. Licata G, Arisi M, Venturini M, Rossi M, Tomasi C, Calzavara-Pinton I, et al. Pretreatment with an Aerosol Foam Containing Calcipotriene and Betamethasone Strongly Improves the Efficacy of Narrow-Band UVB Phototherapy. Dermatol Ther (Heidelb). 2022;12:2161-71.
23. Tzaneva S, Hönigsmann H, Tanew A, Seeber A. A comparison of psoralen plus ultraviolet A (PUVA) monotherapy, tacalcitol plus PUVA and tazarotene plus PUVA in patients with chronic plaque-type psoriasis. Br J Dermatol. 2002;147:748-53.
24. Rivard J, Janiga J, Lim HW. Tacrolimus ointment 0.1% alone and in combination with medium-dose UVA1 in the treatment of palmar or plantar psoriasis. J Drugs Dermatol. 2006;5:505-10.
25. Colombo MD, Cassano N, Bellia G, Vena GA. Cyclosporine Regimens in Plaque Psoriasis: An Overview with Special Emphasis on Dose, Duration, and Old and New Treatment Approaches. Sci World J. 2013;2013:805705.
26. Rudnicka L, Olszewska M, Goldust M, Waśkiel-Burnat A, Warszawik-Hendzel O, Dorożyński P, et al. Efficacy and Safety of Different Formulations of Calcipotriol/Betamethasone Dipropionate in Psoriasis: Gel, Foam, and Ointment. J Clin Med. 2021;10:5589.
27. Hsieh TS, Tsai TF. Combination Therapy for Psoriasis with Methotrexate and Other Oral Disease-Modifying Antirheumatic Drugs: A Systematic Review. Dermatol Ther (Heidelb). 2023;13:891-909.
28. Isnard Bagnis C, Tezenas du Montcel S, Beaufils H, Jouanneau C, Jaudon MC, Maksud P, et al. Long-term renal effects of low-dose cyclosporine in uveitis-treated patients: follow-up study. J Am Soc Nephrol. 2002;13(12):2962-8.
29. Korstanje MJ, van Breda Vriesman CJ, van de Staak WJ. Cyclosporine and methotrexate: a dangerous combination. J Am Acad Dermatol. 1990;23:320-1.
30. Odderskov C, Stengaard-Pedersen K, Ellingsen T, Hornung N. Methotrexate pharmacokinetic is influenced by co-administration of cyclosporin in rheumatoid arthritis patients. Results from a randomized clinical trial. Scand J Clin Lab Invest. 2020;80:185-90.
31. Aydin F, Canturk T, Senturk N, Turanli AY. Methotrexate and ciclosporin combination for the treatment of severe psoriasis. Clin Exp Dermatol. 2006;31:520-4.
32. Clark CM, Kirby B, Morris AD, Davison S, Zaki I, Emerson R, et al. Combination treatment with methotrexate and cyclosporin for severe recalcitrant psoriasis. Br J Dermatol. 1999;141:279-82.
33. Mohanan S, Ramassamy S, Chandrashekar L, Thappa DM. A retrospective analysis of combination methotrexate-cyclosporine therapy in moderate-severe psoriasis. J Dermatolog Treat. 2014;25:50-3.
34. Balak DMW, Gerdes S, Parodi A, Salgado-Boquete L. Long-term Safety of Oral Systemic Therapies for Psoriasis: A Comprehensive Review of the Literature. Dermatol Ther (Heidelb). 2020;10:589-613.
35. Lebwohl M, Menter A, Koo J, Feldman SR. Combination therapy to treat moderate to severe psoriasis. J Am Acad Dermatol. 2004;50:416-30.
36. Kuijpers AL, van Dooren-Greebe JV, van de Kerkhof PC. Failure of combination therapy with acitretin and cyclosporin A in 3 patients with erythrodermic psoriasis. Dermatology. 1997;194:88-90.

37. Menter A, Gelfand JM, Connor C, Armstrong AW, Cordoro KM, Davis DMR, et al. Joint American Academy of Dermatology–National Psoriasis Foundation guidelines of care for the management of psoriasis with systemic nonbiologic therapies. J Am Acad Dermatol. 2020;82:1445-86.
38. Strober BE, Clay Cather J, Cohen D, Crowley JJ, Gordon KB, Gottlieb AB, et al. A Delphi Consensus Approach to Challenging Case Scenarios in Moderate-to-Severe Psoriasis: Part 2. Dermatol Ther (Heidelb). 2012;2:2.
39. Ameen M, Smith HR, Barker JN. Combined mycophenolate mofetil and cyclosporin therapy for severe recalcitrant psoriasis. Clin Exp Dermatol. 2001;26:480-3.
40. Narang T, Kumar S, Handa S, Dogra S. Hydroxyurea and acitretin as a novel combination therapy in severe plaque psoriasis. Br J Dermatol. 2018;179:1212-3.
41. Arora S, Das P, Arora G. Systematic Review and Recommendations to Combine Newer Therapies With Conventional Therapy in Psoriatic Disease. Front Med (Lausanne). 2021;8:696597.
42. Spuls PI, Rozenblit M, Lebwohl M. Retrospective study of the efficacy of narrowband UVB and acitretin. J Dermatolog Treat. 2003;14 Suppl 2:17-20.
43. Orfanos CE, Pullmann H, Sterry W, Künzig M. Retinoid PUVA (RePUVA): systemic combination therapy in psoriasis. Z Hautkr. 1978;53:494-504.
44. Jacobe H, Winterfield L, Kim F, Huet-Adams B, Cayce R. The role of narrowband UV-B plus alefacept combination therapy in the treatment of psoriasis. Arch Dermatol. 2008;144:1067-8; author reply 1068-9.
45. Lebwohl M. Combining the new biologic agents with our current psoriasis armamentarium. J Am Acad Dermatol. 2003;49:S118-124.
46. van Lümig PPM, Menting SP, van den Reek JMPA, Spuls PI, van Riel PLCM, van de Kerkhof PCM, et al. An increased risk of non-melanoma skin cancer during TNF-inhibitor treatment in psoriasis patients compared to rheumatoid arthritis patients probably relates to disease-related factors. J Eur Acad Dermatol Venereol. 2015;29:752-60.
47. Armstrong AW, Bagel J, Van Voorhees AS, Robertson AD, Yamauchi PS. Combining biologic therapies with other systemic treatments in psoriasis: evidence-based, best-practice recommendations from the Medical Board of the National Psoriasis Foundation. JAMA Dermatol. 2015;151:432-8.
48. Lluch-Galcerá JJ, Carrascosa JM, González-Quesada A, Rivera-Díaz R, Sahuquillo-Torralba A, Llamas-Velasco M, et al. Safety of biologic therapy in combination with methotrexate in moderate to severe psoriasis: a cohort study from the BIOBADADERM registry. Br J Dermatol. 2024;190:355-63.
49. Xie Y, Liu Y, Liu Y. Are biologics combined with methotrexate better than biologics monotherapy in psoriasis and psoriatic arthritis: A meta-analysis of randomized controlled trials. Dermatol Ther. 2021;34:e14926.
50. Strik AS, van den Brink GR, Ponsioen C, Mathot R, Löwenberg M, D'Haens GR. Suppression of anti-drug antibodies to infliximab or adalimumab with the addition of an immunomodulator in patients with inflammatory bowel disease. Aliment Pharmacol Ther. 2017;45:1128-34.
51. Mease PJ, Reddy S, Ross S, Lisse JR, Reis P, Griffing K, et al. Evaluating the efficacy of biologics with and without methotrexate in the treatment of psoriatic arthritis: a network meta-analysis. RMD Open. 2024;10:e003423.
52. Atzeni F, Boccassini L, Antivalle M, Salaffi F, Sarzi-Puttini P. Etanercept plus ciclosporin versus etanercept plus methotrexate for maintaining clinical control over psoriatic arthritis: a randomised pilot study. Ann Rheum Dis. 2011;70(4):712-4.
53. Vena GA, Mastrandrea V, Battaglini S, Loconsole F, Buquicchio R, Cassano N. Combination of Etanercept and Twice-Weekly Administration of Cyclosporin in Psoriasis Unsatisfactorily Controlled by Etanercept Monotherapy: A Retrospective Analysis. Eur J Inflamm. 2012;10:239-42.
54. Gyldenløve M, Alinaghi F, Zachariae C, Skov L, Egeberg A. Combination Therapy with Apremilast and Biologics for Psoriasis: A Systematic Review. Am J Clin Dermatol. 2022;23:605-13.
55. Nast A, Spuls PI, van der Kraaij G, Gisondi P, Paul C, Ormerod AD, et al. European S3-Guideline on the systemic treatment of psoriasis vulgaris - Update Apremilast and Secukinumab - EDF in cooperation with EADV and IPC. J Eur Acad Dermatol Venereol. 2017;31:1951-63.
56. Martin A, Thatiparthi A, Liu J, Wu JJ. Interleukin-17 Inhibitor Combination Therapies for the Treatment of Psoriasis: A Systematic Review. J Clin Aesthet Dermatol. 2022;15:S19-31.
57. Polat Ekinci A, Bölük KN, Babuna Kobaner G. Secukinumab and acitretin as a combination therapy for three clinical forms of severe psoriasis in multi-drug refractory patients: A case series of high efficacy and safety profile. Dermatol Ther. 2021;34:e14704.
58. Diotallevi F, Paolinelli M, Radi G, Offidani A. Latest combination therapies in psoriasis: Narrative review of the literature. Dermatol Ther. 2022;35:e15759.

59. Hren MG, Khattri S. Treatment of recalcitrant psoriasis and psoriatic arthritis with a combination of a biologic plus an oral JAK or TYK2 inhibitor: a case series. Ann Rheum Dis. 2024;83:1392-3.
60. Amara S, Patel A, Lebwohl M. Safety and Efficacy of Combination Therapy of Upadacitinib and Biologic Agents for Treatment-Resistant Psoriasis and Psoriatic Arthritis. J Skin. 2024;8:1574-80.
61. Choi CW, Kim BR, Ohn J, Youn SW. The Advantage of Cyclosporine A and Methotrexate Rotational Therapy in Long-Term Systemic Treatment for Chronic Plaque Psoriasis in a Real World Practice. Ann Dermatol. 2017;29:55-60.
62. Ellis CN, Reiter KL, Bandekar RR, Fendrick AM. Cost-effectiveness comparison of therapy for psoriasis with a methotrexate-based regimen versus a rotation regimen of modified cyclosporine and methotrexate. J Am Acad Dermatol. 2002;46:242-50.
63. Tostivint I, du Montcel ST, Jaudon MC, Mallet A, Le Hoang P, Bodaghi B, et al. Renal outcome after ciclosporin-induced nephrotoxicity. Nephrol Dial Transplant. 2007;22:880-5.
64. Micali G, Wilsmann-Theis D, Mallbris L, Gallo G, Marino V, Brault Y, et al. Etanercept reduces symptoms and severity of psoriasis after cessation of cyclosporine therapy: results of the SCORE study. Acta Derm Venereol. 2015;95:57-61.
65. Singh S, Reddy DC, Pandey SS. Topical therapy for psoriasis with the use of augmented beta-methasone and calcipotriene on alternate weeks. J Am Acad Dermatol. 2000;43:61-5.
66. Hudson CP, Kempers S, Menter A, Papp K, Smith S, Sofen H, et al. An open-label, multicenter study of the efficacy and safety of a weekday/weekend treatment regimen with calcitriol ointment 3 microg/g and clobetasol propionate spray 0.05% in the management of plaque psoriasis. Cutis. 2011;88:201-7.
67. Koo J. Systemic sequential therapy of psoriasis: a new paradigm for improved therapeutic results. J Am Acad Dermatol. 1999;41:S25-8.
68. Short MW, Vaughan TK. Sequential therapy using cyclosporine and acitretin for treatment of total body psoriasis. Cutis. 2004;74:185-8.
69. Calzavara-Pinton P, Leone G, Venturini M, Sala R, Colombo D, La Parola IL, et al. A comparative non randomized study of narrow-band (NB) (312 +/- 2 nm) UVB phototherapy versus sequential therapy with oral administration of low-dose Cyclosporin A and NB-UVB phototherapy in patients with severe psoriasis vulgaris. Eur J Dermatol. 2005;15:470-3.
70. Gollins CE, Vincent R, Fahy C, McHugh N, Tillett W. Effectiveness of sequential lines of biologic and targeted small molecule drugs in psoriasis: A systematic review and meta-analysis. Skin Health Dis. 2024;4:e350.
71. Sidhu JK, Matreja PS, Gupta AK, Singh A, Singh S. Head-to-Head Comparison of Tazarotene and Calcitriol with or without Sequential Therapy in Mild-to-Moderate Psoriasis: A Randomized Open-label Study. J Res Pharm Pract. 2024;12:44-8.
72. Tiplica GS, Salavastru CM. Mometasone furoate 0.1% and salicylic acid 5% vs. mometasone furoate 0.1% as sequential local therapy in psoriasis vulgaris. J Eur Acad Dermatol Venereol. 2009;23:905-12.
73. Brodell RT, Bruce S, Hudson CP, Weiss JS, Colón LE, Johnson LA, et al. A multi-center, open-label study to evaluate the safety and efficacy of a sequential treatment regimen of clobetasol propionate 0.05% spray followed by Calcitriol 3 mg/g ointment in the management of plaque psoriasis. J Drugs Dermatol. 2011;10:158-64.

14

Management of Psoriatic Arthritis: Diagnosis and Treatment Options

Ashish Jacob Mathew

■ INTRODUCTION

Psoriatic arthritis (PsA) is a complex, chronic, inflammatory disease characterized by peripheral arthritis, axial disease, enthesitis, and dactylitis. It is observed in nearly a third of patients with psoriasis and has an equal prevalence in both sexes. For the most part, psoriasis precedes the development of PsA. Nonetheless, in 20% of patients, PsA can manifest before psoriasis and in about 15%, skin and musculoskeletal symptoms co-occur.[1,2] Early diagnosis of PsA is paramount to minimizing long-term worse outcomes, including radiographic damage and burden of comorbidities, and initiating appropriate treatment, thus promoting a better quality of life in patients.[3] This could, however, be challenging given the frequency of nonspecific symptoms and the need for reliable diagnostic biomarkers in PsA. Acute phase reactants can often be normal, even in patients with active PsA. Thus, PsA mostly continues to be a clinical diagnosis.[4] Dermatology clinics are among the earliest contact points for diagnosing PsA, and dermatologists have a critical role in recognizing the early symptoms.

The treatment options and outcomes of psoriatic disease have undergone a paradigm change over the past few decades, with targeted therapies playing a vital role.[5] Nonetheless, the complex heterogeneity of psoriatic disease poses significant management challenges in routine care (**Fig. 1**). This chapter engages with the diagnosis and treatment of PsA, detailing the options and complexities of early detection and management.

■ CHARACTERIZATION OF PATIENTS WITH PSORIASIS AT RISK OF DEVELOPING PSORIATIC ARTHRITIS

Conversion of psoriasis to PsA occurs in up to 3% of patients every year. Identifying patients with psoriasis at risk of developing PsA by characterizing clinical, musculoskeletal imaging, and laboratory features, which shape the preclinical stages of the disease, is critical.[6] Musculoskeletal imaging-like ultrasound (MSUS) and magnetic resonance imaging (MRI) have enhanced our understanding of the pathogenesis of PsA to a great extent.[7] The preclinical phases of PsA can be described in three categories:[8-10]

1. *Psoriasis patients with increased risk of PsA*: Individuals with psoriasis who have one or more clinical (presence of arthralgia, severe psoriasis, nail or scalp psoriasis) or genetic risk factors for developing PsA.
2. Individuals with psoriasis who have synovio-entheseal abnormalities in MSUS or MRI but no clinical symptoms.
3. Psoriasis patients and musculoskeletal symptoms that another diagnosis cannot explain.

CHAPTER 14: Management of Psoriatic Arthritis: Diagnosis and Treatment Options

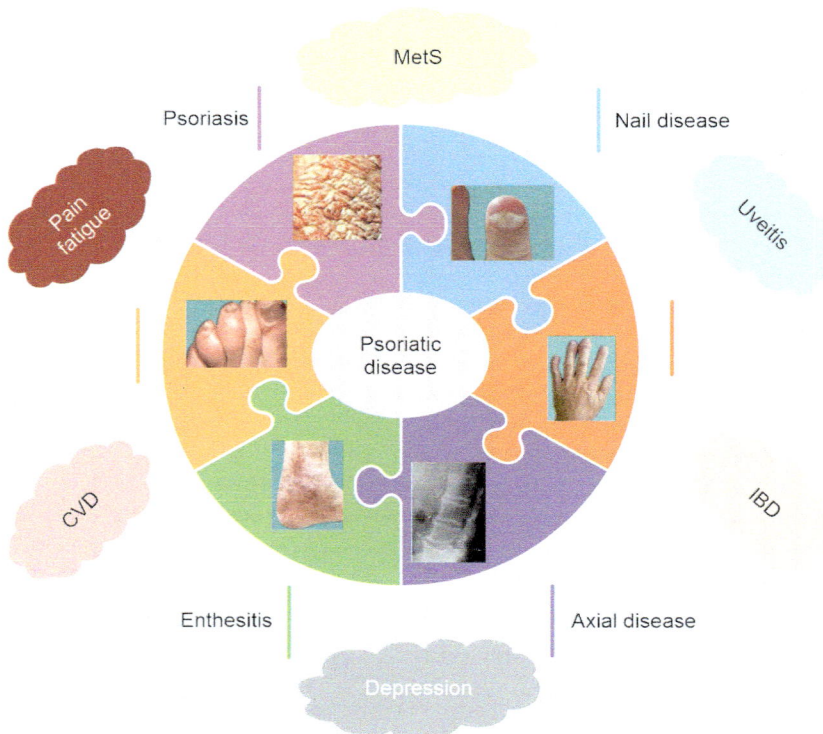

FIG. 1: Clinical domains and associated conditions of psoriatic disease.
(CVD: cardiovascular disease; IBD: inflammatory bowel disease; MetS: metabolic syndrome)

DIAGNOSING PSORIATIC ARTHRITIS

Psoriatic arthritis is a multifaceted disease that involves musculoskeletal and extra-musculoskeletal features that may manifest in combination in a particular patient. The overall disease burden depends on the extent and severity of each clinical domain individually and together.[11] The musculoskeletal domains in PsA include peripheral arthritis, axial disease, enthesitis, and dactylitis.

Identifying the Musculoskeletal Clinical Domains in Psoriatic Arthritis

The involvement of small joints in upper and lower limbs may be asymmetric and initially restricted to a few joints. However, multiple joints may get involved symmetrically with time, resembling features of rheumatoid arthritis (RA). The involvement of distal interphalangeal joints and interphalangeal joints of thumbs, along with the distribution of arthritis, can differentiate between PsA and RA, gouty arthritis, and osteoarthritis.[12] Enthesitis is a common clinical manifestation in patients with PsA that may occur early in its course. However, this feature could be present in other conditions like diabetes, obesity, and metabolic syndrome, which frequently coexist with PsA. Mechanical enthesitis is often observed in elderly individuals. Clinical examination of enthesitis is usually challenging and nonspecific, considering

CHAPTER 14: Management of Psoriatic Arthritis: Diagnosis and Treatment Options

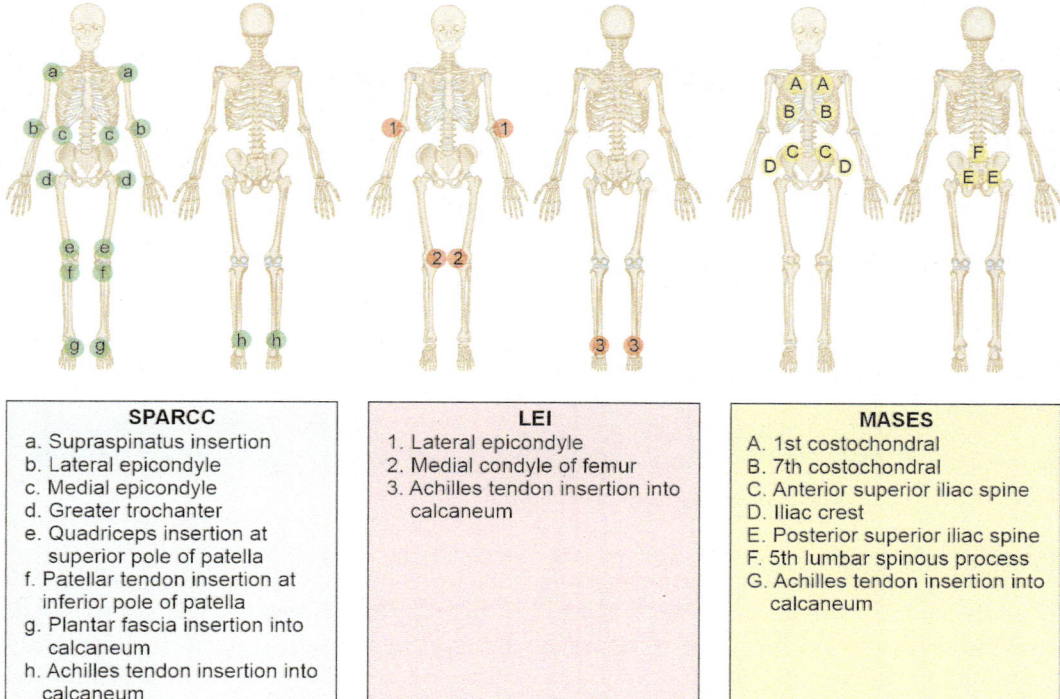

FIG. 2: Validated scoring systems for enthesitis—entheses for scoring.

the proximity of entheses to fibromyalgia tender points. Validated enthesitis scoring systems like the Spondyloarthritis Research Consortium of Canada (SPARCC) and the Leeds Enthesitis Index (LEI) can be used to examine the peripheral entheses[13,14] **(Fig. 2)**. During routine clinical examinations, dermatologists can quickly assess peripheral entheses for swelling or tenderness.

Dactylitis, a uniform swelling of the entire digit following inflammation of the joints, tendons, and soft tissue, can occur in nearly 50% of patients with PsA at some point in the disease course. The digit looks like a sausage due to the inflammation.[15] Examination of the toes is vital in patients with psoriatic disease, as nearly two-thirds of dactylitis occurs in the toes and is asymmetric **(Fig. 3)**. Other diseases like tuberculosis, gouty arthritis, sarcoidosis, and sickle cell disease should be considered differentials of dactylitis.

Axial disease in PsA is the most challenging clinical domain diagnosis. There is a lack of universally accepted definitions for this domain.[16] The physical examination for this domain is identical to that in axial spondyloarthritis. The presence of inflammatory back pain, as defined by the Assessment of Spondyloarthritis International Society (ASAS), performs poorly as a screening tool. This is the only clinical domain that warrants using an MRI of the sacroiliac joints and spine as a prerequisite for diagnosis.[17] Coexisting conditions like degenerative disc disease and diffuse idiopathic skeletal hyperostosis (DISH) are common in patients with PsA and should be considered while interpreting the imaging findings.

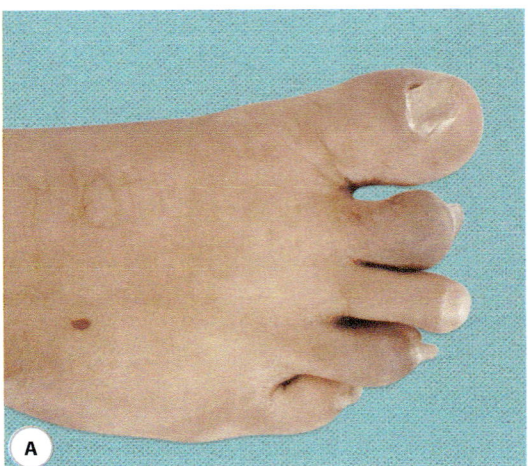 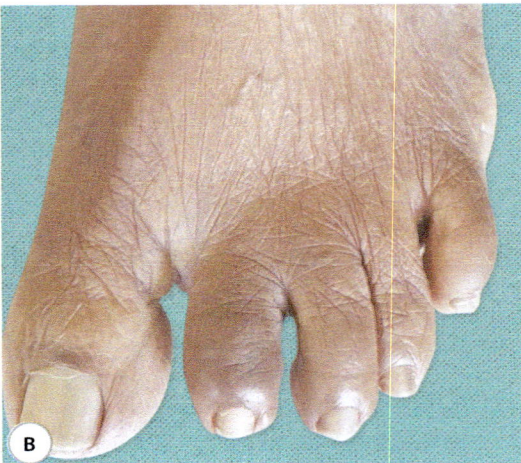

FIGS. 3A AND B: Dactylitis of the second toe in two patients.

A comprehensive clinical examination of all the clinical domains of PsA and a clear understanding of differential diagnoses is crucial in diagnosing PsA and avoiding overtreatment.

Extra-musculoskeletal Features of Psoriatic Arthritis—Not to Be Passed Over

These include the skin and nails, ocular symptoms of uveitis (occasionally asymptomatic), gastrointestinal symptoms suggestive of inflammatory bowel disease (IBD), and comorbidities like obesity, metabolic syndrome, cardiovascular (CV) disease, liver disease, depression, and anxiety. All patients with PsA should be screened for these disorders at regular intervals.[18-20]

Role of Soluble Biomarkers in the Diagnosis of Psoriatic Arthritis

Biomarkers are objectively measurable characteristics that are potential indicators of normal function, disease activity, and therapeutic response. Identifying specific biomarkers can aid in screening and early diagnosis of PsA, especially in patients with nonspecific symptoms. Considering the heterogeneity of the disease, this continues to be an unmet need in PsA. Bone and cartilage turnover markers [cartilage oligomeric metalloproteinase (COMP), matrix metalloproteinase (MMP)] are significantly higher in patients with PsA than those with psoriasis and healthy controls.[21,22]

Imaging in the Diagnosis of Psoriatic Arthritis

Radiographs of the hands, feet, pelvis, and spine must be routinely performed in patients with PsA. They assist in diagnosis and differentiating PsA from other forms of arthritis. A combination of erosive changes and bone proliferation is pathognomonic of PsA. Specific radiological signs, including pencil-in-cup deformities, tuft resorption at terminal phalanges, fluffy periostitis, bone formation at the entheses, asymmetric, paramarginal syndesmophytes, skipping vertebral levels and bulkier than the ones observed in spondyloarthritis are to be noted in patients with PsA. Sacroiliac involvement in PsA can be unilateral.[23]

The MSUS and MRI are very efficacious in the early diagnosis of PsA.[24] These advanced imaging techniques may facilitate early disease classification by integrating the Classification Criteria for Psoriatic Arthritis (CASPAR).[25] Subclinical tenosynovitis, enthesitis, and synovitis in peripheral joints of psoriasis patients with musculoskeletal symptoms not explained by other diagnoses detected by MSUS are now well-recognized as risk factors for the development of PsA, and these patients may warrant a closer follow-up.[26] MSUS can also be used to identify enthesitis accurately in the clinics, especially in women and patients with concomitant fibromyalgia.[27] Of late, studies have looked at ultrasound of fingernails for early detection of enthesitis.[28] These are helpful in better phenotyping of patients with PsA.

■ SCREENING QUESTIONNAIRES FOR PSORIATIC ARTHRITIS: USEFUL TOOLS IN DERMATOLOGY CLINICS

Several screening questionnaires, including the Psoriasis Epidemiology Screening Tool (PEST), the Psoriasis Arthritis Screening and Evaluation (PASE), the Toronto Psoriatic Arthritis Screen (ToPAS), updated ToPAS-II, and the Early ARthritis for Psoriatic patients (EARP) have been developed to be used in dermatology clinics for early identification of PsA. EARP demonstrated the best sensitivity among these questionnaires, and ToPAS II had the highest specificity in diagnosing PsA. These questionnaires, at best, could be used to refer the patient to a rheumatologist for a comprehensive clinical examination.[29,30]

■ MANAGEMENT OF PATIENTS WITH PSORIATIC ARTHRITIS

A comprehensive clinical assessment of the patient gives the treating physician a good understanding of the extent of the disease. Planning the treatment of psoriatic disease is a complex task that must weigh the extent and severity of the clinical domains, comorbidities, and patient preferences, as well as, in resource-poor settings, the availability of drugs and the spending capacity of the patient. Though an array of disease-modifying antirheumatic drugs (DMARDs), both conventional and targeted, is available, the caregiver can often experience starvation in the midst of plenty, considering the diversity of the disease. Shared decision-making and a treat-to-target strategy should be encouraged in routine care for better outcomes.[31]

Multidisciplinary Strategies in the Management of Psoriatic Arthritis

Psoriatic disease is a multifaceted condition that spans multiple specialties. Interdisciplinary strategies are pivotal in providing quality care to patients. The importance of combined dermatology–rheumatology psoriatic disease clinics, with occasional involvement of ophthalmology and gastroenterology, leading to comprehensive assessment, early detection, and a coordinated therapeutic approach, is increasingly recognized globally. This has improved overall outcomes and patient satisfaction and enhanced communication and efficiency between medical specialties.[32-34]

Treat-to-target Strategy in the Management of Psoriatic Arthritis

The treat-to-target strategy in PsA is borrowed from other chronic diseases like diabetes mellitus, hypertension, and hypothyroidism. An ideal "target" to achieve in PsA for improved clinical outcomes and delayed disease progression can be the minimal disease activity (MDA) state. This includes tender and swollen joint counts, the extent of psoriasis by PASI or body surface area, tender enthesitis count, and a Visual Analog Score for patient global disease activity and pain. For a heterogeneous disease with multidomain involvement, MDA, a dichotomous measure, provides a fair representation of other facets of the disease, including the patient's perspective. Other composite indices, which are continuous measures, include the Disease Activity in Psoriatic Arthritis (DAPSA), Psoriatic Arthritis Disease Activity Score (PASDAS), and Composite Psoriatic Disease Activity Index (CPDAI).[35-38]

Overarching Principles of Management

Being a potentially severe disease, managing PsA should be a multidisciplinary task involving rheumatologists and dermatologists. Non-musculoskeletal manifestations, including the skin, eyes, and gastrointestinal tract, and comorbidities, like obesity, metabolic syndrome, CV disease, and depression, should be factored in while choosing the medication in shared decision-making between the patient and the physician. Patients often present with multidomain disease.[39] The availability and efficacy of medicines, patient preferences, and cost should also be reviewed when deciding on the appropriate therapy. The primary objective of treatment should be to augment the health-related quality of life through controlling inflammation and preventing structural damage, thus normalizing function and social participation. The effectiveness of treatment should be monitored by regular disease activity assessment to attain a target of remission or the lowest possible level of disease activity in all the domains.[40]

■ MEDICATIONS FOR THE TREATMENT OF PSORIATIC ARTHRITIS

The availability of medications for treating PsA has exponentially expanded since 2000, following the advent of biologic DMARDs (bDMARDs). These can be broadly classified as conventional synthetic (cs) DMARDs and targeted therapies, including bDMARDs and targeted synthetic DMARDs. For most patients from resource-poor settings, csDMARDs are the readily available and affordable medications. Evidence for the effectiveness of csDMARDs in clinical trials is weak, though data from real-world registries and routine care settings report overall better effectiveness.[41,42]

Adjunctive Treatments

Nonsteroidal anti-inflammatory drugs (NSAIDs) are the first line of treatment for peripheral arthritis, axial disease, enthesitis, and dactylitis. These are effective medications for pain relief and improving function for short periods. Intra-articular glucocorticoids have been the mainstay of initial treatment for active peripheral arthritis. The physician must be cautious of tendon rupture while injecting glucocorticoids at the entheses. These complications are very infrequent with the introduction of MSUS-guided glucocorticoid injections. Generally, oral corticosteroids should be avoided for peripheral manifestations of the disease.[43]

Methotrexate

Methotrexate (MTX) has been one of the most widely used medications for PsA since the 1980s. Findings from the MTX in PsA (MIPA) clinical trial suggest that doses below 15 mg/week may not be effective.[44] Yet another study of etanercept and MTX in combination or monotherapy among patients with PsA (SEAM-PsA) demonstrated comparative numerical effectiveness between the drugs for peripheral arthritis, enthesitis, and skin involvement.[45] Systemic absorption of MTX following oral administration tends to reduce beyond 20 mg/week; hence, higher doses are preferably administered as subcutaneous injections. MTX is also known to reduce antidrug antibody levels and is used along with some biologics. The common adverse events of this medicine are tolerability issues, including nausea, vomiting, diarrhea, and severe fatigue. Laboratory monitoring for hematological and liver parameters should be encouraged among patients initiated on MTX.[46,47]

Sulfasalazine

Sulfasalazine (SSZ) has some effect on peripheral arthritis but no significant benefits on skin, enthesitis and dactylitis.[48,49]

Leflunomide

Leflunomide (LFN) has also demonstrated efficacy in peripheral arthritis endpoints but not in other clinical domains. One of the serious adverse effects of this drug is liver injury, which may be augmented if used concomitantly with MTX. Yet another disadvantage of this drug, primarily reported in Japan, is an increase in pulmonary fibrosis in some patients.[50,51]

Cyclosporine

Cyclosporine A (CsA) is effective for skin psoriasis and peripheral arthritis. Its effectiveness in other domains is weak. CsA warrants laboratory monitoring for renal toxicity, and hypertension can limit its use.[52]

Biologic Disease-modifying Antirheumatic Drugs

Table 1 describes the details of these medications, including their effectiveness in clinical trials for the primary endpoints.[53-70]

■ TREATMENT STRATEGIES BASED ON CLINICAL DOMAINS

Peripheral Arthritis

Nonsteroidal anti-inflammatory drugs and intra-articular glucocorticoids may be considered for short duration. The use of oral glucocorticoids is generally limited to polyarticular forms or as a bridge therapy in PsA, considering the high prevalence of comorbidities and CV risk factors in patients. The use of csDMARDs with early escalation of therapy between 3 and 6 months is universally recommended as the first line of treatment in peripheral arthritis. In resource-limited settings, a combination of csDMARDs (mainly MTX and LFN) may be considered if monotherapy does not provide the desired effect in patients with polyarticular involvement.

There is data to support the use of bDMARDs as first-line therapy for peripheral arthritis, particularly in patients with early disease. There is no difference in efficacy for tumor necrosis factor inhibitor (TNFi), interleukin 17 inhibitor (IL-17i), IL-23i, Janus kinase inhibitor (JAKi) or phosphodiesterase 4 inhibitor (PDE4i) in the management of peripheral arthritis. A combination of cDMARDs and bDMARDs may not be necessary for achieving better response rates, although increased drug survival has been demonstrated in some studies. Two head-to-head randomized clinical trials (RCTs) have compared the efficacy of TNFi with IL-17i, with comparable effects on peripheral arthritis. Another RCT, comparing upadacitinib and adalimumab, showed the superiority of the former only at higher doses than recommended for peripheral arthritis.[71-73]

Axial Disease

Initiation of bDMARDs or JAKis is strongly recommended for patients with axial symptoms who do not respond to NSAIDs.[71-73]

Enthesitis and Dactylitis

Nonsteroidal anti-inflammatory drugs can be used initially for enthesitis. Ultrasound-guided local glucocorticoid injection can be tried in patients with persistent enthesitis. MTX can be used as an option for some patients who continue to have symptomatic enthesitis. bDMARDs and JAKi remain the definitive treatments for enthesitis.[74,75]

TABLE 1: Targeted therapies in the management of patients with psoriatic arthritis (PsA)

Biological therapy	Phase III trial	Year of approval (FDA/EMA)	Dose approved	Primary endpoint period	ACR20 efficacy	Placebo (PBO)	Enthesitis	Dactylitis
TNF inhibitors								
Etanercept	Mease et al. 2000	2002 (FDA) 2000 (EMA)	50 mg SC weekly	12 weeks	73%	13%	–	–
Infliximab	Kavanaugh et al. 2007 IMPACT	2005 (FDA) 1999 (EMA)	Induction: 5 mg/kg IV at weeks 0, 2, and 6 Maintenance: 5 mg/kg IV every 8 weeks	16 weeks	65%	10%	–	–
Adalimumab	Mease et al. 2005 ADEPT	2005 (FDA) 2003 (EMA)	40 mg SC every other week	12 weeks	58%	14%	Mean improvement greater than PBO, but not reaching statistical significance	
Certolizumab pegol	Mease et al. 2014 RAPID PsA	2013 (FDA) 2009 (EMA)	400 mg SC at weeks 0, 2, and 4, then 200 mg every other week	12 weeks	58%	24%	Mean improvement for both enthesitis and dactylitis in doses 200 and 400 mg significantly greater than PBO	
Golimumab (GOL)	Kavanaugh et al. 2012 GO-REVEAL (SC) Kavanaugh et al. 2017 GO-VIBRANT (IV)	2009 (FDA) 2009 (EMA)	50 mg every 4 weeks (SC) 2 mg/kg at weeks 0 and 4, then every 8 weeks (IV)	14 weeks	51% (SC) 75% (IV)	9% (SC) 14% (IV)	MASES Mean ± SD% change from baseline PBO 39.1 ± 76.1 GOL 50 mg 56.3 ± 62.4	Dactylitis score Mean ± SD% change from baseline PBO 57.2 ± 81.2 GOL 50 mg 70.4 ± 59.9
IL-12/23 inhibitor								
Ustekinumab (UST)	McInnes et al. 2013 PSUMMIT-1	2013 (FDA) 2013 (EMA)	45 mg at week 0 and 4, then 45 mg every 12 weeks (SC)	24 weeks	42% (45 mg); 50% (90 mg)	23%	Modified MASES (including plantar fascia) at week 24 PBO 81% UST 45 mg 68.6% ($p = 0.018$) UST 90 mg 60.8% ($p = 0.0002$) Combined UST 64.6% ($p = 0.0006$)	Ordinal scale (0–3) PBO 76% UST 45 mg 56.6% ($p = 0.005$) UST 90 mg 55.8% ($p = 0.004$) Combined UST 56.2% ($p = 0.001$)

Continued

CHAPTER 14: Management of Psoriatic Arthritis: Diagnosis and Treatment Options

Continued

Biological therapy	Phase III trial	Year of approval (FDA/EMA)	Dose approved	Primary endpoint period	ACR20 efficacy	Placebo (PBO)	Enthesitis	Dactylitis
IL-17 inhibitors								
Secukinumab (SEC)	Mease et al. 2015 FUTURE-1	2016 (FDA) 2015 (EMA)	With a SC loading dose: 150 mg/week at weeks 0, 1, 2, 3, and 4, then 150 mg every 4 weeks. Without a loading dose 150 mg SC every 4 weeks. If patient continues to have active psoriasis, to consider a dose of 300 mg every 4 weeks	24 weeks	50% (150 mg)	17.3%	4-point enthesitis index (lateral epicondyle of humerus, proximal Achilles) at week 24. Pooled doses SEC 47.5% PBO 12.8% ($p < 0.05$)	Dactylitis digit count (total score 20). Pooled doses SEC 52.4% PBO 12.8 ($p < 0.05$)
	Mease et al. 2018 FUTURE-5			16 weeks SEC 300 mg with loading dose SEC 150 mg with loading dose SEC 150 mg without loading dose	SEC 150 mg without loading dose 53.2%	23.5%	Enthesitis resolution 16 weeks 41.9% versus 35.4% (PBO)—NS 24 weeks 47.3% versus 34.4% ($p < 0.05$)	Dactylitis resolution 16 weeks 56.3% versus 32.3% (PBO) $p < 0.001$ 24 weeks 61.2% versus 33.9% (PBO) $p < 0.0001$
Ixekizumab (IXE)	Mease et al. 2017 SPIRIT-P1	2017 (FDA) 2018 (EMA)	160 mg at week 0, then 80 mg every 4 weeks (SC)	24 weeks	58%	30%	LEI significant reduction noted only in 2 weekly doses of IXE at week 12 duration	LDI significant reduction noted in both 4 and 2 weekly doses of IXE

Continued

CHAPTER 14: Management of Psoriatic Arthritis: Diagnosis and Treatment Options

Continued

Biological therapy	Phase III trial	Year of approval (FDA/EMA)	Dose approved	Primary endpoint period	ACR20 efficacy	Placebo (PBO)	Enthesitis	Dactylitis
Bimekizumab	McInnes et al. 2023 BE-OPTIMAL (Bio-naive patients) Merola et al. 2023 BE-COMPLETE (previous inadequate response to bDMARDs)	2024 (FDA) 2023 (EMA)	160 mg every 4 weeks (SC) For PsA with moderate-to-severe plaque psoriasis—320 mg (2 doses of 160 mg each) at week 0, 4, 8, 12, 16 and every 8 weeks thereafter After 16 weeks, switch to 160 mg could be considered	16 weeks	Primary endpoint ACR50 at week 16 BE-OPTIMAL 44% BE-COMPLETE 43%	BE-OPTIMAL 10% BE-COMPLETE 7%	Pooled data from BE-OPTIMAL and BE-COMPLETE LEI 50% PBO 35% ($p = 0.008$)	Pooled data from BE-OPTIMAL and BE-COMPLETE LDI 76% PBO 51% ($p = 0.0022$)
IL-23 inhibitors								
Guselkumab (GUS)	Deodhar et al. 2020 DISCOVER-1 (both bio-naive and bio inadequate response patients)	2020 (FDA) 2020 (EMA)	100 mg at weeks 0 and 4, then 100 mg every 8 weeks (SC)	24 weeks	GUS 100 mg q4w 59.4% $p < 0.001$ GUS q8w 52% $p < 0.001$	22.2%	Resolution of enthesitis GUS 100 mg q4w 47.9% PBO 27.3% $p = 0.013$ GUS q8w 40.3% $p = 0.094$	Resolution of dactylitis GUS 100 mg q4w 63.2% p—NS GUS 100 mg q8w 65.3% p—NS PBO 49.1%
Risankizumab (RZB)	Kristensen et al. 2022 KEEPsAKE-1	2022 (FDA) 2022 (EMA)	150 mg SC week 0, 4, and every 12 weeks thereafter	24 weeks	RZB 150 mg 57.3% $p < 0.001$	33.5%	RZB 150 mg 48.4% PBO 34.8% $p < 0.001$	RZB 150 mg 68.1% PBO 51% $p < 0.001$

Continued

CHAPTER 14: Management of Psoriatic Arthritis: Diagnosis and Treatment Options

Continued

Biological therapy	Phase III trial	Year of approval (FDA/EMA)	Dose approved	Primary endpoint period	ACR20 efficacy	Placebo (PBO)	Enthesitis	Dactylitis
Costimulatory blockade								
Abatacept	Mease et al. 2017 ASTRAEA	2017 (FDA) 2017 (EMA)	125 mg weekly (SC) 500 mg (<60 kg) 750 mg (60–100 kg) 1,000 mg (>100 kg) At weeks 0, 2, 4, then every 4 weeks (IV)	24 weeks	57.3% $p < 0.001$	33.5%	LEI Resolution 48.4% PBO 34.8% $p < 0.001$	LDI Resolution 68.1% PBO 51% $p < 0.001$
Targeted synthetic DMARDs								
Apremilast (APR)	Kavanaugh et al. 2014 PALACE-1	2014 (FDA)	Dosage titration (days 1–5), then 30 mg twice daily (PO)	16 weeks	39.8%	19%	Mean change in MASES at week 24 APR 30 mg −1.7 ± 0.29 ($p = 0.03$) PBO −0.8 ± 0.31 $p = 0.03$	Mean change in dactylitis severity score at week 24 APR 30 mg −1.8 ± 0.27 PBO −1.3 ± 0.27 p—NS
Tofacitinib (Tofa)	Mease PJ, et al. 2017 OPAL Broaden	2017 (FDA)	5 mg twice daily	12 weeks	50%	33%	Mean change in LEI at 12 weeks Tofa 5 mg −8 ± 0.2 PBO −4 ± 0.2 p—NS	Mean change in dactylitis severity score Tofa 5 mg −3.5 ± 1.0 PBO −2.0 ± 1.1 p—NS
Upadacitinib (UPA)	SELECT-PsA 1	2021 (FDA)	15 mg once daily	12 weeks	71%	36%	Resolution of LEI at week 24 UPA 15 mg Percentage points difference with PBO $p < 0.001$	Resolution of LDI at week 24 UPA 15 mg Percentage points difference with PBO p—NS

(bDMARDs: biologic disease-modifying antirheumatic drugs; EMA: European Medicines Agency; FDA: Food and Drug Administration; IL: interleukin; IV: intravenous; LDI: Leeds Dactylitis Index; LEI: Leeds Enthesitis Index; MASES: Maastricht Ankylosing Spondylitis Enthesitis Score; SC: subcutaneous; TNF: tumor necrosis factor)

Related Conditions

These include IBD (Crohn's disease and ulcerative colitis) and noninfectious anterior uveitis. MTX and SSZ have been used for IBD. bDMARDs, including TNFi, IL-12/IL-23i, IL-23i, and JAKi have demonstrated proven efficacy for IBD. MTX can be used as the first-line agent for uveitis, followed by TNFi (mostly adalimumab), which is recommended. Etanercept is not recommended for use in uveitis.[76]

Comorbidities

Table 2 highlights the use of DMARDs in patients with comorbidities.

Switching and Tapering of Biologic DMARDs

Switching within the class once or to another bDMARD or JAKi may be considered in patients who have an inadequate response to a bDMARD or a JAKi. A total discontinuation of a bDMARD or a JAKi is generally not recommended. However, a dose reduction or spacing of treatment interval may be considered in patients who attain long-term remission.[77]

Difficult to Treat and Complex to Manage Psoriatic Arthritis

Despite the array of treatment options for PsA, many patients do not attain minimal disease activity. There could be several reasons for this, including the complex phenotype of the disease, ineffectiveness or loss of effect of multiple therapies, adverse effects associated with medications, comorbidities, varied effectiveness of drugs on different clinical domains, and concomitant fibromyalgia and/or chronic widespread pain. Difficult-to-treat (D2T) refers to patients of PsA who are resistant or refractory to various medications. This could be due to the ineffectiveness or loss of effect of multiple therapies or the differential effectiveness of drugs across the clinical phenotypes in PsA. Complex-to-manage encompasses a more extensive conundrum. These include adverse effects associated with medications, comorbidities, co-existing

TABLE 2: Usefulness of DMARDs in patients with comorbidities

Comorbidity	MTX/LEF	TNFi	IL-17i	IL-12/IL-23i	JAKi	PDE4i
High CV risk						
Congestive heart failure						
Obesity						
MASLD						
Depression or anxiety						
Active viral hepatitis						
HIV						
Tuberculosis						
Malignancy						
Demyelinating disease						
Active infection						

(CV: cardiovascular; HIV: human immunodeficiency virus; IL: interleukin; JAKi: Janus kinase inhibitor; LEF: leflunomide; MASLD: metabolic dysfunction associated steatotic liver disease; MTX: methotrexate; PDE4i: phosphodiesterase 4 inhibitor; TNFi: tumor necrosis factor inhibitor)

Note: Red: Contraindicated; Green: Can be prescribed; Amber: Can be administered with caution.

medical conditions, fatigue, work impairment, concomitant fibromyalgia and/or chronic pain syndrome, as well as region-specific challenges, including infections and access to medications. An ongoing project by GRAPPA is in the process of creating more specific definitions for these states of the disease, which will have implications for management in routine care.[78-80]

CONCLUSION

Management of PsA continues to be a challenging task in routine care. With the addition of newer treatment targets, the chronic complications of the disease are dwindling. The availability of generic JAKi in resource-poor settings has revolutionized the outcome of psoriatic disease over the past few years. Refinements in outcome measurement tools need to be considered for accurately measuring the burden of the disease. Regional disparities, including socioeconomic and cultural aspects, must be regarded while discussing the patient's options. Multidisciplinary clinics must be encouraged in the management of psoriatic disease.

TAKE HOME MESSAGE

- Psoriatic arthritis is a multi-faceted immune-mediated inflammatory disease with a heterogeneous phenotype.
- Early detection and treatment can considerably reduce the burden of disease and radiological structural damage.
- Multidisciplinary clinics should be encouraged for early detection and optimal management of psoriatic comorbidities and related conditions.
- Treat-to-target using composite disease measures should be routinely applied while managing psoriatic arthritis.
- Conventional and biologic disease-modifying anti-rheumatic drugs should be initiated in a shared decision-making process, keeping the clinical domains in mind.

REFERENCES

1. Ritchlin CT, Colbert RA, Gladman DD. Psoriatic arthritis. N Engl J Med. 2017;376:957-70.
2. FitzGerald O, Ogdie A, Chandran V, Coates LC, Kavanaugh A, Tillett W, et al. Psoriatic arthritis. Nat Rev Dis Primers. 2021;7(1):59.
3. Haroon M, Gallagher P, FitzGerald O. Diagnostic delay of more than 6 months contributes to poor radiographic and functional outcome in psoriatic arthritis. Ann Rheum Dis. 2015;74:1045-50.
4. Rida MA, Chandran V. Challenges in the clinical diagnosis of psoriatic arthritis. Clin Immunol. 2020;214:108390.
5. Coates LC, Helliwell PS. Psoriatic arthritis: state of the art review. Clin Med (Lond). 2017;17:65-70.
6. Scher JU, Ogdie A, Merola FJ, Ritchlin C. Preventing psoriatic arthritis: focusing on patients with psoriasis at increased risk of transition. Nat Rev Rheumatol. 2019;15:153-66.
7. Mathew AJ, Østergaard M, Eder L. Imaging in psoriatic arthritis: Status and recent advances. Best Pract Clin Rheumatol. 2021;35:101690.
8. Perez-Chada LM, Haberman RH, Chandran V, Rosen CF, Ritchlin C, Eder L, et al. Consensus terminology for preclinical phases of psoriatic arthritis for use in research studies: results from a Delphi consensus study. Nat Rev Rheumatol. 2021;17:238-43.
9. Ciccia F, Gandolfo S, Caporali R, Scher JU. Understanding the spectrum from preclinical psoriatic arthritis to early diagnosis of the disease. Lancet Rheumatol. 2024;S2665-9913(24)00268-6.
10. Eder L, Polacheck A, Rosen RF, Chandran V, Cook R, Gladman DD. The development of psoriatic arthritis in patients with psoriasis is preceded by a period of nonspecific musculoskeletal symptoms: A prospective cohort study. Arthritis Rheumatol. 2017;69:622-29.
11. Takeshita J, Grewal S, Langan SM, Mehta NM, Ogdie A, Voorhees ABS, et al. Psoriasis and comorbid diseases: Implications for management. J Am Dermatol. 2017;76:393-403.
12. Saalfeld W, Mixon AM, Zelie J, Lydon EJ. Differentiating psoriatic arthritis from

osteoarthritis and rheumatoid arthritis: A narrative review and guide for advanced practice providers. Rheumatol Ther. 2021;8:1493-517.
13. Araujo EG, Schett G. Enthesitis in psoriatic arthritis (Part 1): pathophysiology. Rheumatology (Oxford). 2020;59(Suppl1):i10-4.
14. Helliwell PS. Assessment of enthesitis in psoriatic arthritis. J Rheumatol. 2019;46:869-70.
15. Kaeley GS, Eder L, Aydin SZ, Gutierrez M, Bakewell C. Dactylitis: A hallmark of psoriatic arthritis. Semin Arthritis Rheum. 2018;48:263-73.
16. Gottlieb AB, Merola JF. Axial psoriatic arthritis: An update for dermatologists. J Am Acad Dermatol. 2021;84:92-101.
17. Pascu LS, Sârbu N, Brădeanu AV, Stan DJ, Matei MN, Sârbu ML, et al. MRI findings in axial psoriatic spondyloarthritis. Diagnostics (Basel). 2023;13:1342.
18. Monteleone G, Moscardelli A, Colella A, Marafini I, Salvatori S. Immune-mediated inflammatory diseases: common and different pathogenic and clinical features. Autoimmune Rev. 2023;22:103410.
19. Mattay SS, Zamani M, Saturno D, Loftus Jr EV, Ciorba MA, Yarur A, et al. Risk of major cardiovascular events in immune-mediated inflammatory disorders on biologics and small molecules: Network meta-analysis. Clin Gastroenterol Hetpal. 2024;22:961-70.
20. Gupta S, Syrimi Z, Hughes DM, Zhao SS. Comorbidities in psoriatic arthritis: a systematic review and meta-analysis. Rheumatol Int. 2021;41:275-84.
21. Pennington SR, FitzGerald O. Early origins of psoriatic arthritis: Clinical, genetic and molecular biomarkers of progression from psoriasis to psoriatic arthritis. Front Med (Lausanne). 2021;8:723944.
22. Cretu D, Gao L, Liang K, Soosaipillai A, Diamandis EP, Chandran V. Differentiating psoriatic arthritis from psoriasis without psoriatic arthritis using novel serum biomarkers. Arthritis Care Res (Hoboken). 2018;70:454-61.
23. Mathew AJ, Østergaard M, Eder L. Imaging in psoratic arthritis: status and recent advances. Best Pract Res Clin Rheumatol. 2021;35:101690.
24. Mathew AJ, Coates LC, Danda D, Conaghan PG. Psoriatic arthritis: lessons from imaging studies and implications for therapy. Expert Rev Clin Immunol. 2017;13:133-42.
25. Felbo SK, Terslev L, Østergaard M. Imaging in peripheral and axial psoriatic arthritis: contributions to diagnosis, follow-up, prognosis and knowledge of pathogenesis. Clin Exp Rheumatol. 2018;36(Suppl 114):24-34.
26. Zabotti A, De Marco G, Gossec L, Baraliakos X, Aletaha D, Iagnocco A. EULAR points to consider for the definition of clinical and imaging features suspicious of progression from psoriasis to psoriatic arthritis. Ann Rheum Dis. 2023;82:1162-70.
27. Polachek A, Furer V, Zureik M, Nevo S, Mendel L, Levartovsky D, et al. Role of ultrasound for assessment of psoriatic arthritis patients with fibromyalgia. Ann Rheum Dis. 2021;80:1553-58.
28. Agache M, Popescu CC, Enache L, Dumitrescu BM, Codreanu C. Nail ultrasound in psoriasis and psoriatic arthritis – A narrative review. Diagnostics (Bassel). 2023;13:2236.
29. Haddad A, Feld J, Zisman D. The performance of psoriatic arthritis screening questionnaires in patients with psoriasis. J Rheumatol. 2019;46:1643-45.
30. Mishra S, Kancharla H, Dogra S, Sharma A. Comparison of four validated psoriatic arthritis screening tools in diagnosing psoriatic arthritis in patients with psoriasis (COMPAQ study). Br J Dermatol. 2017;176:765-70.
31. Van den Bosch F, Coates L. Clinical management of psoriatic arthritis. Lancet. 2018;391:2285-94.
32. Klavdianou K, Stavropoulou M, Panagakis P, Papoutsaki M, Panagiotopoulos A, Koutsianas C, et al. Patient characteristics, treatment patterns and disease outcomes in patients with psoriatic arthritis followed in a combined Dermatology-Rheumatology clinic: a retrospective real-world study. Rheumatol Int. 2022;42:1035-41.
33. Jadon DR, Helliwell PS. The role of the multidisciplinary team in the management of psoriatic arthritis. Musculoskeletal Care. 2022;(Supp 1): S32-40.
34. Brazzelli V, Bobbio Pallavicini F, Maggi P, Chętko L, Isoletta E, Giuli ND, et al. A multidisciplinary dermatology-gastroenterology-rheumatology (DER.RE.GA) unit for the care of patients with immune-mediated inflammatory diseases: analysis of the first 5 years from the dermatologist's perspective. Front Med (Lausanne). 2023;10:1290018.
35. Ortolan A, Lorenzin M, Cozzi G, Scagnellato L, Favero M, Striani G, et al. Treat-to-target in real-life psoriatic arthritis patients: achieving minimal disease activity with bDMARDs/ tsDMARDs and potential barriers. Semin Arthritis Rheum. 2023;62:152237.
36. Hackett S, Coates LC. Outcome measures in psoriatic arthritis: where next? Musculoskeletal Care. 2022;20 (Suppl 1):S22-S31.
37. Coates LC. Outcome measures in psoriatic arthritis. Rheum Dis Clin North Am. 2015;41:699-710.

38. Kasiem FR, Kok MR, Luime JJ, Tchetverikov L, Korswagen LA, Denissen NHAM, et al. Construct validity and responsiveness of feasible composite disease activity measures for use in daily clinical practice in patients with psoriatic arthritis. RMD Open. 2023;9:e002972.
39. Ogdie A, Hur P, Liu M, Rebello S, McLean RR, Dube B, et al. Effect of multidomain disease presentations on patients with psoriatic arthritis in the Corrona Psoriatic Arthritis/ Spondyloarthritis registry. J Rheumatol. 2021;48:698-706.
40. Ayan G, Ribeiro A, Macit B, Proft F. Pharmacological treatment strategies in psoriatic arthritis. Clin Ther. 2023;45:826-40.
41. Kharouf F, Gladman DD. Advances in the management of psoriatic arthritis in adults. BMJ. 2024;387:e081860.
42. Hsieh TS, Tsai TF. Combination of methotrexate with oral disease-modifying antirheumatic drug in psoriatic arthritis: a systematic review. Immunotherapy. 2024;16:115-30.
43. Eder L, Chandran V, Ueng J, Bhella S, Lee KA, Rahman P, et al. Predictors of response to intra-articular steroid injection in psoriatic arthritis. Rheumatology (Oxford). 2010;49:1367-73.
44. Kingsley GH, Kowalczyk A, Taylor H, Ibrahim F, Packham JC, McHugh NJ, et al. A randomized placebo-controlled trial of methotrexate in psoriatic arthritis. Rheumatology (Oxford). 2012;51:1368-77.
45. Mease PJ, Gladman DD, Collier DH, Ritchlin CT, Helliwell PS, Liu L, et al. Etanercept and methotrexate as monotherapy or in combination for psoriatic arthritis: Primary results from a randomized, controlled phase III trial. Arthritis Rheum. 2019;71:1112-24.
46. Cronstein BN, Aune TM. Methotrexate and its mechanisms of action in inflammatory arthritis. Nat Rev Rheumatol. 2020;16:145-54.
47. Coates LC, Merola JF, Grieb SM, Mease PJ, Duffin KC. Methotrexate in psoriasis and psoriatic arthritis. J Rheumatol Suppl. 2020;96:31-5.
48. Gupta AK, Grober JS, Hamilton TA, Ellis CN, Siegel MT, Voorhees JJ, et al. Sulfasalazine therapy for psoriatic arthritis: a double blind, placebo controlled trial. Clinical Trial. 1995;22:894-8.
49. Jacobs ME, Pouw JN, Welsing P, Radstake TRDJ, Leijten EFA. First-line csDMARD monotherapy drug retention in psoriatic arthritis: methotrexate outperforms sulfasalazine. Rheumatology (Oxford). 2021;60:780-84.
50. Lopez-Medina C, Schiotis R, Collantes-Estévez. Leflunomide in the treatment of psoriatic arthritis. 2022;4:e230-31.
51. Haroon M, Batool S, Asif S, Hashmi F, Ullah S. Combination of methotrexate and leflunomide is safe and has good drug retention among patients with psoriatic arthritis. J Rheumatol. 2021;48: 1624-26.
52. Soriano A, Pipitone N, Salvarani C. Cyclosporine in psoriatic arthropathy. Clin Exp Rheumatol. 2015;33:S101-3.
53. Ruyssen-Witrand A, Perry R, Watkins C, Braileanu G, Kumar G, Kiri S, et al. Efficacy and safety of biologics in psoriatic arthritis: a systematic literature review and network meta-analysis. RMD Open. 2020;6:e0001117.
54. Mease PJ, Goffe BS, Metz J, VanderStoep A, Finck B, Burge DJ. Etanercept in the treatment of psoriatic arthritis and psoriasis: a randomised trial. Lancet. 2000;356:385-90.
55. Kavanaugh A, Krueger GG, Beutler A, Guzzo C, Zhou B, Dooley LT, et al. Infliximab maintains a high degree of clinical response in patients with active psoriatic arthritis through 1 year of treatment: results from the IMPACT 2 trial. Ann Rheum Dis. 2007;66:498-505.
56. Mease PJ, Gladman DD, Ritchlin CT, Ruderman EM, Steinfeld SD, Choy EHS, et al. Adalimumab for the treatment of patients with moderately to severely active psoriatic arthritis: results of a double-blind, randomized, placebo-controlled trial. Arthritis Rheum. 2005;52:3279-89.
57. Mease PJ, Fleischmann R, Deodhar AA, Wollenhaupt J, Khraishi M, Kielar D, et al. Effect of certolizumab pegol on signs and symptoms in patients with psoriatic arthritis: 24-week results of a phase -3 double-blind randomised placebo-controlled study (RAPID-PsA). Ann Rheum Dis. 2014;73:48-55.
58. Kavanaugh A, van der Heijde D, McInnes IB, Mease P, Krueger GG, Gladman DD, et al. Golimumab in psoriatic arthritis: one-year clinical efficacy, radiographic, and safety results from a phase III, randomized, placebo-controlled trial. Arthritis Rheum. 2012;64:2504-17.
59. Kavanaugh A, Husni ME, Harrison DD, Kim L, Lo KH, Leu JH, et al. Safety and efficacy of intravenous golimumab in patients with active psoriatic arthritis: Results through week twenty-four of the GO-VIBRANT study. Arthritis Rheumatol. 2017;69:2151-61.
60. McInnes IB, Kavanaugh A, Gottlieb AB, Puig L, Rahman P, Ritchlin C, et al. Efficacy and safety of ustekinumab in patients with active psoriatic arthritis: 1 year results of the phase 3, multicentre, double-blind, placebo-controlled PSUMMIT 1 trial. Lancet. 2013;382:780-9.

61. Mease PJ, McInnes IB, Kirkham B, Kavanaugh A, Rahman P, van der Heijde D, et al. Secukinumab inhibition of interleukin-17A in patients with psoriatic arthritis. N Engl J Med. 2015;373:1329-39.
62. Mease PJ, van der Heijde D, Landewé R, Mpofu S, Rahman P, Tahir H, et al. Secukinumab improves active psoriatic arthritis symptoms and inhibits radiographic progression: primary results from the randomised, double-blind, phase III FUTURE 5 study. Ann Rheum Dis. 2018;77:890-7.
63. Mease PJ, van der Heijde D, Ritchlin CT, Okada M, Cuchacovich RS, Shuler CL, et al. Ixekizumab, an interleukin-17A specific monoclonal antibody, for the treatment of biologic-naive patients with active psoriatic arthritis: results from the 24-week randomised, double-blind, placebo-controlled and active (adalimumab)-controlled period of the phase III trial SPIRIT-P1. Ann Rheum Dis. 2017;76:79-87.
64. McInnes IB, Asahina A, Coates LC, Landewé R, Merola JF, Ritchlin CT, et al. Bimekizumab in patients with psoriatic arthritis, naive to biologic treatment: a randomised, double-blind, placebo-controlled, phase 3 trial (BE OPTIMAL). The Lancet. 2023;401:25-37.
65. Deodhar A, Helliwell PS, Boehncke WH, Kollmeier AP, Hsia EC, Subramanian RA, et al. Guselkumab in patients with active psoriatic arthritis who were biologic-naive or had previously received TNFα inhibitor treatment (DISCOVER-1): a double-blind, randomised, placebo-controlled phase 3 trial. Lancet. 2020;395:1115-25.
66. Kristensen LE, Keiserman M, Papp K, McCasland L, White D, Lu W, et al. Efficacy and safety of risankizumab for active psoriatic arthritis: 24-week results from the randomised, double-blind, phase 3 KEEPsAKE 1 trial. Ann Rheum Dis. 2022;81:225-31.
67. Mease PJ, Gottlieb AB, van der Heijde D, FitzGerald O, Johnsen A, Nys M, et al. Efficacy and safety of abatacept, a T-cell modulator, in a randomised, double-blind, placebo-controlled, phase III study in psoriatic arthritis. Ann Rheum Dis. 2017;76:1550-8.
68. Kavanaugh A, Mease PJ, Gomez-Reino JJ, Adebajo AO, Wollenhaupt J, Gladman DD, et al. Treatment of psoriatic arthritis in a phase 3 randomised, placebo-controlled trial with apremilast, an oral phosphodiesterase 4 inhibitor. Ann Rheum Dis. 2014;73:1020-6.
69. Mease P, Hall S, FitzGerald O, van der Heijde D, Merola JF, Avila-Zapata F, et al. Tofacitinib or adalimumab versus placebo for psoriatic arthritis. N Eng J Med. 2017;377:1537-50.
70. McInnes IB, Anderson JK, Magrey M, Merola JF, Liu Y, Kishimoto M, et al. Trial of Upadacitinib and Adalimumab for Psoriatic Arthritis. N Engl J Med. 2021;384:1227-39.
71. Coates LC, Soriano ER, Corp N, Bertheussen H, Duffin KC, Campanholo CB, et al. Group for research and assessment of psoriasis and psoriatic arthritis (GRAPPA): updated treatment recommendations for psoriatic arthritis 2021. Nat Rev Rheumatol. 2022;18:465-79.
72. Gossec L, Kerschbaumer A, Ferreira RJO, Aletaha D, Baraliakos X, Bertheussen H, et al. EULAR recommendations for the management of psoriatic arthritis with pharmacological therapies: 2023 update. Ann Rheum Dis. 2024;83:706-19.
73. Coates LC, Gossec L. The updated GRAPPA and EULAR recommendations for the management of psoriatic arthritis: Similarities and differences. Joint Bone Spine. 2023;90:105469
74. Eder L, Mathew AJ, Carron P, Bertheussen H, Cañete JD, Azem M, et al. Management of enthesitis in patients with psoriatic arthritis: An updated literature review informing the 2021 GRAPPA treatment guidelines. J Rheumatol. 2023;50:258-64.
75. Palominos PE, Fernández-Ávla DG, Coates LC, Adebajo A, Toukap AN, Abogamal A, et al. Management of dactylitis in patients with psoriatic arthritis: an updated literature review informing the 2021 GRAPPA treatment recommendations. J Rheumatol. 2023;50:265-78.
76. Jadon DR, Corp N, van der Windt DA, Coates LC, Soriano ER, Kavanaugh A, et al. Management of concomitant inflammatory bowel disease or uveitis in patients with psoriatic arthritis: An updated review informing the 2021 GRAPPA treatment recommendations. J Rheumatol. 2023;50:438-50.
77. Merola JF, Lockshin B, Mody EA. Switching biologics in the treatment of psoriatic arthritis. Semin Arthritis Rheum. 2017;47:29-37.
78. Singla S, Ribeiro A, Torgutalp M, Mease PJ, Proft F. Difficult-to-treat psoriatic arthritis (D2T PsA): a scoping literature review informing a GRAPPA research project. RMD Open. 2024;10:e003809.
79. Kumthekar A, Ashrafi M, Deodhar A. Difficult to treat psoriatic arthritis — how should we manage? Clin Rheumatol. 2023;42:2251-65.
80. Ribeiro AL, Singla S, Chandran V, Chronis N, Liao W, Lindsay C, et al. Deciphering difficult-to-treat psoriatic arthritis (D2T-PsA): a GRAPPA perspective from an international survey of healthcare professionals. Rheum Adv Pract. 2024;8:rkae074.

15

Pustular Psoriasis

Sudip Das, SK Shahriar Ahmed

■ INTRODUCTION

Pustular psoriasis (PP) is a chronic, multisystemic, autoinflammatory disease, which presents with widespread, macroscopic, aseptic pustules. Its clinical course is extremely variable, diverse, and unexpected. Its heterogeneous, cutaneous, and extracutaneous symptoms pose considerable challenges to the timely diagnosis and treatment. It was first reported by Leo Ritter von Zumbusch in 1910.[1] Dysregulation of the interleukin-36 (IL-36) signaling cascade pathway plays a key role in the pathogenesis of PP. The altered expression of various IL-36 pathway constituents has been shown to cause excess production of inflammatory cytokines and neutrophil recruitment in the epidermis.[2] The associated morbidity is high, which can lead to a significant impact on quality of life (QoL) or life-threatening emergencies. In 2017, the European Rare and Severe Psoriasis Expert Network (ERASPEN) defined generalized pustular psoriasis (GPP) as primary, sterile, macroscopically visible pustules on nonacral skin. GPP subclassifiers are (1) with or without systemic inflammation, (2) with or without plaque psoriasis, and (3) either relapsing (>1 episode) or persistent (>3 months).

According to ERASPEN, a diagnosis of GPP can be made only when the condition has relapsed at least once or has persisted for >3 months.[3] There is a dearth of GPP data in India. Nonetheless, GPP is regarded as a rare disease due to its extremely low incidence and frequency. Globally, the prevalence of GPP can be estimated as 1–7 cases per million persons. However, data are variable, and estimations range from 1.76 cases per million in France to 7.46 cases per million in Japan, and 180 cases per million in Italy.[4-6] Although GPP can manifest at any age, from infancy to old age, the typical age at diagnosis is approximately 50 years old. GPP patients generally have a majority of females. Patients with the *IL36RN* mutation are more prone to experience early-onset GPP.[7-10]

■ EPIDEMIOLOGY

Pustular psoriasis is a rare entity. It shows a bimodal age distribution. The condition typically manifests in the adult age-group between the ages of 40 and 50 years, while in the pediatric age-group, it typically manifests in infancy. Asians tend to be more affected than Caucasians. It is more predominant in the women population. Roughly 1% of all clinical cases of psoriasis are pustular variations.[11,10] The association with plaque psoriasis ranges from 25% to 30% to 65% of cases.[12,13] Genetic studies of the various forms of PP reveal differences from plaque psoriasis. In PP, *IL36RN* mutations are the most frequently observed. The genes encoding the IL-36 family are located in chromosome 2q13. Mutations in the *AP1S3* and *CARD14* genes were found in some patients.

TYPES

Generalized:
- *von Zumbusch subtype*: Diffuse generalized pustular eruption with associated systemic symptoms (fevers, arthralgias, etc.)
- *Annular subtype*: Annular lesions with pustules along the advancing edge
- *Exanthematic subtype*: Acute pustular eruption without systemic symptoms that resolves after a few days
- *Impetigo herpetiformis*: PP occurring during pregnancy

Localized:
- *Acrodermatitis continua of Hallopeau*: Pustules affecting the fingers, toes, and nail beds
- *Palmoplantar psoriasis*: Pustules affecting the palms and soles

PATHOGENESIS

When keratinocyte comes under stress in a genetically predisposed person due to a certain triggering factor, a chain of inflammatory events gets started. Possible triggers for GPP flares include withdrawal of corticosteroids, exposure to certain medications (lithium, iodine, penicillin, interferon-alpha, etc.), stress, infection, pregnancy, phototherapy, vaccination, and hypocalcemia. Loss-of-function mutations have been implicated in *IL36RN*, which encodes an IL-36 receptor antagonist (IL-36Ra).[2] Both PP and chronic plaque psoriasis display overexpression of IL-1, IL-17, IL-23, IL-36, tumor necrosis factor alpha (TNF-α), and interferon gamma (IFN-γ). The expression levels of IL-1, IL-1RN, IL-36, IL-36, IL-36, and IL-36Ra are more intense in the pustular form. IL-36 has four subgroups (IL-36α, IL-36β, IL-36γ, IL-36Ra) and they come under family of IL-1.[14] The corresponding receptors are named as follows: For IL-36 α and β, IL-1Rrp2 and IL-1RAcp receptors, expressed in monocytes, T and B lymphocytes; for IL-36γ, the receptors are the same but expressed in keratinocytes epithelial cells; for IL-36Ra, the receptors are IL-1Rrp2 and SIGIRR, expressed by keratinocytes, monocytes, and dendritic cells.[15] Complexes of host DNA debris, and LL-37 are released from keratinocytes when they come under stress. It triggers the plasmacytoid dendritic cells. IL-36 acts on its receptor and activates intracellular pathways for the transcription of proinflammatory cytokines. It is possible that IL-36-Ser18 induces hyperkeratosis and CXCL8 production and regulates the production of CXCL1, CXCL10, and CCL20 by keratinocytes. Neutrophil elastase, calpain, proteinase-3, and cathepsin G help in the procession and activation of different subgroups of IL-36. In vitro, stimulation of human keratinocytes with different cytokines increases gene expression of several chemokines to T-lymphocytes (CCL20, CCL5, CCL2, CCL17, and CCL22), and neutrophils (CXCL8, CCL20, and CXCL1) and macrophages (CCL3, CCL4, CCL5, CCL2, CCL17, and CCL22). IL-36 has been shown to activate the vascular endothelium, resulting in notable edema of the papillary dermis, red blood cell extravasation, and the extravasation of other cells, including eosinophils.[16]

HISTOPATHOLOGY

Many of the histopathological features of PP mimic that of psoriasis vulgaris, including parakeratosis, hyperkeratosis, elongation of the rete ridges, reduced stratum granulosum, and suprapapillary thinning of epidermis. Neutrophilic infiltration at stratum corneum (Munro's microabscess) and stratum spinosum or granulosum (spongiform pustules of Kogoj) is more prominent in PP than in other variants of psoriasis vulgaris.

CLINICAL FEATURES

According to the 2018 Japanese Dermatological Association (JDA) diagnostic criteria for GPP, patients with all of the following features can

be definitively diagnosed with GPP, while those with features 2 and 3 would be suspected of having GPP.[17]
- Systemic symptoms such as fever and fatigue
- Systemic or extensive flush accompanied by multiple sterile pustules
- Neutrophilic subcorneal pustules histopathologically characterized by Kogoj's spongiform pustules
- Recurrence of these clinical and histological findings

Numerous isolated or confluent superficial, yellowish pustules on an erythematous background are the hallmarks of PP. Both localized and widespread pustulosis are possible. A thorough examination of the skin on the entire body should be done to rule out any other causes of or plaques that are the initial stage of PP. Symptoms such as fever, headaches, joint discomfort, and leukocytosis are common in the generalized von Zumbusch subtype presentation. However, the exanthematic subtype does not exhibit systemic signs but manifests as an abrupt pustular eruption. The annular subtype is more commonly observed in youngsters around the expanding edge of annular lesions with pustules. The finger, toe, and nailbeds are affected in acrodermatitis continua of Hallopeau. Palmoplantar psoriasis, which can be seen as part of SAPHO syndrome, affects the palms and soles.

DIFFERENTIAL DIAGNOSIS

Differential diagnosis is given as follows:
- Acute generalized exanthematous pustulosis
- Drug eruption reaction
- Impetigo
- Dermatitis herpetiformis
- Infected eczema
- Erythroderma
- Acute cutaneous lupus
- Dyshidrotic eczema
- Disseminated herpes simplex virus
- Pemphigus vulgaris
- Pemphigus foliaceus

COMPLICATION

The complications include:
- Septicemia, commonly in the generalized form
- Dyselectrolytemia
- Hypocalcemia
- Acid–base imbalance
- Hyperthermia
- Acute liver injury
- Acute renal failure
- Malnutrition

MANAGEMENT

The first step in treatment of PP is to identify the cause and address it properly. We have to keep it mind that von Zumbusch subtype is a medical emergency and it requires hospital admission. Proper aseptic environment, maintaining fluid–electrolyte and acid–base balance and thermoregulation are utmost necessary. Systemic symptoms including fever, joint pain, and secondary infection (if any) will require proper treatment with antipyretics, anti-inflammatory medications, and antibiotics.

Complete blood count (CBC), serum calcium level, liver function test, erythrocyte sedimentation rate (ESR), C-reactive protein (CRP), renal function test, blood culture, serology profile, screening for tuberculosis, and punch biopsy are done. Cultures to be done from weeping lesions: To exclude primary or secondary infections. Topical treatments such as steroids, calcipotriene (calcipotriol), and tacrolimus should be considered as maintenance or adjuvant therapy. Methotrexate, cyclosporine, and systemic retinoids (acitretin, isotretinoin) are considered first-line in adult patients. Second-line treatment includes TNF-α inhibitors (e.g., etanercept, adalimumab, and infliximab) and IL-17 inhibitors (ixekizumab, secukinumab, and brodalumab).[18,19]

Biologics may be considered over nonbiologics, as initial therapy, if two of the following three criteria are fulfilled:
1. Patients with a flare affecting ≥5% of the body surface area (BSA)
2. Patients with Generalized Pustular Psoriasis Physician Global Assessment (GPPGA) total score ≥3
3. Patients with significant impact on psychological/social function [e.g., Dermatology Life Quality Index (DLQI) ≥ 10]

Guselkumab, an IL-23 monoclonal antibody, is the first biological therapy to have demonstrated moderate efficacy and a good safety profile in Japanese patients with GPP.[19] TNF-α inhibitor, IL-17 inhibitor have shown mixed results in GPP.[19-21] IL-1 inhibitors anakinra have been proved efficacious in randomized placebo-controlled trials. The novel IL-36 receptor inhibitor spesolimab is an effective treatment of GPP.[2] It was approved in GPP by the Food and Drug Administration (FDA) in March 2024. The efficacy of spesolimab in patients with GPP was demonstrated regardless of the presence of *IL36RN* mutation. However, it is more effective in de novo cases of GPP than PP, which develops from earlier plaque psoriasis. In a phase 2, multicenter, double-blind, placebo-controlled trial done by Bachelez et al. at the end of week 1, total of 54% in the spesolimab group had a pustulation subscore of 0 (complete pustular clearance), as compared to 6% in the placebo group after receiving a single 900-mg intravenous dose of spesolimab. In addition, 43% achieved a GPPGA total score of 0 or 1 in the spesolimab group, compared to 11% in the placebo group. Rapid control of skin symptoms, within a week of treatment, is now a feasible treatment aim based on the recent results with IL-36 inhibitors.[22] Morita et al. aimed to assess the efficacy and safety of spesolimab for GPP flare prevention in a multicenter, randomized, placebo-controlled, phase 2b trial. They found that high-dose (600 mg loading dose followed by 300 mg every 4 weeks) spesolimab is superior to moderate (600 mg loading dose followed by 300 mg every 12 weeks) to low doses (300 mg loading dose followed by 150 mg every 12 weeks) in GPP flare prevention, significantly reducing the risk of a GPP flare and flare occurrence over 48 weeks.[23] Adverse events such as infection, asthenia and fatigue, nausea and vomiting, headache, pruritus, and infusion site hematoma, and bruising were noticed in the spesolimab group.[22] Imsidolimab showed efficacy in an open-label study that involved eight patients experiencing a GPP flare and is presently progressing into a phase 3 clinical trial.[24] There are also case reports of GPP exhibiting a positive response to IL-1 inhibition with anakinra, canakinumab, and gevokizumab.[25,26]

In the second and third trimesters, biologics—apart from certolizumab pegol—are actively transported across the placenta; the effects of this on the development of the newborn have not been well researched. For the first 6 months of life, live vaccinations should not be given to newborns whose mothers are receiving biological therapy after 16 weeks of pregnancy. Systemic steroids could be used in life-threatening emergencies and should be tapered as soon as possible.[25-28]

Treatment for children with GPP involves acitretin, corticosteroids, methotrexate, and cyclosporine and is much the same as for adults **(Flowchart 1)**. Although the safety of biologics in children has not been well established, they can be cautiously considered for severe/refractory cases with switching/discontinuation of biologics at the earliest.[29]

CHAPTER 15: Pustular Psoriasis

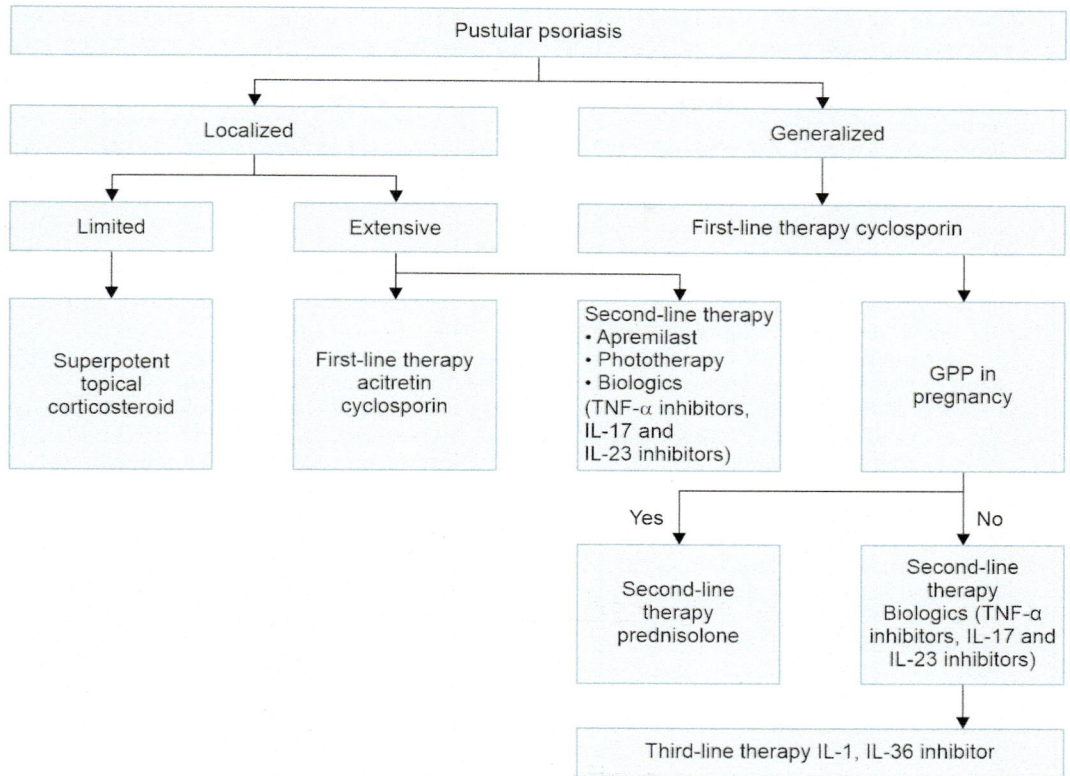

FLOWCHART 1: Treatment algorithm in pustular psoriasis.
(GPP: generalized pustular psoriasis; IL-17: interleukin 17; TNF-α: tumor necrosis factor alpha)

TAKE HOME MESSAGE

- Pustular psoriasis is different from plaque psoriasis, can arise de Novo associated with IL 36 RN gene.
- No prior history of psoriasis is essential.

REFERENCES

1. Zumbusch LR. Psoriasis und pustulöses Exanthem. Archiv für Dermatol Syph. 1910;99:335-46.
2. Bachelez H, Choon SE, Marrakchi S, Burden AD, Tsai TF, Morita A, et al. Inhibition of the Interleukin-36 Pathway for the Treatment of Generalized Pustular Psoriasis. N Engl J Med. 2019;380(10):981-3.
3. Navarini AA, Burden AD, Capon F, Mrowietz U, Puig L, Köks S, et al.; ERASPEN Network. European consensus statement on phenotypes of pustular psoriasis. J Eur Acad Dermatol Venereol. 2017;31(11):1792-9.
4. Ly K, Beck KM, Smith MP, Thibodeaux Q, Bhutani T. Diagnosis and screening of patients with generalized pustular psoriasis. Psoriasis (Auckl). 2019;9:37-42.
5. Zheng M, Jullien D, Eyerich K. The prevalence and disease characteristics of generalized pustular psoriasis. Am J Clin Dermatol. 2022;23(Suppl 1):5-12.
6. Reynolds KA, Pithadia DJ, Lee EB, Clarey D, Liao W, Wu JJ. Generalized pustular psoriasis: a review of the pathophysiology, clinical manifestations, diagnosis, and treatment. Cutis. 2022;110(2 Suppl):19-25.

7. Marrakchi S, Puig L. Pathophysiology of generalized pustular psoriasis. Am J Clin Dermatol. 2022;23(Suppl 1):13-9.
8. Zhou J, Luo Q, Cheng Y, Wen X, Liu J. An update on genetic basis of generalized pustular psoriasis (Review). Int J Mol Med. 2021;47(6):118.
9. von dem Borne PA, Jonkman MF, van Doorn R. Complete remission of skin lesions in a patient with subcorneal pustular dermatosis (Sneddon–Wilkinson disease) treated with antimyeloma therapy: association with disappearance of M protein. Br J Dermatol. 2017;176(5):1341-4.
10. Boehner A, Navarini AA, Eyerich K. Generalized pustular psoriasis–a model disease for specific targeted immunotherapy, systematic review. Exp Dermatol. 2018;27(10):1067-77.
11. Komatsuda S, Kamata M, Chijiwa C, Namiki K, Fukaya S, Hayashi K, et al. Gastrointestinal bleeding with severe mucosal involvement in a patient with generalized pustular psoriasis without IL36RN mutation. Br J Dermatol. 2019;46(1):73-5.
12. Baker H, Ryan TJ. Generalized Pustular Psoriasis. A clinical and epidemiological study of 104 cases. Br J Dermatol. 1968;80:771-93.
13. Gooderham MJ, Voorhees AS, Lebwohl MG. An update on generalized pustular psoriasis. Expert Rev Clin Immunol. 2019;15:907-19.
14. Twelves S, Mostafa A, Dand N, Burri E, Farkas K, Wilson R, et al. Clinical and genetic differences between pustular psoriasis sub-types. J Allergy Clin Immunol. 2019;143:1021-6.
15. Furue K, Yamamura K, Tsuji G, Mitoma C, Uchi H, Nakahara T, et al. Highlighting Interleukin-36 Signaling in Plaque Psoriasis and Pustular Psoriasis. Acta Derm Venereol. 2018;98:5-13.
16. Gabay C, Towne JE. Regulation and function of interleukin-36 cytokines in homeostasis and pathological conditions. J Leukoc Biol. 2015;97:645-52.
17. Fujita H, Terui T, Hayama K, Akiyama M, Ikeda S, Mabuchi T, et al. Japanese guidelines for the management and treatment of generalized pustular psoriasis: The new pathogenesis and treatment of GPP. J Dermatology. 2018;45(11):1235-70.
18. Terui T, Kobayashi S, Okubo Y, Murakami M, Zheng R, Morishima H, et al. Efficacy and safety of guselkumab in Japanese patients with palmoplantar pustulosis: a phase 3 randomized clinical trial. JAMA Dermatol. 2019;155:1153-61.
19. Mrowietz U, Bachelez H, Burden AD, Rissler M, Sieder C, Orsenigo R, et al. Secukinumab for moderate-to-severe palmoplantar pustular psoriasis: results of the 2PRECISE study. J Am Acad Dermatol. 2019;80:1344-52.
20. Pinter A, Wilsmann-Theis D, Peitsch WK, Mössner R. Interleukin-17 receptor A blockade with brodalumab in palmoplantar pustular psoriasis: report on four cases. J Dermatol. 2019;46:426-30.
21. Bissonnette R, Poulin Y, Bolduc C, Maari C, Provost N, Syrotuik J, et al. Etanercept in the treatment of palmoplantar pustulosis. J Drugs Dermatol. 2008;7:940-6.
22. Bachelez H, Choon SE, Marrakchi S, Burden AD, Tsai TF, Morita A, et al.; Effisayil 1 Trial Investigators. Trial of spesolimab for generalized pustular psoriasis. N Engl J Med. 2021;385(26):2431-40.
23. Morita A, Strober B, Burden AD, Choon SE, Anadkat MJ, Marrakchi S, et al. Efficacy and safety of subcutaneous spesolimab for the prevention of generalised pustular psoriasis flares (Effisayil 2): an international, multicentre, randomised, placebo-controlled trial. Lancet. 2023;402(10412):1541-51.
24. Warren RB, Reich A, Kaszuba A, Placek W, Griffiths CEM, Zhou J, et al. Imsidolimab, an anti-interleukin-36 receptor monoclonal antibody, for the treatment of generalized pustular psoriasis: results from the phase II GALLOP trial. Br J Dermatol. 2023;189(2):161-9.
25. Hüffmeier U, Wätzold M, Mohr J, Schön MP, Mössner R. Successful therapy with anakinra in a patient with generalized pustular psoriasis carrying IL36RN mutations. Br J Dermatol. 2014;170(1):202-4.
26. Skendros P, Papagoras C, Lefaki I, Giatromanolaki A, Kotsianidis I, Speletas M, et al. Successful response in a case of severe pustular psoriasis after interleukin-1β inhibition. Br J Dermatol. 2017;176(1):212-5.
27. Seishima M, Fujii K, Mizutani Y. Generalized Pustular Psoriasis in Pregnancy: Current and Future Treatments. Am J Clin Dermatol. 2022;23(5):661-71.
28. Smith CH, Yiu ZZN, Bale T, Burden AD, Coates LC, Edwards W, et al.; British Association of Dermatologists' Clinical Standards Unit. British Association of Dermatologists guidelines for biologic therapy for psoriasis 2020: a rapid update. Br J Dermatol. 2020;183(4):628-37.
29. Saeki H, Terui T, Morita A, Sano S, Imafuku S, Asahina A, et al.; Biologics Review Committee of the Japanese Dermatological Association for Psoriasis. Japanese guidance for use of biologics for psoriasis (the 2019 version). J Dermatol. 2020;47(3):201-22.

16. Special Considerations in Psoriasis Management: Pregnancy, Children, and Elderly Patients

Neena Khanna, Sachin Gupta

CLINICAL CASE SCENARIO

Anita, a 30-year-old female is a known case of psoriasis and was being managed on adalimumab injections. Upon discovering her pregnancy, she stopped all treatment due to fear about potential risks to her child. As a result, her psoriasis has significantly flared. Anita is now deeply concerned about the effects of psoriasis treatment drugs for her unborn baby and is anxious about finding safe treatment alternatives. This situation highlights the complex decisions faced in pregnant patients with psoriasis, where we must balance effective disease management against potential risks to their pregnancy.

INTRODUCTION

Though the treatment of psoriasis is decided based on severity of involvement, impact on patient's quality of life, and other underlying comorbidities, it needs to be modified in vulnerable populations such as pregnant women, children, and the elderly. These groups experience unique challenges due to physiological changes, varying pharmacokinetic responses to treatments, and distinct psychosocial impacts. For example, Anita's case presents the urgent need for treatment options that ensure both the efficacy of treatment and the safety of the mother and fetus. This chapter will talk about management of psoriasis in these vulnerable groups, discussing the importance of personalized treatment plans that address the specific needs and potential risks associated with each group.

PSORIASIS IN PREGNANCY

Psoriasis during pregnancy necessitates special consideration due to the potential impact of the disease and its treatment on both maternal and fetal health. During pregnancy, the immune system undergoes shift from a Th1-dominant (proinflammatory) to a Th2-dominant (anti-inflammatory) state to accommodate the fetus. This immunological adaptation can variably affect psoriasis, an autoimmune skin condition. Approximately 55% of pregnant women with psoriasis experience an improvement in severity of psoriasis due to reduced proinflammatory responses, while around 21% may see a worsening, likely influenced by hormonal fluctuations and individual immune responses.[1]

Psoriasis, particularly when severe, is linked to increased risks for adverse pregnancy outcomes such as preterm and low-birth-weight neonates.[2] These complications are due to systemic inflammation that characterizes active psoriasis. Managing psoriasis during pregnancy therefore demands careful consideration of treatment options to mitigate potential risks to fetal development as also avoiding teratogenic medications like methotrexate and retinoids.

Treatment Strategies during Pregnancy

Managing psoriasis during pregnancy requires a strategic approach that prioritizes safety while effectively controlling the disease. Treatment in pregnant patients, similar to nonpregnant individuals, is categorized into topical therapy, phototherapy, and systemic therapy. Topical treatments, including emollients and low to medium potency topical corticosteroids (TCS), are the first-line choice for localized disease due to minimal systemic absorption. For more extensive or resistant psoriasis, phototherapy, particularly narrowband UVB (NBUVB), is preferred due to its safety profile. Systemic therapies are generally reserved for severe cases, with some agents like cyclosporine considered under strict medical supervision due to potential risks to the fetus.

Topical Treatments

Mild-to-moderate psoriasis in pregnant patients is predominantly managed using topical agents due to their safety profile and minimal systemic absorption.[3] Recommended treatments include:

- *Moisturizers and emollients*: Essential for maintaining skin hydration and barrier function, which is particularly important due to skin sensitivity during pregnancy.
- *TCS creams*: Low- to mid-potency TCS are generally safe during pregnancy when used on limited body surface area and for restricted duration. Evidence-based guidelines suggest these as the preferable options, and more potent corticosteroids be reserved as second-line treatments, applied briefly and under strict supervision.[4]
- *Other topical agents*: Vitamin D analogs, such as calcipotriene, are generally deemed safe for localized treatment of plaques without the systemic side effects often associated with steroid use.[5] However, their application should be limited to small surface areas, and practical measures like avoiding occlusive dressings can help prevent systemic absorption and reduce toxicity risks. The use of coal tar is debated due to potential carcinogenic effects, but it is considered possibly safe in the second and third trimesters if used cautiously.[6]

Phototherapy

Phototherapy, specifically NBUVB at 311 nm, is considered a second-line treatment for managing psoriasis in pregnant women when topical therapies are inadequate. For those unable to access NBUVB, broadband UVB (290–320 nm) or targeted UVB laser treatments (308 nm excimer laser) can be used. Recognized for its safety, phototherapy effectively treats moderate-to-severe cases of psoriasis without the complications associated with systemic medications.

During phototherapy, patients should use emollients or low- to medium-potency TCS to manage side effects like skin dryness and pruritus. Special care is needed to prevent melasma exacerbation, commonly triggered by UV exposure, by protecting the face during sessions. Additionally, UV light may reduce serum folate levels; thus, supplementing folic acid is essential to prevent potential fetal neural tube defects and ensure maternal and fetal safety.[7]

Systemic Treatments

The use of systemic medications during pregnancy is generally limited due to potential risks to fetal development. However, in cases of severe psoriasis where topical management or phototherapy is inadequate, certain systemic treatments may be considered.

- *Cyclosporine*: This is occasionally used as a short-term treatment option for severe psoriasis due to its relatively favorable profile concerning fetal development at low doses. It should be prescribed at the lowest effective dose and for the shortest duration possible.

- **Biologics**: Biologic therapies offer a targeted approach and may be considered in severe cases of psoriasis that do not respond to other treatments. Certolizumab pegol, a tumor necrosis factor (TNF) inhibitor with minimal placental transfer, is often regarded as a safer option during pregnancy, particularly in the third trimester. It is crucial to carefully evaluate the risk–benefit profile of continuing treatment into the later stages of pregnancy. Other biologics, such as infliximab and adalimumab, should be considered only when the benefits significantly outweigh the risks. These agents should be used with caution, and their use is typically advised against during the third trimester due to the risk of fetal immunosuppression (**Table 1**).[8]

Avoided Treatments

Several psoriasis treatments are contraindicated during pregnancy due to their teratogenic effects, including topical tazarotene, methotrexate, and acitretin.

- *Tazarotene*: Tazarotene is known for its teratogenic effects in animal studies and is classified as category X, suggesting it should be avoided during pregnancy.[9] Despite its low systemic absorption when used topically, tazarotene requires careful consideration due to the potential risks involved.
- *Methotrexate*: A folate antagonist, methotrexate is teratogenic and should not be used in pregnant or lactating women. Conception should be avoided *for 3 months* after the last dose due to the drug's persistence in the liver.
- *Acitretin*: Contraindicated in pregnancy, acitretin significantly increases the risk of severe congenital anomalies. It can be metabolized to etretinate, which remains in body fat for up to 52 months. Therefore, pregnancy should be avoided for *3 years* after the last dose.

Conclusion

Managing psoriasis in pregnancy requires prioritizing both maternal and fetal safety. Treatment typically begins with low-risk topical therapies as first-line options, followed by phototherapy as a second-line treatment if needed. Systemic therapies are reserved for severe cases and require careful consideration. Patients should ideally plan pregnancy during remission, but if not feasible, selecting medications with the best fetal safety profiles is essential. Those on systemic treatments

TABLE 1: Biologic treatment guidelines for pregnancy and prepregnancy planning

Biologic	Placental transfer	Recommendations during pregnancy planning	Recommendations during pregnancy
Certolizumab pegol	Low or negligible	Generally safe, first-line therapy if biological required	Preferred first-line option if systemic therapy needed
Adalimumab	Moderate to high	Advised effective contraception method	Consider stopping in second or third trimester
Infliximab			
Etanercept			
Ustekinumab	Unknown	Advised effective contraception method	Insufficient data
Secukinumab			
Ixekizumab			
Tildrakizumab			

should be advised about the necessary discontinuation period before conception.

PSORIASIS IN CHILDREN

Managing psoriasis in children presents unique challenges due to their sensitive skin, less mature immune systems, the psychological impact of the disease, and limited data available on the safety and efficacy of many treatments for this age-group. The less mature immune system in children not only influences the presentation and course of psoriasis but also affects their response to treatments that modulate immune function, necessitating a cautious approach when prescribing immunosuppressive or biologic therapies.

Topical Therapies

The first line of treatment in pediatric psoriasis involves topical agents due to their safety, efficacy, and minimal systemic effects. These treatments are less likely to cause systemic side effects and can effectively manage localized symptoms.
- *TCS*: Widely used for their anti-inflammatory properties, they vary in potency and formulation to suit different parts of the body. Care is required to avoid side effects such as skin thinning and hypothalamic–pituitary–adrenal (HPA) axis suppression.
- *Vitamin D analogs*: Compounds such as calcipotriol help normalize skin cell growth and are useful in reducing plaques but must be used cautiously to prevent systemic absorption and hypercalcemia.
- *Topical calcineurin inhibitors*: Although not approved for psoriasis by all regulatory bodies, they can be effective for facial and intertriginous psoriasis without the risk of atrophy associated with steroids.

Phototherapy

Phototherapy is recommended for children whose psoriasis is extensive enough that topical treatments alone are insufficient. NBUVB phototherapy is the most common form used for children, due to its safety profile and effectiveness.[10] Excimer laser is an option for localized plaques and reduces the risk of exposure to healthy skin.

Systemic Therapies

Systemic therapies are considered when psoriasis is severe or when other treatments fail to control the disease effectively. These include traditional systemic agents like methotrexate and cyclosporine, which require careful monitoring for side effects such as liver toxicity and hypertension.[11] Biologic therapies, targeting specific components of the immune system, offer a more targeted approach and are increasingly used in severe cases due to their efficacy and potentially safer profiles compared to traditional systemic treatment **(Table 2)**.[12]
- *Methotrexate*: Methotrexate, a well-established systemic treatment, is often used for extensive psoriasis and associated arthritis in children. Administered weekly, either orally or subcutaneously, methotrexate works by inhibiting DNA synthesis, reducing inflammation. Its efficacy is well-documented; however, it requires regular monitoring of liver function and blood counts due to risks of hepatotoxicity and bone marrow suppression.
- *Cyclosporine*: Cyclosporine acts rapidly and is used for severe psoriasis flare-ups. Its mode of action involves suppressing the immune system to reduce the inflammation associated with psoriasis. Despite its effectiveness, cyclosporine's use in children is limited to short courses due to potential side effects, including nephrotoxicity and hypertension, necessitating frequent monitoring of renal function and blood pressure.
- *Biologics*: Biologics target specific parts of the immune system believed to play a key role in the inflammation that drives

CHAPTER 16: Special Considerations in Psoriasis Management: Pregnancy, Children, and...

TABLE 2: Systemic and biologic treatments for pediatric psoriasis

Drug name	Dosage and administration	Important side effects	Monitoring recommendations
Methotrexate	0.2–0.7 mg/kg weekly (oral or subcutaneous)	Hepatotoxicity, bone marrow suppression, gastrointestinal upset	CBC, liver function tests every 2–3 months
Cyclosporine	2–5 mg/kg daily in divided doses (oral)	Nephrotoxicity, hypertension, gum hyperplasia, hirsutism	Blood pressure, renal function every 2 weeks
Acitretin	0.1–1 mg/kg daily (oral)	Teratogenicity, hyperlipidemia, hepatotoxicity, dryness of skin and mucous membranes	Lipid profile, liver function tests, pregnancy test for females of childbearing age
Etanercept	FDA-approved for ≥4 years age—0.8 mg/kg (maximum 50 mg) weekly for 3 months, then adjust as needed	Injection site reactions, infections, potential for autoantibodies	TB screening before initiation, monitor for infections
Adalimumab	EMA-approved ≥4 years (not approved by FDA)—0.8 mg/kg (maximum 40 mg) every other week after an initial double dose	Injection site reactions, infections, potential for autoantibodies	TB screening before initiation, monitor for infections
Secukinumab	FDA-approved for ≥6 years age—weight-based dosing; loading dose then monthly (subcutaneous)	Increased risk of infection, exacerbation of inflammatory bowel disease	TB screening, monitor for infections
Ustekinumab	FDA-approved for ≥12 years age—weight-based dosing every 12 weeks after initial doses at weeks 0 and 4	Injection site reactions, infections, potential for autoantibodies	TB screening, monitor for infections
Ixekizumab	FDA-approved for ages ≥6 years age—weight-based dosing; given every 2–4 weeks initially then every 4 weeks (subcutaneous)	Increased risk of infection, exacerbation of inflammatory bowel disease	TB screening, monitor for infections

(CBC: complete blood count; FDA: Food and Drug Administration; TB: tuberculosis)

psoriasis. These drugs offer a targeted approach and are considered for use in children with severe psoriasis who have not responded adequately to traditional systemic treatments.

- *Etanercept*: Etanercept, a TNF inhibitor, is approved for children aged 4 and older. It works by blocking the action of tumor necrosis factor alpha (TNF-α), a substance in the body that causes inflammation in psoriatic plaques. It is administered via weekly subcutaneous injections and is known for its safety and efficacy, although regular monitoring for infections is necessary.
- *Adalimumab*: Adalimumab, another TNF inhibitor, is effective in treating both psoriasis and psoriatic arthritis. Like etanercept, it is administered through subcutaneous injections every other week. While it is not Food and Drug Administration (FDA)-approved for use in children under 4, it is commonly used off-label in pediatric

populations. Monitoring for infections and tuberculosis screening is required before initiation.
- *Ustekinumab*: Ustekinumab, which targets the interleukin 12 (IL-12) and IL-23, is approved for use in children 12 years and older. This biologic is administered every 12 weeks following two initial doses at weeks 0 and 4. It has been shown to be effective in reducing psoriatic lesions with a good safety profile, though it necessitates monitoring for infections.
- *Secukinumab and ixekizumab*: Secukinumab and ixekizumab are IL-17 inhibitors used in children 6 years and older. These medications are given by subcutaneous injection and are effective for treating moderate-to-severe plaque psoriasis. As with other biologics, the potential for increased infection risk exists, and regular follow-up is essential to monitor for adverse effects.

Conclusion

In pediatric psoriasis, treatment prioritizes safety and minimizing systemic exposure. Topical therapies and NBUVB phototherapy are first-line treatments due to their favorable safety profiles. Systemic therapies, including methotrexate and cyclosporine, are reserved for severe cases and require careful monitoring. Biologics, such as etanercept and adalimumab, provide effective options for children, with approvals based on age. Regular follow-up and monitoring are crucial to manage potential side effects and ensure optimal outcomes in this vulnerable population.

■ PSORIASIS IN THE ELDERLY

The aging significantly affects both the presentation and management of psoriasis in elderly patients. Aging skin exhibits decreased cell turnover, reduced collagen production, and diminished sebaceous and sweat gland activity, exacerbating dryness and scaling. Additionally, skin thinning in elderly individuals can alter psoriatic plaque appearance and increase sensitivity to trauma and medications.

Elderly patients often have multiple comorbidities such as cardiovascular disease, diabetes, and arthritis, complicating psoriasis management. These conditions can influence treatment choices due to potential drug interactions and side effects. Polypharmacy, common in this age-group, heightens the risk of adverse drug reactions, especially with systemic treatments requiring careful monitoring and dose adjustment.

Furthermore, immunosenescence, the gradual decline of the immune system with age, increases the risk of infections. Systemic psoriasis treatments, which are immunosuppressive, can exacerbate this risk, making elderly patients particularly vulnerable to infection.[13]

Topical Therapies

Topical treatments remain the cornerstone for managing mild-to-moderate psoriasis in the elderly due to their minimal systemic effects. However, care must be taken with topical steroids to avoid skin thinning, which can be more pronounced in elderly patients.

Systemic Therapies

In elderly patients, systemic therapies must be administered with caution due to increased susceptibility to adverse effects and potential comorbidities. Methotrexate should be used at lower doses to minimize the risk of myelosuppression, considering factors like poor bone marrow reserve, renal impairment, and folate depletion. Caution is also advised when used alongside other antifolate medications due to synergistic adverse effects.

Cyclosporine poses significant nephrotoxicity risks, particularly in elderly patients with reduced renal function. Its metabolism via cytochrome P450 3A4 (CYP3A4) necessitates careful consideration of drug interactions, as concurrent use of nephrotoxic drugs should be avoided. Regular follow-ups are essential due to higher adverse reaction rates compared to methotrexate.

Acitretin is advantageous in the elderly due to its nonimmunosuppressant action, eliminating teratogenicity concerns. However, it can cause xerosis and alter liver enzymes and lipid levels, necessitating stringent follow-ups. Lower doses are often effective in elderly patients. Apremilast, a newer phosphodiesterase-4 inhibitor, is effective and well tolerated in the elderly, with no need for dosage modification even in cases of mild-to-moderate renal impairment.

Biologic Therapies

Biologics, particularly TNF-α inhibitors, are extensively used in elderly psoriasis patients but carry a higher infection risk, which can sometimes be fatal. Good prebiologic workup, immunization, and regular monitoring are crucial. Studies indicate similar efficacy between elderly and younger patients using TNF-α inhibitors, though elderly patients experience higher rates of adverse effects.[14]

While etanercept is commonly prescribed, newer IL-17 and IL-23 inhibitors, such as secukinumab and ustekinumab, are emerging as promising alternatives due to their efficacy and comparable safety profiles.[15] Nonetheless, higher rates of adverse effects and treatment discontinuation in the elderly necessitate careful patient selection and individualized treatment plans. Further research is warranted to thoroughly assess the long-term safety and efficacy of these newer biologics in older populations. Regular follow-up and patient education remain critical, ensuring that biologic therapy effectively manages psoriasis while maintaining safety in this vulnerable age-group.

Conclusion

In elderly patients with psoriasis, treatment typically starts with topical therapies to minimize systemic exposure, progressing to systemic treatments like lower doses of methotrexate or cyclosporine when necessary. In cases where these are insufficient or unsuitable, biologic therapies, such as TNF-α inhibitors and the newer IL-17 and IL-23 inhibitors, are considered, ensuring all treatments are closely monitored for efficacy and potential side effects due to the heightened risk of adverse reactions in this age-group.

TAKE HOME MESSAGE

- Psoriasis management requires special consideration for pregnant women, children, and the elderly. Pregnancy poses risks to the fetus, the elderly face challenges due to comorbidities and drug interactions, and children require different dosing and treatments due to their unique disease characteristics and responses.
- *Pregnancy*: Use safer, nonsystemic treatments like topical therapies and phototherapy primarily, avoiding teratogenic medications such as methotrexate and retinoids. Certolizumab pegol is preferred among biologics due to minimal placental transfer.
- *Pediatrics*: Prefer treatments with minimal systemic effects, like topical agents and NBUVB phototherapy. For severe cases, systemic therapies such as methotrexate and cyclosporine can be used with careful monitoring. Approved biologics include etanercept (age ≥4 years), adalimumab (age ≥4 years by EMA), secukinumab and ixekizumab (age ≥6 years), and ustekinumab (age ≥4 years).
- *Elderly*: Topical therapies are preferred for their safety, while systemic treatments like methotrexate and cyclosporine are used cautiously at lower doses. Biologics, including TNF-α and IL-17 inhibitors, offer effective options but require close monitoring due to increased infection risks.

REFERENCES

1. Raychaudhuri SP, Navare T, Gross J, Raychaudhuri SK. Clinical course of psoriasis during pregnancy. Int J Dermatol. 2003;42(7):518-20.
2. Cohen-Barak E, Nachum Z, Rozenman D, Ziv M. Pregnancy outcomes in women with moderate-to-severe psoriasis. J Eur Acad Dermatol Venereol. 2011;25(9):1041-7.
3. Bae YS, Van Voorhees AS, Hsu S, Korman NJ, Lebwohl MG, Young M, et al.; National Psoriasis Foundation. Review of treatment options for psoriasis in pregnant or lactating women: from the Medical Board of the National Psoriasis Foundation. J Am Acad Dermatol. 2012;67(3):459-77.
4. Chi CC, Kirtschig G, Aberer W, Gabbud JP, Lipozenčić J, Kárpáti S, et al. Evidence-based (S3) guideline on topical corticosteroids in pregnancy. Br J Dermatol. 2011;165(5):943-52.
5. Murase JE, Heller MM, Butler DC. Safety of dermatologic medications in pregnancy and lactation: Part I. Pregnancy. J Am Acad Dermatol. 2014;70(3):401.e1-415.
6. Franssen ME, van der Wilt GJ, de Jong PC, Bos RP, Arnold WP. A retrospective study of the teratogenicity of dermatological coal tar products. Acta Derm Venereol. 1999;79(5):390-1.
7. Balakirski G, Gerdes S, Beissert S, Ochsendorf F, von Kiedrowski R, Wilsmann-Theis D. Therapy of psoriasis during pregnancy and breast-feeding. J Dtsch Dermatol Ges. 2022;20:653-83.
8. Owczarek W, Walecka I, Lesiak A, Czajkowski R, Reich A, Zerda I, et al. The use of biological drugs in psoriasis patients prior to pregnancy, during pregnancy and lactation: a review of current clinical guidelines. Postepy Dermatol Alergol. 2020;37(6):821-30.
9. Vena GA, Cassano N, Bellia G, Colombo D. Psoriasis in pregnancy: challenges and solutions. Psoriasis (Auckl). 2015;5:83-95.
10. Crall CS, Rork JF, Delano S, Huang JT. Phototherapy in children: Considerations and indications. Clin Dermatol. 2016;34(5):633-9.
11. Napolitano M, Megna M, Balato A, Ayala F, Lembo S, Villani A, et al. Systemic treatment of pediatric psoriasis: A review. Dermatol Ther (Heidelb). 2016;6(2):125-42.
12. Menter A, Cordoro KM, Davis DMR, Kroshinsky D, Paller AS, Armstrong AW, et al. Joint American Academy of Dermatology-National Psoriasis Foundation guidelines of care for the management and treatment of psoriasis in pediatric patients. J Am Acad Dermatol. 2020;82(1):161-201.
13. Caruso C, Buffa S, Candore G, Colonna-Romano G, Dunn-Walters D, Kipling D, et al. Mechanisms of immunosenescence. Immun Ageing. 2009;6:10.
14. Neema S, Kothari R, Rout A, Mani S, Bhatt S, Sandhu S. Systemic treatment of psoriasis in special population. Indian J Dermatol Venereol Leprol. 2023;1-8.
15. Sandhu VK, Ighani A, Fleming P, Lynde CW. Biologic treatment in elderly patients with psoriasis: A systematic review. J Cutan Med Surg. 2020;24(2):174-86.

17. Psoriasis and Quality of Life: Impact on Patients' Daily Lives and Mental Health

Sanjeev Handa, Sukhdeep Singh, Tarun Narang

■ INTRODUCTION

Psoriasis is a chronic, inflammatory dermatosis affecting 2% of world population with a significant detrimental impact on quality of life (QoL). It has a similar impact on QoL as ischemic heart disease, diabetes, cancer, and depression.[1] Low QoL in psoriasis can be attributed to chronic recurrent nature of disease, fear of unexpected relapses, and lack of cure.

■ LINK BETWEEN PSYCHIATRIC DISORDERS AND PSORIASIS

Impairments in QoL seem to be associated with development of psychiatric disorders. Psychiatric disorders especially depressive disorders are common in patients with psoriasis. Although psoriasis does not directly involve central nervous system (CNS), psychiatry morbidity may stem from complex interplay of stress, physical discomfort, disfigurement inherent to psoriasis as well as emotional response to the condition and perceived stigma.[2] An increased risk for depression, anxiety, and suicidality associated with greater psoriasis severity has been reported.[3] Various other psychiatric disorders like eating disorders, somatoform disorders, sleep disorders, and sexual disorders have been found to have increased prevalence in psoriasis. Previous studies reported a lower prevalence of psychiatric disorders in psoriasis (24.7–36.7%), most of these were based on assessment of psychiatric symptoms rather than psychiatric disorders.[4-6] A study which was based on both self-assessment and clinician-administered evaluations found a higher prevalence of psychiatric disorders (41.7%) especially depressive disorders in mild-to-moderate psoriasis.[2] Chronic low-grade depression or dysthymia was the most common diagnosis which may have been missed or underestimated in other studies. There was also only a modest correlation between results of self-assessment and clinician-administered evaluations indicating that psychiatric disorders may not be obvious to clinicians unless investigated.[2]

■ EMERGING ROLE OF CYTOKINES IN DEPRESSION ASSOCIATED WITH PSORIASIS

Chronic inflammation in psoriasis has been considered as a trigger for depression. Psoriatic plaques have increased nerve fiber density and abnormal expression of various neuropeptides. Inflammatory pathway which includes tumor necrosis factor alpha (TNF-α), interferon gamma (IFN-γ), other type-1 cytokines, and interleukin 17 (IL-17) pathway strongly delineates the pathophysiologic mechanisms of psoriasis and depression.[7] IL-21, IL-17, and T helper 17 (Th17) subsets, and transforming growth factor beta (TGF-β) are also found in patients of major depression.[7]

In animal models of multiple sclerosis, Th17 cells have been shown to cause neuronal cell death, most of the data linking psoriasis and depression has been extrapolated from those models.[8] Cohort studies have shown that psoriasis patients who have increased levels of IL-17A also have increased risk of depression and anxiety.[8] Numerous studies have also shown the increased levels of proinflammatory cytokines like TNF-α and IL-6 in major depression with fluctuation of their levels influencing mood.[8] Therefore, the striking similarity between psoriatic inflammation and neuroinflammation leads to depression.

■ FACTORS AFFECTING QUALITY OF LIFE IN PSORIASIS PATIENTS

Quality of life includes all factors that impact an individual's life, representing how well personal hopes align with real-life experiences. Health-related quality of life (HRQOL) focuses solely on health aspects, such as psychological, social, and physical well-being. The domains like employment and daily activities are most severely affected ones.

- *Age and gender*: Two studies have shown a negative impact on QoL in younger patients with moderate-to-severe psoriasis.[9,10] Older patients with longer disease duration had more difficulties in social functioning and impairment in QoL.[11] Gupta et al. reported that severity of psoriasis was not related to age or gender.[10] A recent study by Joseph et al. found statistically significant high scores in females for questions related to personal relations.[12]
- *Marital status*: Studies have shown no significant association between marital status and QoL.[12]
- *Location of lesions*: Lesions on visible site, over face, neck, sensitive regions like genitals, palmoplantar regions causing difficulty in daily activities are expected to have higher impairment in QoL. However, a recent review concluded that no one region affected by psoriasis predicts significantly better or worse QoL than another; all psoriatic regions predict decreased QoL.[13]
- *Symptoms like itching and pain*: These symptoms interfere with self-care and are associated with low QoL. Chronic pruritus leads to sleep disturbances, disruption of social relationships, higher anxiety and depression and lower QoL.
- Presence of comorbidities like psoriatic arthritis and other comorbidities
- *Duration of disease*: Older patients with longer disease duration had more difficulties in social functioning and impairment in QoL.[14] However, a study from US population showed no correlation between duration of disease and QoL demonstrating that patients do not adapt over time.
- *Body surface area*: A strong correlation has been observed between Psoriasis Area and Severity Index (PASI) scores and QoL scores with PASI > 18 having higher physical disability and mental stress rating.[15] Increased body surface area can lead to increased financial burden leading to impairment in QoL.

■ TOOLS TO MEASURE QUALITY OF LIFE AND PSYCHIATRIC COMORBIDITIES IN PSORIASIS

Various tools can be used to measure the impact on QoL in psoriasis ranging from general and skin specific tools to psoriasis specific measures. The most common skin specific measure used is Dermatology Life Quality Index (DLQI).

- The *DLQI* is a 10-item questionnaire designed to assess the impact of skin disease on QoL and disability.[16] It covers various life aspects, such as symptoms, self-perception, activities, relationships, and treatment effects. Patients rate how much their skin disease affects them, with options ranging from "very much" to "not at all". Each response is scored from 0 to 3, resulting in a total score out of 30, where a higher score indicates greater impairment of QoL. In a study of patients with mild-to-moderate psoriasis, analysis of DLQI scores was done for possible evaluation of underlying psychiatric disorder.[17] It was found that out of 104 patients of psoriasis with mean DLQI score of 6.85, 47 patients had at least one psychiatric disorder, out of which depressive disorder was most common (39.4%).[17] About 7% patients had more than one psychiatric disorder. Using regression analysis, it was revealed that symptoms and feelings domain of DLQI predicted a psychiatric disorder more often than other domains, even though the mean scores across each heading of DLQI were significantly more in group with any diagnosed psychiatric disorder.[17] This suggests that feelings and reactions to symptoms of disease are main contributor of impaired QoL in patients with mild-to-moderate psoriasis. Therefore, DLQI may serve as a screening tool for psychiatric disorders especially depressive disorder in mild-to-moderate psoriasis requiring need-based referral to psychiatric services.

- *Psoriasis Index of Quality of Life (PSORIQOL)*: It is a 25-item tool with yes/no responses, created through interviews to evaluate an individual's ability to meet their needs.
- *Psoriasis Life Stress Inventory (PLSI)*: It is a 15-item questionnaire to assess psychological stress and coping strategies ranging from 0 to 45.
- *Psoriasis Disability Index (PDI)*: It is a 15-question survey that measures how psoriasis affects daily activities, work, personal relationships, leisure, and treatment. Each question can be answered with "Not at all" (0), "A little" (1), "A lot" (2), or "Very much" (3). A higher total score means a greater impact on QoL.
- *Modified Patient Health Questionnaire 9 (PHQ-9)*: A major barrier to diagnosis of depression in primary care is lack of simple and rapid screening instruments available in local language. A rapid modified questionnaire with dichotomous responses based on first four questions of PHQ-9 in Hindi language was developed and its performance assessed by receiver operator curve analysis.[17] A cut of two items had a sensitivity of 70% and specificity of 76% in predicting depressive disorder in psoriasis, these patients can be evaluated more thoroughly and managed accordingly.[17] This is important because screening for depressive disorders in psoriasis patients should take into account dysthymic states as well which are much more common and cause morbidity.
- *Perceived Stress Scale (PSS)*: It includes 10 questions related to perceived stress of person in last 1 month with each item scored from 0 (never) to 4 (very often). Final score ranges from 0 to 40 with categorization into low stress (0–13), moderate stress (14–26), and high perceived stress (27–40).[18] In a study, 90% patients of psoriasis were found to have moderate level of stress on PSS.[19]
- *PHQ-4*: It is a self-reported 4-item screening tool with first two items for depression and other two for measuring anxiety. Each item ranges from 0 to 3 with total score ranging from 0 to 12 categorized into normal, mild, moderate, and severe.[20] In a study, 12.3% of participants reported mild-to-moderate anxiety and depression on this scale.[19]

STRATEGIES TO IMPROVE QUALITY OF LIFE IN PSORIASIS

- *Effective pharmacological management*: Effective management of psoriasis is crucial for improving the QoL. Treatment options include topical treatments,

CHAPTER 17: Psoriasis and Quality of Life: Impact on Patients' Daily Lives and Mental Health

TABLE 1: Effect of pharmacological treatments in quality of life (QoL) in psoriasis	
Treatment	**Outcomes**
Etanercept	Improvement in DLQI by 65–70% compared to placebo[21]
Infliximab	Median percentage improvement in DLQI scores of 84.0% and 91.0%, in 3 mg/kg and 5 mg/kg group, respectively[22]
Clobetasol propionate foam (clobetasol foam) 0.05%	Greater improvement in QoL compared to other topical therapies in non-scalp regions[23]
Cyclosporin	Intermittent short courses improve QoL and improve itch and severity of disease[24]
Combination of topical calcipotriol and betamethasone versus topical calcipotriol alone	Combination more effective in terms of QoL than monotherapy[25]
Methotrexate versus cyclosporine	Difference in QoL was comparable in both groups[26]
(DLQI: Dermatology Life Quality Index)	

phototherapy, systemic medications, and biologics. Different pharmacological treatments have varying effects on QoL **(Table 1)**.

- *Counseling of patients*: It improves mental and psychological condition. It should aim at encouraging active coping strategies, restructuring negative thoughts about disease, expressing emotions, and seeking social support and distracting themselves by engaging in various activities. Improvement of PASI and attaining remission is not enough, patient education along with supportive therapy are equally important. The patient needs to be counseled regarding noncontagious nature of disease, relapsing-remitting course, and exacerbating factors like stress, alcohol, smoking, coping with the disease.

  Studies have shown that developing a support system, including friends, family, counselors, and doctors, lessens the negative impact of QoL, reducing depression and social discomfort.[27]

- *Lifestyle modifications*: These include intervention strategies promoting health such as yoga, relaxation, meditation, biofeedback, cognitive–behavioral therapies and spirituality. Bed rest for short duration can be useful in patients of erythrodermic and pustular psoriasis. Various dietary supplements like evening primrose oil, turmeric have been used historically to control disease. Apart from this, dietary supplementation with oily fish such as salmon, sardine, mackerel rich in n-3 fatty acids is a useful adjunct in psoriasis due to immunomodulatory therapies. Other lifestyle modifications like cessation of smoking and alcohol should be encouraged.

■ TREATMENT OF DEPRESSION RELATED TO PSORIASIS

In psoriasis, depression occurs secondary to metabolic inflammation, therefore improving inflammation in psoriasis with targeted biologics should improve depression. The highest clinical efficacy with fastest onset of action can be achieved with IL-17 inhibitors particularly brodalumab and the IL-17A and F antibody, bimekizumab followed by IL-23 antagonists.[28] Among TNF inhibitors, etanercept has been associated with sustained significant reduction in anxiety and depression in patients of psoriasis.[29] Other TNF antagonists like infliximab have shown antidepressant effects in other inflammatory disorders like rheumatoid arthritis.[29]

CONCLUSION

Psoriasis profoundly impacts the QoL, affecting not just physical health but also psychological and social well-being. While the severity and manifestation of the disease vary among individuals, the chronic and visible nature of psoriasis often leads to significant emotional distress and social stigma. Effective management strategies, including appropriate pharmacological treatments, psychological support, and lifestyle modifications, are crucial for improving the QoL for those affected. Patient education and advocacy play vital roles in reducing stigma and promoting a better understanding of the disease.

TAKE HOME MESSAGE

- Psoriasis significantly affects quality of life, impacting not only physical health but also psychological and social well-being.
- The chronic and visible nature of psoriasis can lead to emotional distress and social stigma.
- Effective management strategies—including appropriate medications, psychological support, and lifestyle changes—are essential for enhancing the quality of life for those affected.
- Regular assessment of quality of life and mental health is crucial to tailor interventions and improve outcomes for psoriasis patients.
- Patient education and advocacy play vital roles in reducing stigma and promoting a better understanding of the disease.

REFERENCES

1. Finlay AY, Kelly SE. Psoriasis—An index of disability. Clin Exp Dermatol. 1987;12:8-11.
2. Singh SM, Narang T, Dogra S, Verma AK, Gupta S, Handa S. Psychiatric morbidity in patients with psoriasis. Cutis. 2016;97(2):107-12.
3. Suija K, Kalda R, Maaroos HI. Patients with depressive disorder, their co-morbidity, visiting rate and disability in relation to self-evaluation of physical and mental health: a cross-sectional study in family practice. BMC Fam Pract. 2009;10:38.
4. Mattoo S, Handa S, Kaur I, Gupta N, Malhotra R. Psychiatric morbidity in psoriasis: prevalence and correlates in India. Ger J Psychiatry. 2005;8:17-22.
5. Mattoo SK, Handa S, Kaur I, Gupta N, Malhotra R. Psychiatric morbidity in vitiligo and psoriasis: a comparative study from India. J Dermatol. 2001;28:424-32.
6. Mehta V, Malhotra S. Psychiatric evaluation of patients with psoriasis vulgaris and chronic urticaria. Ger J Psychiatry. 2007;10:104-10.
7. Aleem D, Tohid H. Pro-inflammatory Cytokines, Biomarkers, Genetics and the Immune System: A Mechanistic Approach of Depression and Psoriasis. Rev Colomb Psiquiatr (Engl Ed). 2018;47(3):177-86.
8. Zafiriou E, Daponte AI, Siokas V, Tsigalou C, Dardiotis E, Bogdanos DP. Depression and Obesity in Patients With Psoriasis and Psoriatic Arthritis: Is IL-17-Mediated Immune Dysregulation the Connecting Link? Front Immunol. 2021;12:699848.
9. López-Estebaranz JL, Sánchez-Carazo JL, Sulleiro S. Effect of a family history of psoriasis and age on comorbidities and quality of life in patients with moderate to severe psoriasis: Results from the ARIZONA study. J Dermatol. 2016;4:395-401.
10. Gupta MA, Gupta AK. Age and gender differences in the impact of psoriasis on quality of life. Int J Dermatol. 1995;34:700-3.
11. Ograczyk A, Miniszewska J, Kępska A, Zalewska-Janowska A. Itch, disease coping strategies and quality of life in psoriasis patients. Postep Dermatol Alergol. 2014;31:299-304.
12. Joseph DM, Binitha MP, Jithu V, Vasudevan B, Jishna P. Determinants of quality of life in patients with psoriasis attending the dermatology outpatient clinic in a tertiary care center: A cross-sectional study. J Skin Sex Transm Dis. 2021;3:156-61.
13. Nabieva K, Vender R. Quality of Life and Body Region Affected by Psoriasis: A Systematic Review. Actas Dermosifiliogr. 2023;114(1):33-8.
14. Gelfand JM, Feldman SR, Stern RS, Thomas J, Rolstad T, Margolis DJ. Determinants of quality of life in patients with psoriasis: A study from the US population. J Am Acad Dermatol. 2004;51:704-8.

15. Rakhesh SV, D'Souza M, Sahai A. Quality of life in psoriasis: A study from south India. Indian J Dermatol Venereol Leprol. 2008;74(6):600-6.
16. Finlay AY, Khan G. Dermatology Life Quality Index (DLQI)—a simple practical measure for routine clinical use. Clin Exp Dermatol. 1994;19:210-6.
17. Singh SM, Narang T, Dogra S, Verma AK, Gupta S, Handa S. An analysis of dermatological quality-of-life scores in relation to psychiatric morbidity in psoriasis. Indian Dermatol Online J. 2016;7:208-9.
18. Cohen S, Kamarak T, Mermelstein R. A global measure of perceived stress. J Health Soc Behav. 1983;24:386-96.
19. Kaur R, Sharma S, Das K, Narang T. Stress and Quality of Life in Psoriasis. Nurs Midwifery Res J. 2022;18(3):147-56.
20. Spitzer RL, Williams JW, Kroenke K. Primary Care Evaluation of Mental Disorders. Patient Health Questionnaire. Pfizer Inc. [online] Available from https://med.stanford.edu/fastlab/research/imapp/msrs/_jcr_content/main/accordion/accordion_content3/download_256324296/file.res/PHQ9%20id%20date%2008.03.pdf [Last accessed January 2025].
21. Krueger GG, Langley RG, Finlay AY, Griffiths CE, Woolley JM, Lalla D, et al. Patient-reported outcomes of psoriasis improvement with etanercept therapy: results of a randomized phase III trial. Br J Dermatol. 2005;153:1192-9.
22. Feldman SR, Gordon KB, Bala M, Evans R, Li S, Dooley LT, et al. Infliximab treatment results in significant improvement in the quality of life of patients with severe psoriasis: a double-blind placebo-controlled trial. Br J Dermatol. 2005;152:954-60.
23. Gottlieb AB, Ford RO, Spellman MC. The efficacy and tolerability of clobetasol propionate foam 0.05% in the treatment of mild to moderate plaque-type psoriasis of nonscalp regions. J Cutan Med Surg. 2003;7:185-92.
24. Salek MS, Finlay AY, Lewis JJ, Sumner MI. Quality of life and clinical outcome in psoriasis patients using intermittent cyclosporine (Neoral) Qual Life Res. 2004;13:91-5.
25. van de Kerkhof PC. The impact of a two-compound product containing calcipotriol and betamethasone dipropionate (Daivobet/Dovobet) on the quality of life in patients with psoriasis vulgaris: a randomized controlled trial. Br J Dermatol. 2004;151:663-8.
26. Heydendael VM, Spuls PI, Opmeer BC, de Borgie CA, Reitsma JB, Goldschmidt WF, et al. Methotrexate versus cyclosporine in moderate-to-severe chronic plaque psoriasis. N Engl J Med. 2003;349:658-65.
27. Janowski K, Steuden S, Pietrzak A, Krasowska D, Kaczmarek L, Gradus I, et al. Social support and adaptation to the disease in men and women with psoriasis. Arch Dermatol Res. 2012;304:421-32.
28. Mrowietz U, Sümbül M, Gerdes S. Depression, a major comorbidity of psoriatic disease, is caused by metabolic inflammation. J Eur Acad Dermatol Venereol. 2023;37(9):1731-8.
29. Uzzan S, Azab AN. Anti-TNF-α Compounds as a Treatment for Depression. Molecules. 2021;26(8):2368.

18. Psoriasis and Dermatology Practice: Clinical Pearls and Best Practices for Patient Management

Manjeet Naresh Ramteke

■ OVERVIEW OF PSORIASIS AND DERMATOLOGY PRACTICE

Psoriasis is chronic multisystem, autoimmune and inflammatory disorder. It is multifactorial disease with a complex pathogenesis, which results from the interaction between numerous external and internal factors. The global prevalence of psoriasis is about 0.09–11.4% as per the World Health Organization (WHO).[1] Psoriasis presents with a wide range of clinical manifestations including individual lesions varying from pinpoint to large plaques, which can progress into generalized forms. The lesions reflect the complex pathophysiological mechanisms involved in psoriasis, such as uncontrolled proliferation of keratinocytes and angiogenesis, inflammation and dysregulation of immune response. In addition to skin symptoms, there are abnormalities in nails, joint involvement, ocular disorders, metabolic syndrome, cardiovascular disease, type 2 diabetes, obesity, Crohn's disease, mental health disease, etc. in patients of psoriasis.[2] There is availability of vast range of therapeutic agents right from topicals, phototherapy, and systemic drugs, but there remains no definitive cure. Despite the great therapeutic variety, treatment selection is still based on clinical factors (patients and psoriasis' characteristics) and not on genetic ones. Most of the practitioners are still using the principle of *one size fits all* of traditional medicine. But many dermatological disorders including psoriasis are polygenic, complex, and multifactorial. And so the approach is changing from traditional one to personalized or individual's medicine. The current therapy selection process for patients with psoriasis is mostly empirical and lacks accuracy. Many factors contribute to therapy selection, including a physician's experience with psoriasis treatment, as well as clinical phenotypic features, comorbidities, patient preferences, pharmaceutical marketing strategies, and financial or payor restraints.[3] From a patient's point of view, it is a difficult and puzzling experience for them as there is a cycle of therapy changes in case of failure to respond adequately and getting a proper treatment, which gives adequate benefit. With the advent of new agents like biologics and small molecules, it has revolutionized the treatment of moderate-to-severe disease, demonstrating superior efficacy and safety profiles to conventional oral therapies and achieving complete or almost complete skin clearance.

■ EFFECTIVE COMMUNICATION WITH PSORIASIS PATIENTS: HEALTH LITERACY AND CULTURAL COMPETENCE

Effective communication between a psoriatic patient and his physician is important for enhancing treatment outcomes and successful dermatological care. A large interest has developed in the area of physician–patient communication in the last decade. It has also been included in the curriculum of medical education. Increased interest in physician–patient communication has evolved for better possible care for patient and family. Also it is fulfilling professional expectations of being a good doctor, decreasing the likelihood of malpractice claims, and maintaining a successful practice.[4] Studies also indicate that the ability to communicate honestly and empathically with patients has a powerful effect on the success of a medical practice.[5] There are lot of unique communication challenges in dermatology. Patients are frustrated because of chronic skin problems, which cannot be cured but only controlled. Patients come to the dermatologist for unrealistic expectations for improving their looks. The scheduled visits are brief with relatively short period of time in dermatology practice.

Steps to improve physician–patient communication are as follows:[6]

1. *Use open body language*: Sit with the patient with good eye contact.
2. *Ask open-ended questions*: Avoid yes or no queries.
3. *Respect the patient*: Learn about patient's personal preferences, limitations, and cultural background and take them into account when deciding on treatment plan.
4. *Involve the patient*: Take their feedback and involve them in the management of the patient for increased compliance.
5. *Address patient discomfort*: Discuss what patient feels and do not jump into writing a new medication.
6. *Acknowledge emotions*: Showing empathy, address patient's emotions.
7. *Coordinate care*: Work with other specialty doctors, ancillary and support services so they are aware of your patient's dermatology needs.
8. *Offer guidance*: Give the patient the directions they need for successful management of their condition.
9. *Invite questions*: Ask what questions the patient have.
10. *Provide information*: Give information as much as you can for patient's condition, care, and prognosis.
11. *Simplify electronic records*: Electronic records should be clear and understandable, which will help patient understand their treatment.

Understanding the knowledge, attitude, and practice (KAP) of individuals toward psoriasis is crucial in order to provide efficient management and support.[7] Knowledge analysis reveals that many people have a limited understanding of the underlying causes and triggers of psoriasis. Some misconceptions include associating it with poor hygiene or contagiousness, leading to social stigmatization. Attitude analysis often reveals negative emotions such as embarrassment, shame, and low self-esteem, affecting the mental well-being of individuals living with psoriasis. In terms of practice, findings indicate that adherence to treatment regimens can be a challenge due to the inconvenience or side effects of medications.[8]

Health literacy (HL) is defined as a patient's ability to seek, process, understand, and use health information.[9] It comprises a range of skills from reading and writing in health settings and having the language and confidence to discuss health to "critical" skills, which enable people to "exert greater control over life events and situations".[10] Poor HL creates barriers to understand one's health, illness, and treatment fully. Since limited HL is associated with poorer patient–physician communication, health-related skills, health outcomes, and treatment adherence, high levels of HL may be a helpful approach to improve self-management skills, treatment adherence, and quality of life.[11] HL is an essential factor required for effective self-management of chronic conditions such as psoriasis. People with psoriasis have lower HL as compared to other chronic skin disorders and overall heath outcome. A study by Avazeh et al. showed that medication adherence was influenced by several factors such as age, treatment type, satisfaction with treatment, experience of adverse effects, and most importantly HL.[9] And thus, patients with higher overall HL had better medication adherence. HL for people living with psoriasis can be increased by effective communication and teaching. Patient should receive written and verbal communication about psoriasis and its treatment in plain, nonmedical language. Support from peer groups and fellow patients can be taken, who can also be positive role models. Teaching in the form of hearing, seeing, and doing in their approach should be advocated. Also techniques such as "Teach-Back" in which patients are asked to assume the role of teacher and explain back the concepts they learned, can be used to ensure clear communication and also to build patient HL.[11] The use of internet as well as traditional sources of information like specialist professionals and peers should be emphasized for acquiring knowledge.

Dermatologists worldwide should be aware of the changing demographics of the population and associated healthcare diversities based on sex, race, ethnicity, socioeconomic status, disability, religion, and sexual orientation. Because of these diversities, cultural competence is becoming important especially in healthcare delivery. Cultural competence is loosely defined as the ability to understand, appreciate, and interact with people from cultures or belief systems different from one's own. It is also described as the acquisition of knowledge, interactional skills, and innovation in order to provide quality healthcare to diverse populations.[12] It is an overall approach of having an open mind, feeling empathy, and being accommodating to patients from all walks of life.[13] Cultural competent healthcare provider improves overall health outcome by establishing rapport and engaging in shared decision-making between the patient and physician in a manner that is respectful of a patient's values, goals, health needs, and cultural background and thus improving patient's satisfaction, and, ultimately, health outcome.[14] The goal of healthcare in dermatology is holistic. Cultural competence can be practised by the healthcare provider in their day-to-day interaction with patients by speaking in their local language, exercising cultural sensitivity with respect, empathy, and curiosity, being mindful of religion and spirituality, and considering skin's psychological impact. Patient's benefits of cultural competence are increased trust and mutual respect between the patient and provider, which also improves HL. Healthcare benefits of cultural competence include reduction in medical error, numbers of necessary treatments, and numbers of missed clinical visits, and also improvement in efficiency of care while community benefits are that it reduced health disparities in the patient population, includes all the members from the community and also involves the provider in the community.[15] The concept of cultural competence is a less ventured area in India. This concept became highly relevant in the coronavirus disease 2019 (COVID-19) pandemic era where the literature showed that cultural diversity is an important challenge to equitable distribution of healthcare services and accessibility.[16] There is existence of many cultures and subcultures in India, which becomes a challenge to practice cultural competence; and also limited time and resources, reluctance, or failed efforts in recognizing the cultural impacts on health, and incompetent leadership to highlight the importance of culture are other limitations in cultural competence. Also, with so many healthcare streams in India, the perspective of disease, its causes, and treatment approaches also change. This concept of cultural competence applies to psoriasis too, in fact to all the dermatological disorders where there would be differences in the epidemiology, clinical features, genetic predisposition, as well as treatment response. It is thus important to administer quality patient care and improve health outcomes and most importantly, the basic principles of professionalism are achieved.

CLINICAL PEARLS IN PSORIASIS MANAGEMENT: DIAGNOSIS, TREATMENT, AND FOLLOW-UP

Diagnosis of psoriasis is usually made by clinical morphology and site of lesions. Histopathology is rarely required but may help to differentiate psoriasis from another dermatosis if the diagnosis is not easy. The two histologic criteria as the "ñ sign," in which (1) the tilde represents a wavy laminar, parakeratotic, and separated stratum corneum and (2) the n denotes epidermal hyperplasia and regularly elongated rete ridges.[17] The extent and severity of psoriasis can be measured using the Psoriasis Area and Severity Index (PASI) but has limitation of high interobserver variability. Recently biomarkers like genetic, soluble, tissue-associated biomarkers, etc., that help in diagnosis and prognosis, assess who can develop severe form of disease and comorbidities, and also predict the response to various therapeutic interventions in psoriasis have been developed, but there are no approved biomarkers as of now.[18] A nail clipping may be performed to diagnose nail psoriasis. Imaging and/or referral to a rheumatologist should be performed in all patients with isolated nail psoriasis to evaluate for early arthritic changes. It is important to evaluate the various domains of disease for psoriasis patients, such as synovitis, enthesitis, dactylitis, and skin and nail disease.

The treatment of psoriasis should address both psychosocial and clinical manifestations of the disease as well as the extent of the disease, relevant comorbidities, and the effect of the disease on patients' quality of life. Treatment can vary from topical to systemic, with biological therapies as the last resort therapy but also with the highest efficiency.[19] Emollients and moisturizers may help in improving barrier function and retain the hydration of the stratum corneum. Topical potent corticosteroid with vitamin D or a vitamin D analog once daily for 4 weeks should be used for trunk and limb involvement. Ultra high- and high-potency (class 1–3) corticosteroids use for up to 4 weeks is generally safe with minimal risk of skin atrophy.[20] One study found that application of topical clobetasol led to a greater treatment response in African American skin compared to Caucasian skin, suggesting a different approach in patient with skin of color.[21] Topical corticosteroid should not be used for >12 weeks for nail disease, as it can result in bone atrophy with persistent use.[22] For maintenance treatment, vitamin D analogs, topical retinoids, and calcineurin inhibitors can be used. Proactive treatment is topical treatment (twice weekly) of areas which are clinically quiescent but are usually involved in recurrence, and can be a good strategy during maintenance.[23] Newer topical treatments like tapinarof, roflumilast, crisaborole, and tofacitinib are recently developed, which can be used for plaque psoriasis and intertriginous areas. Advise about the proper use and application of topical treatments should be given by healthcare professional.

Ultraviolet (UV) light-based therapies, which include narrowband and broadband UVB, UVA in conjunction with photosensitizing agents, targeted UVB treatments such as with an excimer laser are different modes of phototherapy. Narrowband UVB (NBUVB) can be used in plaque psoriasis as well as guttate psoriasis and can safely be given to children, pregnant and lactating females, and even older patients.[24] It can be used safely in patients with comorbidities who have contraindication for systemic treatment. It is recommended to be given thrice weekly for maximum response.

CHAPTER 18: Psoriasis and Dermatology Practice: Clinical Pearls and Best Practices for...

Application of a thin layer of emollient, such as petrolatum, is recommended before NBUVB treatment sessions, as this increases treatment effectiveness in psoriasis and also reduces UV-induced erythema.[25] Vitamin D analogs can be used in conjunction with phototherapy but should be applied after the phototherapy treatment to avoid inactivation by UVA and blocking UVB radiation.[26]

Systemic drugs are used in extensive psoriasis, the involvement of nails and psoriatic arthritis (PsA). Routine blood, liver functions, and renal functions should be monitored in patients on systemic therapy. Methotrexate (MTX), cyclosporine, acitretin, and small molecules, like apremilast and tofacitinib are possible systemic options. MTX is currently the first line of therapy in psoriasis, proven effective for chronic lesions, while also being indicated in the long-term medication of severe forms such as erythrodermic and pustular psoriasis. Cyclosporin is a potent immunosuppressant, rapid-acting medication for severe, recalcitrant disease, acute flares, and erythroderma but total length of therapy should not go beyond 1 year[27] and combination of cyclosporin with phototherapy is contraindicated. Acitretin, a second-generation retinoid, is administered specifically for the treatment of moderate-to-severe psoriasis, aside from generalized pustular, erythrodermic psoriasis and nail psoriasis. Being nonimmunosuppressive, it can be given in psoriasis patient on highly active antiretroviral therapy treatment of human immunodeficiency virus (HIV) and can also be combined with phototherapy for more efficacy. The efficacy of acitretin is dose-dependent, and the response varies from patient to patient.[28] Apremilast has demonstrated a modest efficacy in chronic plaque psoriasis, but has good efficacy in scalp, palmoplantar, nail psoriasis as well as PsA. It can be combined with other nonbiologic and biologic treatment. Tofacitinib can be considered for treatment of moderate-to-severe psoriasis but is not currently Food and Drug Administration (FDA) approved for that indication.[27] Tofacitinib can be used with MTX and should not be combined with potent immunosuppressants, such as azathioprine and cyclosporine, or with biologics used for psoriasis.[27] Practical challenge with conventional systemics is durations of therapy due to concerns of toxicity. An expert consensus from India suggests that the patients can be continued on treatment with strict monitoring protocols or can be considered for discontinuation or tailoring of therapy if sustained remission has been maintained for 6 months.[28] Biologic agents available in India are tumor necrosis factor alpha (TNF-α) inhibitors (adalimumab, etanercept, infliximab) and interleukin 17 (IL-17) inhibitors (secukinumab). Biologic therapy is reserved to psoriatic patients who satisfy the disease severity criteria while also presenting active PsA, those who have persistent or rapidly relapsing psoriasis (described as a reduction in PASI score <50% of the baseline in the following 3 months after completing systemic nonbiologic therapy), or in individuals in whom Dermatology Life Quality Index (DLQI) score improvement is lower than 5 points from the baseline at the start of therapy, after at least 6 month of nonbiologic therapy or when patients develop intolerances or have contraindications for classic systemic therapies.[29] Before starting any biological agent, the patient should be worked up for tuberculosis and hepatitis and must be monitored regularly after starting. Compared with lower-weight patients, overweight or obese patients are less likely to respond to TNF-α inhibitors. Secukinumab is recommended as a monotherapy treatment option in adult patients with moderate-to-severe plaque psoriasis. Dual biologic therapy is an off-label treatment and is not officially approved by the US FDA, and can be used in patients with psoriasis and PsA.[30] Concomitant

MTX reduces the immunogenicity and augments the efficacy of biologic therapies for psoriasis.[31] Live vaccines are to be avoided in people taking biological agents. Importance of patient education should be emphasized as psoriasis is a complex and multisystem disease.

Patient should be assessed for response to treatment by noting a reduction in baseline disease severity score (PASI) and improvement in physical, social, and psychological functioning at follow-up. Patients should be regularly followed up for screening of diabetes, hypertension (HTN), dyslipidemia as well as complications of psoriasis. Summarized, a yearly standard fasting lipid profile and at least 3-yearly fasting blood glucose measurement are recommended.[32] A cohort BIOBADADERM study stated that the incidence of adverse events (AEs) in patients with psoriasis who are treated with systemic agents varies over time and appears to be highest in the first year of treatment, regardless of the medication used.[33] Thus, regular monitoring along with testing of patient who are on any systemic therapy should be advised for the first year. Less intense and evenly spaced assessments and testing are recommended after the first year of treatment. Patients are advised to maintain healthy weight and should be encouraged to spend some time outdoor for sunlight. Infection is a known trigger for flares in psoriatic disease, so as far as possible should be prevented. Patient with moderate-to-severe psoriasis is associated with 5-year reduced life expectancy as compared to people without psoriasis.[31] One study showed that people who have psoriasis on >10% of their bodies have an increased mortality risk—or risk of death—compared to general population.[34] Thus, psoriasis patients with body surface area involvement of greater than 10% should be targeted for preventative health interventions.

■ BEST PRACTICES FOR PSORIASIS PATIENT MANAGEMENT: MULTIDISCIPLINARY CARE AND PATIENT EDUCATION

Psoriasis is a T cell-mediated autoimmune chronic inflammatory condition, which affects skin, nails, and joints. As it is associated with multiple comorbidities like diabetes mellitus (DM), HTN, obesity, hyperlipidemia, severe mental health issues, and numerous triggering factors like stress, alcohol, smoking, infections, and drugs, a multidisciplinary approach to patient care and patient education of the condition is crucial for holistic and effective management. The need for multidisciplinary management is reinforced by consensus among experts for patient satisfaction and overall healthcare.

Multidisciplinary care involved many specialists including dermatologist, rheumatologist, physician, psychiatrist, dietician, and physiotherapist. Dermatologist are the primary specialist in diagnosing and treating majority of psoriasis patients with topical, oral immunosuppressants and biologics. PsA can have severe impact on quality of life with late catastrophic consequences, and since most skin lesions developed before arthritis with 30% of patients having PsA at the time of presentation, they play a crucial role in early diagnosis and treatment, and early referral to a rheumatologist prevents catastrophic consequences of late PsA.[35,36] PsA can have varied presentation and can mimic other causes of arthritis, thus a rheumatologist involvement is essential for early diagnosis and timely management of PsA to prevent irreversible joint damage.[37] A physician plays a role in screening and managing comorbidities, which are commonly associated with psoriasis.[35] Psoriasis being a chronic disease has high incidence of mental health issues including depression and anxiety, which further can worsen the condition. A psychiatrist can address the psychological impact of the disease. Cognitive–behavioral therapy and counseling can improve the quality of life.[38] A dietician should be involved in dietary counseling to address obesity, a metabolic syndrome. The consumption of foods like yogurts, fish rich in omega-3 polyunsaturated fatty acids, fruits, vegetables as well as pre- and probiotic provide potential benefit.[39] A physiotherapist can help maintain joint mobility and alleviate pain in patient with PsA. Exercise programs can also support weight loss and overall health improvement.

Educating patients about the autoimmune and chronic nature of the disease and helping them understand that it is not curable but symptoms can be managed effectively is crucial and awareness regarding the potential triggers of the condition, like stress, alcohol smoking, drugs, and skin injury, should be provided. Patients should understand regarding the consistency with the prescribed treatment, even if the lesions improve. Clear instructions of how to take medicines and when to seek follow-up can enhance the treatment adherence. Etiopathogenesis of psoriasis is associated with metabolic syndrome and is also linked with multiple potential triggers including stress, alcohol intake, smoking, etc. Patients should be educated to avoid taking stress and follow cessation of smoking, excessive alcohol consumption not only aggravate the lesions it can also react with systemic medications and increases the likelihood of hepatotoxicity. Patients should be encouraged for intake of healthy diet containing fruits, green vegetables, yogurts, omega 3 fatty acids-rich foods, fish oil, and avoid consumption of processed foods rich in sugar and saturated fatty acids.[39,40] Mental health should be supported for early recognition of mental health issues. Patients also need to be educated about signs and symptoms of anxiety and depression. They should also be provided easy access to support groups and counseling services. And finally, self-care practices, daily use of moisturizers, and avoidance of harsh soaps and body wash should be encouraged.

Integrating disease management and proper patient education regarding the disease ensures that all the aspect of the condition and its impact in the patient's quality of life are addressed effectively. Collaborative management leads to overall improvement of disease management, higher patients' satisfaction which eventually improves the quality of patient's life and effective management of comorbid conditions improved the long-term health outcomes.

CONCLUSION

In managing psoriasis, a nuanced understanding of the condition, paired with clinical expertise, is essential to providing effective care. The best practices outlined throughout this chapter highlight the importance of individualized treatment plans that consider both the severity of the disease and the unique needs of each patient. Advances in both pharmacological and non-pharmacological treatments offer new hope, but successful management often requires a multidisciplinary approach involving education, emotional support, and consistent follow-up. By integrating clinical pearls and evidence-based strategies, dermatologists can improve patient outcomes, reduce the physical and psychological burden of the disease, and help patients achieve long-term control of their psoriasis. Ultimately, a holistic approach, focused on both physical and mental well-being, will remain the cornerstone of effective psoriasis management in dermatology practice.

CHAPTER 18: Psoriasis and Dermatology Practice: Clinical Pearls and Best Practices for...

> **TAKE HOME MESSAGE**
>
> Effective psoriasis management requires a patient-centered, individualized approach. Understanding the diversity of presentations and treatment options—ranging from topical therapies to biologics—is crucial for tailoring interventions that optimize outcomes. Key clinical pearls, such as early intervention, addressing comorbidities, and providing ongoing education and emotional support, can significantly enhance patient care. With continuous advancements in dermatology, staying informed about the latest evidence and treatment modalities will enable dermatologists to provide the best care possible, ultimately improving both the physical and psychological well-being of patients with psoriasis.

REFERENCES

1. Oon HH, Tan C, Aw DCW, Chong WS, Koh HY, Leung YY, et al. 2023 guidelines on the management of psoriasis by the Dermatological Society of Singapore. Ann Acad Med Singap. 2024;53(9):562-77.
2. Bu J, Ding R, Zhou L, Chen X, Shen E. Epidemiology of Psoriasis and Comorbid Diseases: A Narrative Review. Front Immunol. 2022;13:880201.
3. Ritchlin C, Pennington S, Reynolds N, FitzGerald O. Moving Toward Precision Medicine in Psoriasis and Psoriatic Arthritis. J Rheumatol Suppl. 2020;96:19-24.
4. Nguyen TV, Hong J, Prose NS. Compassionate care: Enhancing physician–patient communication and education in dermatology. J Am Acad Dermatol. 2013;68(3):353.e1-353.e8.
5. Forster HP, Schwartz J, DeRenzo E. Reducing legal risk by practicing patient-centered medicine. Arch Intern Med. 2002;162(11):1217-9.
6. Palmer WJ. (2018). 11 steps to improving doctor-patient communication. [online] Available from https://www.dermatologytimes.com/view/11-steps-improving-doctor-patient-communication [Last accessed January 2025].
7. Grodner C, Kluger N, Fougerousse AC, Cinotti E, Lacarrubba F, Quiles-Tsimaratos N, et al. Tattooing and psoriasis: dermatologists' knowledge, attitudes and practices. An international study. J Eur Acad Dermatol Venereol. 2019;33(1):e38-e40.
8. Tian J, Zhang L, Zhao X, Yang L. Knowledge, attitude, and practice of psoriasis patients toward their diseases: a web-based, cross-sectional study. Front Med (Lausanne). 2024;11:1288423.
9. Avazeh Y, Rezaei S, Bastani P, Mehralian G. Health literacy and medication adherence in psoriasis patients: a survey in Iran. BMC Prim Care. 2022;23(1):113.
10. Rowlands G. Health literacy and psoriasis: putting the patient at the centre of care. Br J Dermatol. 2019;180(6):1299-300.
11. Larsen MH, Strumse YAS, Borge CR, Osborne R, Andersen MH, Wahl AK. Health literacy: a new piece of the puzzle in psoriasis care? A cross-sectional study. Br J Dermatol. 2019;180(6):1506-16.
12. McKesey J, Berger TG, Lim HW, McMichael AJ, Torres A, Pandya AG. Cultural competence for the 21st century dermatologist practicing in the United States. J Am Acad Dermatol. 2017;77(6):1159-69.
13. Bilcha K. Cultural Competence in Dermatology. Pract Dermatol. 2021.
14. Betancourt JR. Cultural competency: providing quality care to diverse populations. Consult Pharm. 2006;21(12):988-95.
15. American Hospital Association. (2025). Becoming a Culturally Competent Health Care Organization. [online] Available from https://www.aha.org/ahahret-guides/2013-06-18-becoming-culturally-competent-health-care-organization [Last accessed January 2025].
16. Balachandran P, Karuveettil V, Janakiram C. Development and validation of cultural competence assessment tool for healthcare professionals, India. Front Public Health. 2022;10:919386.
17. Camporro ÁF, Roncero-Riesco M, Revelles-Peñas L, Nebreda DR, Estenaga Á, Díaz de la Pinta J, et al. The ñ Sign: A Visual Clue for the Histopathologic Diagnosis of Psoriasis. JAMA Dermatol. 2022;158(4):451-2.
18. Kar BR, Sathishkumar D, Tahiliani S, Parthasarathi A, Neema S, Ganguly S, et al. Biomarkers in Psoriasis: The Future of Personalised Treatment. Indian J Dermatol. 2024;69(3):256.
19. Mihu C, Neag MA, Bocşan IC, Melincovici CS, Vesa ŞC, Ionescu C, et al. Novel concepts in psoriasis: histopathology and markers related to modern treatment approaches. Rom J Morphol Embryol. 2022;62(4):897.
20. Castela E, Archier E, Devaux S, Gallini A, Aractingi S, Cribier B, et al. Topical corticosteroids in plaque psoriasis: a systematic review of risk of adrenal axis suppression and skin atrophy. J Eur Acad Dermatol Venereol. 2012;26 Suppl 3:47-51.
21. Lili L, Klopot A, Readhead B, Baida G, Dudley J, Budunova I. Transcriptomic Network Interactions

in Human Skin Treated with Topical Glucocorticoid Clobetasol Propionate. J Invest Dermatol. 2019; 139(11):2281-91.
22. Rigopoulos D, Gregoriou S, Daniel I CR, Belyayeva H, Larios G, Verra P, et al. Treatment of Nail Psoriasis with a Two-Compound Formulation of Calcipotriol plus Betamethasone Dipropionate Ointment. Dermatology. 2009;218(4):338-41.
23. Ito K, Koga M, Shibayama Y, Tatematsu S, Nakayama J, Imafuku S. Proactive treatment with calcipotriol reduces recurrence of plaque psoriasis. J Dermatol. 2016;43(4):402-5.
24. Nair PA, Badri T. Psoriasis. In: StatPearls [Internet]. Treasure Island (FL): StatPearls Publishing; 2024.
25. Abdallah M, Ahmed El-Khateeb E, Abdel-Rahman S. The influence of psoriatic plaques pretreatment with crude coal tar vs. petrolatum on the efficacy of narrow-band ultraviolet B: a half-vs.-half intra-individual double-blinded comparative study Photodermatol Photoimmunol Photomed. 2011; 27(5):226-30.
26. Elmets CA, Lim HW, Stoff B, Connor C, Cordoro KM, Lebwohl M, et al. Joint American Academy of Dermatology-National Psoriasis Foundation guidelines of care for the management and treatment of psoriasis with phototherapy. J Am Acad Dermatol. 2019;81(3):775-804.
27. Menter A, Gelfand JM, Connor C, Armstrong AW, Cordoro KM, Davis DMR, et al. Joint American Academy of Dermatology–National Psoriasis Foundation guidelines of care for the management of psoriasis with systemic nonbiologic therapies. J Am Acad Dermatol. 2020;82(6):1445-86.
28. Rajagopalan M, Chatterjee M, De A, Dogra S, Ganguly S, Kar B, et al. Systemic Management of Psoriasis Patients in Indian Scenario: An Expert Consensus. Indian Dermatol Online J. 2021;12(5):674-82.
29. Timis T, Florian I, Vesa S, Mitrea DR, Orasan R. An updated guide in the management of psoriasis for every practitioner. Int J Clin Pract. 2021;75(8):e14290.
30. Thibodeaux Q, Ly K, Reddy V, Smith MP, Liao W. Dual biologic therapy for recalcitrant psoriasis and psoriatic arthritis. JAAD Case Rep. 2019;5(10):928-30.
31. Strober B. (2014). 10 Clinical Pearls in Psoriasis. [online] Available from https://mauiderm.com/10-clinical-pearls-in-psoriasis/ [Last accessed January 2025].
32. DeCoster E, Alves de Medeiros A, Bostoen J, Stockman A, van Geel N, Lapeere H, et al. A multileveled approach in psoriasis assessment and follow-up: A proposal for a tailored guide for the dermatological practice. J Dermatol Treat. 2016;27(4):298-310.
33. Descalzo MA, Carretero G, Ferrándiz C, Rivera R, Daudén E, Gómez-García F, et al.; Biobadaderm Study Group. Change over time in the rates of adverse events in patients receiving systemic therapy for psoriasis: A cohort study. J Am Acad Dermatol. 2018;78(4):798-800.
34. Noe M, Shin D, Wan M, Gelfand J. Objective Measures of Psoriasis Severity Predict Mortality: A Prospective Population-Based Cohort Study. J Invest Dermatol. 2018;138(1):228-30.
35. Zheng Y, Zheng M. A multidisciplinary team for the diagnosis and management of psoriatic arthritis. Chin Med J (Engl). 2021;134(12):1387-9.
36. Menter A, Strober BE, Kaplan DH, Kivelevitch D, Prater EF, Stoff B, et al. Joint AAD-NPF guidelines of care for the management and treatment of psoriasis with biologics. J Am Acad Dermatol. 2019;80(4):1029-72.
37. Gossec L, Kerschbaumer A, Ferreira RJO, Aletaha D, Baraliakos X, Bertheussen H, et al. EULAR recommendations for the management of psoriatic arthritis with pharmacological therapies: 2023 update. Ann Rheum Dis. 2024;83(6):706-19.
38. Ferreira BIRC, Abreu JLPDC, Reis JPGD, Figueiredo AMDC. Psoriasis and Associated Psychiatric Disorders: A Systematic Review on Etiopathogenesis and Clinical Correlation. J Clin Aesthet Dermatol. 2016;9(6):36.
39. Musumeci ML, Nasca MR, Boscaglia S, Micali G. The role of lifestyle and nutrition in psoriasis: Current status of knowledge and interventions. Dermatol Ther. 2022;35(9):e15685.
40. Obradors M, Blanch C, Comellas M, Figueras M, Lizan L. Health-related quality of life in patients with psoriasis: a systematic review of the European literature. Qual Life Res. 2016;25(11):2739-54.

19

Patient Education and Support: Strategies for Improving Patient Adherence and Self-management

Satyaki Ganguly, Akshay Sankar Peethambaran

■ INTRODUCTION

Psoriasis is a common chronic inflammatory disease, which involves skin and joints and is characterized by erythematous, scaly papules and plaques.[1] It significantly lowers the patient's quality of life and causes severe morbidity. Psoriasis has a multifaceted effect on a patient's interpersonal, physical, and psychological well-being, and it mostly depends on how the patient perceives their situation. Psoriasis patients frequently attribute a significant negative impact on overall quality of life due to the disease as well as its treatment. Individuals with psoriasis may experience significant psychosocial problems, including significant disapproval, isolation from society, and inequity. Psoriasis patients have a wide range of treatment options, from straightforward topical treatments to potentially harmful oral medications; however, there is no known cure. For the majority of patients, treatment is necessary for the rest of their lives.[2]

Since over 90% of patients with psoriasis have a chronic illness with periodic exacerbations, medication adherence or compliance and self-management including lifestyle modification are as important as pharmacotherapy for both effective disease management and a decrease in clinical severity.[1] Compliance in the medical field refers to how closely a person's actions match health-related advice. This includes the patient's capacity to keep clinic appointments on time, take medication as directed, modify their lifestyle as advised, and finish recommended tests. Medication adherence can be defined as the percentage difference between the number of therapeutic "doses" prescribed to the patient and the number of "doses" taken by the patient. Medication adherence, as stated here, would typically range from 0 to 100%. Patient adherence and self-management, in turn, are dependent on effective counseling and involvement of the patient in his or her treatment. Unfortunately, this is often the most neglected part of psoriasis management. As a result, patients often give up and stop treatment, neglect, go "doctor shopping", seek care from alternative systems of medicine, and even quacks, leading to poor quality of life, frequent exacerbations, increased complications, and morbidity.

■ THE EXTENT OF THE PROBLEM

Medication adherence: The overall mean medication adherence among psoriasis patients is around 60.6%. Patients with lower Dermatology Life Quality Index (DLQI) showed higher medication adherence.[2]

The three primary categories of factors influencing compliance are as follows. These include variables related to disease distribution, treatment, and society.[2]

1. *Disease distribution factors*: Facial lesions and more than three body areas involvement showed association with lower medication adherence.[2]
2. *Societal factors*: Patients who are married, employed, and those who did not have to pay for medications showed higher medication adherence. Alcohol and smoking showed an association with lower medication adherence.[2]
3. *Treatment-related factors*: Compared to topical treatment, oral therapy had substantially lower compliance. Even though using oral medication should be simpler and requires less time, compliance with combined therapy was comparable to that with topical treatment. Patient confidence in a combination of oral and topical treatment regimens is demonstrated by higher drug adherence rates. However, the increased volume of topical medications resulted in decreased adherence. Patients starting treatment for the first time, patients who did not develop an adverse effect, and those prescribed once-daily medications as opposed to twice-daily medication showed higher medication adherence.[2]

PROBLEMS FACED

Inadequate treatment adherence, a prevalent issue in medicine, could account for suboptimal therapy results. Topical therapy is frequently cited by psoriasis patients as one of the worst aspects of their disease. People with more severe psoriasis either in terms of the degree of involvement or the impact on their quality of life are less likely to take their medications as prescribed compared to those with less severe disease. Patients usually express dissatisfaction with available therapy alternatives. This creates a vicious loop in which patients may be less motivated to follow their treatment plans if they have more skin lesions, lower quality of life, and low treatment satisfaction. The consumption of their medication may be further influenced by depressive, hopeless, or helpless feelings.[3]

- *Problems faced with topical treatment*: Most psoriasis patients initiate being treated with a topical medication. Although many patients show early enthusiasm for topical treatments, treatment outcomes are frequently unsatisfactory, leading to disappointment for both patients and physicians. During a patient's treatment journey, this could result in multiple shifts to different topical medicines, systemic drugs, and different medical practitioners entirely.[3]

    There are various possible reasons for these suboptimal results, some of them are as follows.[3]
    - Inability to understand instructions
    - Ineffectiveness of the medication
    - Patients' dislike of the product's consistency; topical medications are often difficult and time-consuming to apply.
    - Adverse effects that force an early stop to the treatment
    - Lack or loss of motivation and underlying depression

- *Problems faced with systemic treatment*: It may be necessary to add phototherapy if topical medications are not feasible or effective enough. If phototherapy proves to be ineffective, impractical, or impossible, systemic treatment with conventional or biological agents needs to be taken into account. Although systemic therapy is a reasonable early choice for some people with more extensive disease and substantial quality-of-life considerations, the order of these options for treatment suggests starting treatment with safer approaches for patients having mild-to-moderate illness.[3]

The following are the causes of the patients' inadequate adherence to systemic therapy:
- Side effects or fear of it
- Perceived ineffectiveness over prolonged duration
- Repeated recurrences
- Cost
- Pill burden

CONSEQUENCES OF NONCOMPLIANCE

Improved compliance is linked to better health outcomes, while poor adherence is related to worse prognosis, more hospitalizations, impaired functioning, increased risk of morbidity and even death from disease-related complications, and substantially larger healthcare expenses. In fact, rather than an impairment of corticosteroid receptor activity, poor adherence could be the cause of tachyphylaxis seen in clinical practice.[3]

METHODS TO IMPROVE

When choosing a treatment, psoriasis patients place a greater emphasis on process characteristics (such as treatment location, mode of delivery, frequency, duration, and cost) than on outcome characteristics. Treatment preferences are influenced by working position and sociodemographic traits. Interestingly, women valued treatment frequency more than men did, whereas men were more preoccupied with the possibility of symptom alleviation. Compared to younger patients, older participants were concerned about more serious adverse effects but judged the possibility of improvement to be less important. Lastly, compared to patients who were not employed, patients who worked a full-time job placed a higher importance on the duration of response, the location of therapy, and the frequency of treatment.[1]

Psoriasis management success is dependent upon patient adherence over an extended period, in addition to a physician's accurate diagnosis and proper treatment recommendations.

Better results could arise from increasing patient adherence, as suggested by the recommendations listed below:[3]
- Physician–patient relationship
- Patient preference
- Patient education
- Adjusting the treatment regimen
- Assessing adherence

Physician–Patient Relationship

Adherence is primarily determined by the relationship between the physician and the patient. The probability of compliance will improve when a doctor speaks understandably, promotes candid communication between the patient and the provider, allows patients to participate in their care, and establishes a welcoming and productive atmosphere. Patient perceptions of doctors' care for their well-being, the clarity of their answers, as well as the accuracy of the information they receive in response to their inquiries all correlate with patient satisfaction. Patient satisfaction is greatly increased when medical professionals use the patient's own words and language and thereby the treatment compliance. When doctors inquire about their patient's mental health and allow them to discuss psychosocial issues, the patients seem happier. In patients with psoriasis, where interpersonal connection issues may take precedence over skin complaints, this may be especially crucial.

Patient Preference

Predicting a person's preferences for a treatment plan is frequently challenging. Applying topical treatments for more extensive psoriasis when the individual has numerous lesions will be impossible and ultimately futile. It is important to pay attention to providing a regimen that benefits. Only patients who pay close attention to treatment may find it feasible to apply several drugs at different times on different days. Dosing straightforward regimens, such as using a single medication twice a day, have a higher probability of being effective. Inquiring about the patient's preferred pharmaceutical route from the range of potential therapies can enhance compliance. Better compliance among patients and therapeutic outcomes may be attained with the use of personalized dosage devices and clear instructions. A practical illustration of the proper administration of these medications will be beneficial to the patients. Family members may help with treatment, aid in remembering dosage regimens, and act as a support system, helping them promote treatment compliance, especially for the parents in case of children, spouse, and caregivers in case of elderly.

Patient Education

Enhancing psoriasis management, therapy, and compliance requires a strong focus on patient education. Patients should feel that the dangers, advantages, and available options have been sufficiently disclosed to them. Assess the patient's understanding, allow them to ask questions, and provide them with adequate information they may use at home. Essential steps that need to be included in the visit include providing written instructions that are easy to follow and contact information in case there are any issues.

Adjusting the Treatment Regimen

There is possibly a propensity to employ stronger or more complicated therapies when individuals do not respond to topical therapy. This might backfire if the patient thought the treatment was too hazardous or the regimen was too complicated, which led to the initial treatment's ineffectiveness. On the other hand, a low threshold for prescribing more effective systemic medications rather than topical medications may convince the despairing patient to continue treatment. Early institution of treatment, which is more effective in achieving early remission and better clearance, may in turn improve compliance.

The impression of therapeutic load may be lessened by scheduling a follow-up appointment soon after starting treatment. Compliance is increased by more frequent visits and interactions with the provider. An increasing improvement should be anticipated as the patient learns more about the doctor's interest in compliance.

Assessing Adherence

It is difficult to evaluate patients' compliance. Treatment diaries and self-reports by patients are frequently erroneous. The clinician may gain insight into existing patterns of compliance by asking a few standard, nonjudgmental questions.

Lastly, the detection of depression/psychiatric comorbidity associated with psoriasis and treatment of the same will improve compliance and outcome. Further, public awareness is important to prevent improper treatment by quacks, resulting in bad treatment outcomes and complications, a situation not uncommon in India.

■ CONCLUSION

Medication adherence is a complicated problem with numerous components. It is essential that doctors and medical support personnel promote adherence, and they should be equipped with techniques and resources to help with compliance. Better compliance can lead to better therapeutic outcomes, which will improve psoriasis patients' healthcare and life conditions.

CHAPTER 19: Patient Education and Support: Strategies for Improving Patient...

> **TAKE HOME MESSAGE**
>
> Since psoriasis is a chronic disorder with no known cure, medication adherence and self-management is as important as pharmacotherapy. Counseling plays a vital role in improving medication adherence and self-management. Medication adherence or compliance depends on area of involvement, type of treatment prescribed and individual patient characteristics. Early institution of more effective therapy and more effective physician-patient communication can result in better adherence.

REFERENCES

1. Belinchón I, Rivera R, Blanch C, Comellas M, Lizán L. Adherence, satisfaction and preferences for treatment in patients with psoriasis in the European Union: a systematic review of the literature. Patient Prefer Adherence. 2016;10: 2357-67.
2. Zaghloul SS, Goodfield MJD. Objective Assessment of Compliance With Psoriasis Treatment. Arch Dermatol. 2004;140:408-14.
3. Feldman SR, Horn EJ, Balkrishnan R, Basra MK, Finlay AY, McCoy D, et al. Psoriasis: Improving adherence to topical therapy. J Am Acad Dermatol. 2008;59:1009-16.

20 Case Studies in Psoriasis Management: Real-World Applications of Psoriasis Diagnosis and Treatment

Shekhar Neema, Siddharth Mani

■ INTRODUCTION

Psoriasis is a T-cell-mediated disorder with an uncertain cause, mainly impacting the skin, nails, and joints. It can develop at any age, though it typically shows two peaks: The first between 16 and 22 years of age, and the second between 57 and 60 years.[1] The average age of onset is around 33 years. In India, psoriasis prevalence has been reported to be between 0.4 and 2.2% in different studies.[2]

Psoriasis treatment depends on its severity, which is assessed by the extent of skin involvement, impact on quality of life, and any related comorbid conditions. Treatment options range from topical therapies and phototherapy to conventional systemic medications, small molecule drugs, and biologic therapies. Presence of comorbidities and concomitant systemic diseases play an important role in choice of therapy.[3]

Herein we report the management of psoriasis in such complicated real-life scenarios.

■ SCENARIO 1: PSORIASIS WITH LATENT TUBERCULOSIS

Case: A 38-year-old male with a known history of hypothyroidism presented with multiple red, raised lesions across the body for the past 8 years. The condition has followed a relapsing and remitting course, with exacerbations typically occurring in winter. The patient reports pain over multiple small joints and experiences early morning stiffness lasting approximately 60 minutes.

On examination, multiple well-defined and polysized erythematous plaques with loosely adherent silvery-white scales were noted involving 40% body surface area. Both Auspitz sign and Grattage test were positive. Scalp involvement included well-defined erythematous and scaly plaques that extended beyond the scalp margins **(Fig. 1)**. Nail examination revealed coarse pitting. Musculoskeletal examination showed dactylitis of left third finger, enthesitis of tendo-Achilles right and tenderness involving distal interphalangeal joints.

Diagnosed with psoriasis vulgaris and psoriatic arthritis, the patient underwent baseline investigations which were within normal limits. In view of severe psoriasis and psoriatic arthritis, individual was planned for biologic therapy.

For biologic therapy evaluation, a chest X-ray was normal; however, the Mantoux test was 23 mm **(Fig. 2)**, and interferon-γ release assay (IGRA) was positive, indicating latent tuberculosis. The patient was initiated on antitubercular prophylaxis with capsule rifampicin 600 mg once daily and tablet isoniazid 300 mg once daily for 3 months. 22 weeks after starting latent tuberculosis infection (LTBI) prophylactic therapy, the patient began treatment with injection secukinumab 300 mg/week.

CHAPTER 20: Case Studies in Psoriasis Management: Real-World Applications...

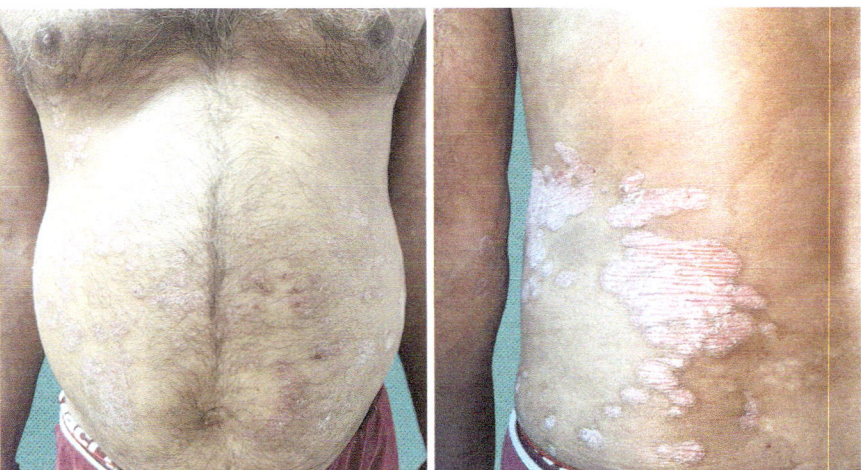

FIG. 1: Multiple well-defined, polysized erythematous plaques with loosely adherent silvery-white scales present over trunk and back.

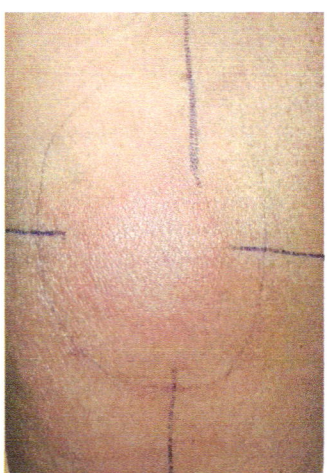

FIG. 2: Positive Mantoux reaction.

Management Pearl

- India has a high prevalence of tuberculosis and LTBI is common in the general population. LTBI can progress to active tuberculosis in almost 10% patients and the risk increases with immunosuppression.[4] This predisposes patients of psoriasis on systemic therapy for the development of active tuberculosis. In the study by Neema et al. out of 105 patients of psoriasis requiring systemic therapy who were evaluated for tuberculosis, 31 were positive for LTBI and two had active tuberculosis.[5]
- *Testing for LTBI*: Reactivation of LTBI is a concern in a patient planned for immunosuppressive therapy. Even though both tuberculin skin test (TST) and IGRA are being used, most authors prefer IGRA over TST for LTBI. However, it is to be kept in mind that IGRA is useful only in LTBI diagnosis. Diagnosis of active tuberculosis requires different sets of investigations. Certain authors also prefer the use of both TST and IGRA rather than two-step testing (TST followed by IGRA) or IGRA alone for the diagnosis of LTBI, especially in patients with a high risk of reactivation.[6] The abovementioned study found discordance in 60.7% (17/28) of patients tested with IGRA and TST. Hence, they recommended that the positivity on either test should prompt further evaluation and treatment decisions should be taken considering the risk-benefit ratio of treatment rather than test results alone. Similar pattern of testing has also been recommended in a cohort study conducted in Spain which showed that a dual screening

strategy with TST and IGRA before tumor necrosis factor inhibitor (TNFi) treatment is more effective. Compared to one single screening test, dual screening can detect more LTBI patients.[7] However, in resource, poor setting TST can be used as first-line test for LTBI and IGRA can be done in following scenarios:
- When results from TST are indeterminate.
- When TST is positive and there is need to increase the acceptability of treatment.
- To follow-up patients who are on biological therapy, when TST is of limited value.

- While most of the dermatologists are confident in using topical agents and narrowband ultraviolet B (NBUVB) for psoriasis with LTBI, administration of biologics is fraught with risks. The confusion further deepens when the standard textbooks mention regarding testing for LTBI while not mentioning about the use of biologics during the time when the patient is on LTBI prophylaxis. The authors preferred interleukin-17 (IL-17) inhibitor over TNF-α inhibitor due to following evidence:
  - The risk of reactivation of tuberculosis is high with TNFis. Various studies have confirmed that anti-TNF-α therapy is associated with 25 times risk of activation of LTBI, depending on the clinical setting and the agent used as has been shown in various studies.[8,9] Most authors either avoid the use of TNFi in LTBI setting or wait for completion of LTBI prophylaxis therapy which defeats the purpose of its use, as the patients have severe psoriasis which necessitates early institution of therapy. Hence, certain authors advocate the use of TNFi after 3-4 weeks of starting LTBI therapy.[10,11] If the condition is urgent, TNFi and preventive treatment can be initiated simultaneously after thorough evaluation.[12] However, this approach is not practiced by many considering the high risk involved with TNFi.
  - Interleukin-17 inhibitors on the other hand pose low to no risk of reactivation of tuberculosis. Even though testing for LTBI is recommended, the biologic can be started simultaneously with LTBI prophylaxis.
  - In a recently conducted multicentric retrospective study, a total of 405 patients having severe plaque psoriasis with concurrent LTBI were included; complete/incomplete/no chemoprophylaxis was administered due to various reasons in 62.2, 10.1, and 27.7% of patients, respectively.
  - Either IL-17i or IL-23i was started in these patients despite having LTBI and irrespective of chemoprophylaxis status. Only one patient who was on ixekizumab developed active tuberculosis while other patients did not show any such conversion. Hence making IL-17 or IL-23 inhibitors the preferred choice over TNF antagonists in patients with LTBI specially for those who are considered at higher risk for developing complications related to chemoprophylaxis, avoiding this preventive strategy.[12]

SCENARIO 2: PSORIASIS IN PREGNANCY

Case: A 33-year-old female with a 2-year history of psoriasis and psoriatic arthritis presented with multiple erythematous, scaly plaques on the scalp, trunk, and limbs, along with joint pain in the small joints of both hands, morning stiffness, dactylitis, and enthesitis. Grattage and Auspitz signs were positive. Baseline investigations, LTBI, rheumatoid factor, and anti-cyclic citrullinated peptide

CHAPTER 20: Case Studies in Psoriasis Management: Real-World Applications...

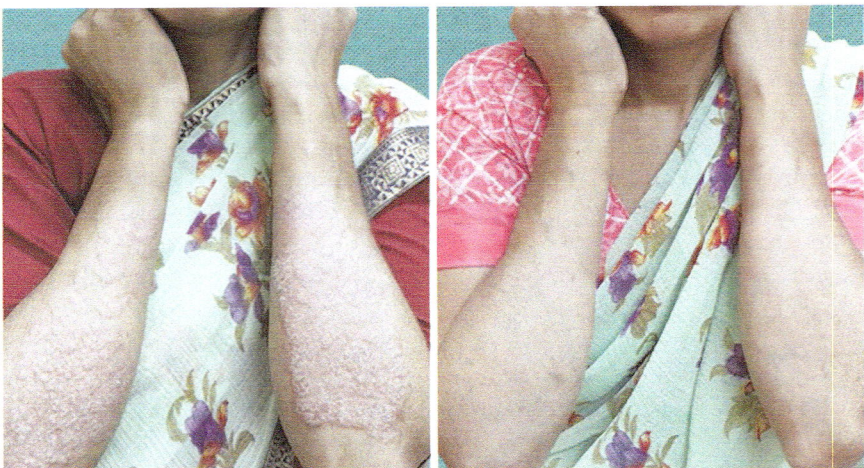

FIG. 3: Pre- and post-etanercept (5 weeks) in a case of psoriasis in pregnancy.

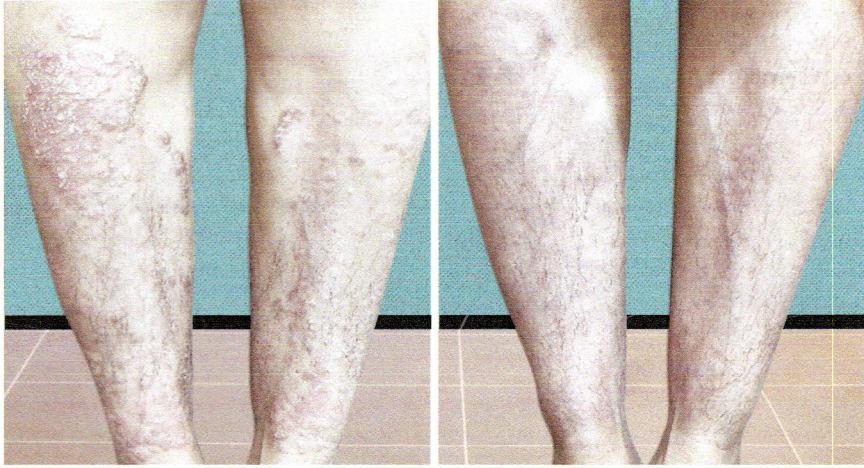

FIG. 4: Pre- and post-etanercept (5 weeks) in a case of psoriasis in pregnancy.

(anti-CCP) antibodies were negative. Due to intolerance to methotrexate and apremilast, she was started on adalimumab, which reduced her Psoriasis Area and Severity Index (PASI) score from 18.4–6 and alleviated joint pain after six doses. Before the seventh dose, she tested positive on a urine pregnancy test, leading to the discontinuation of biologics. She was transitioned to NBUVB therapy and topicals. After a flare at 12 weeks of pregnancy, etanercept was initiated and continued until 30 weeks. She delivered at 36 weeks, with live vaccines for the newborn deferred for 6 months due to prior biologic exposure **(Figs. 3 and 4)**.

Management Pearl

- Pregnancy shifts maternal immune response from a Th1 to a Th2 profile. The progression of psoriasis during pregnancy is variable: Around 55% of patients experience improvement, 23% see a worsening of symptoms, and the remainder remain stable. Psoriatic arthritis may also be triggered postpartum in 30-40% of cases.[13,14] Pregnancy outcomes in patients with psoriasis can be less favorable, with an increased risk of preterm birth, low birth weight, recurrent miscarriage, and a higher rate of cesarean delivery. Fetal risk is influenced by the activity of the mother's disease.[15] Managing severe psoriasis during pregnancy is challenging due to medication safety concerns, primarily due to potential effects on fetal organ development. Clinical scenarios requiring management include the following:

- *Unplanned pregnancy*: If a patient becomes pregnant unexpectedly while on systemic antipsoriatic treatment, the medication should be discontinued, and the patient should be counseled on potential risks and referred to an obstetrician for further care. Teratogenic drugs such as methotrexate and acitretin are contraindicated in pregnancy, whereas cyclosporine and apremilast are safer options. Most biologics have favorable outcomes in pregnancy, and the risk-benefit ratio should be discussed with the patient.[16]
- *Planned pregnancy*: For patients planning to conceive, pregnancy should ideally begin when psoriasis is well-controlled. Treatments should be adjusted to topical options and NBUVB before conception. As NBUVB can lower folic acid levels, folic acid supplementation is recommended to minimize neural tube defect risks.[17]
- *Disease onset or flare during pregnancy*: In cases of new-onset severe psoriasis, such as generalized pustular or erythrodermic psoriasis, or a flare of preexisting disease, systemic therapy may be necessary. Stable chronic plaque psoriasis can often be managed with topicals and NBUVB.

Cyclosporine may be used if the disease is unstable or resistant to initial treatments. For generalized pustular psoriasis in pregnancy—a particularly difficult condition—treatment with cyclosporine, oral steroids, or a combination may be effective.[18] Infliximab and secukinumab have also been used successfully in some cases.[19,20]

- *Biologics in pregnancy*: While drugs such as cyclosporine and apremilast are category C drugs and methotrexate and acitretin are category X drugs, most of the biologics have been placed as category B drugs making them reasonably safer option. In the recently published meta-analysis of fetal and maternal outcomes after maternal biologic use during conception and pregnancy, 11,752 pregnancies exposed to biologics were studied and compared with disease-matched controls and disease-free pregnancies. The prevalence of congenital malformation, preterm delivery, neonatal infection, low birth rate, and small for gestation age remained similar in each of the groups.[21]

Fetal exposure to biologics correlates with the placental transport of immunoglobulins. In the first trimester, fetal immunoglobulin levels are low, but by the third trimester, they reach levels nearly equal to those in the mother. This increased transfer of biologics across the placenta in late pregnancy can potentially weaken the newborn's immune response, making it advisable to discontinue biologics before term and avoid live vaccinations for the infant in the first 6 months. TNF-α inhibitors are generally regarded as safe during the first half of pregnancy. Various monoclonal antibodies have different affinities for Fc receptors. Immunoglobulin G1 (IgG1) antibodies (adalimumab/infliximab/secukinumab/ustekinumab/guselkumab/tildrakizumab/risankizumab) followed by IgG4 antibodies (ixekizumab) and IgG3 and IgG2 (brodalumab) are most easily transmissible. Etanercept has low affinity owing to being fusion protein. Certolizumab pegol, a pegylated antibody fragment (Fab) that lacks the Fc region, is not actively transported across the placenta by the FcRn receptor and is therefore considered safe for use in pregnant women.[22,23]

■ SCENARIO 3: PSORIASIS WITH HEPATITIS

Case: A 31-year-old male presented with 2-year history of multiple red, raised, scaly lesions over the body and scalp. The lesions had a history of waxing and waning, with new lesions occurring primarily in winter. The patient reported a history of physical and mental stress, depressive symptoms, and alcohol intake for the past 10 years (120–180 mL of whiskey twice weekly).

There was no history of joint pain, early morning stiffness, pus-filled lesions, oral or genital ulcers, fever, sore throat, drug intake prior to the onset of lesions, chest pain, palpitations, or syncope.

On examination, 30–40% of the body surface area, including the scalp, was involved with well-defined erythematous scaly plaques that had loosely adherent silvery-white scales. Grattage test and Auspitz sign were positive. Dermoscopy revealed multiple red regular dots with white scales. The PASI score was 18.2. Nails, as well as oral and genital mucosa, were normal.

Laboratory investigations showed elevated liver enzymes [serum glutamic oxaloacetic transaminase (SGOT): 250 IU/L, serum glutamate pyruvate transaminase (SGPT): 234 IU/L, and γ-glutamyl transferase (GGT): 126 IU/L]. Other hematological and biochemical parameters were normal. Chest X-ray was normal. The patient tested negative for human immunodeficiency virus (HIV), venereal disease research laboratory (VDRL), and anti-hepatitis C virus (anti-HCV), but was hepatitis B surface antigen (HBsAg) positive with anti-HBe positive and HBV DNA levels over 2,000 IU/mL.

The patient did not respond to treatment with apremilast. He was started on prophylactic antiviral therapy (tenofovir with entecavir) for hepatitis B and managed with topical treatments and NBUVB therapy for 4 weeks. Later, he was given etanercept 50 mg subcutaneously once a week for 5 months, to which he responded well **(Figs. 5 and 6)**.

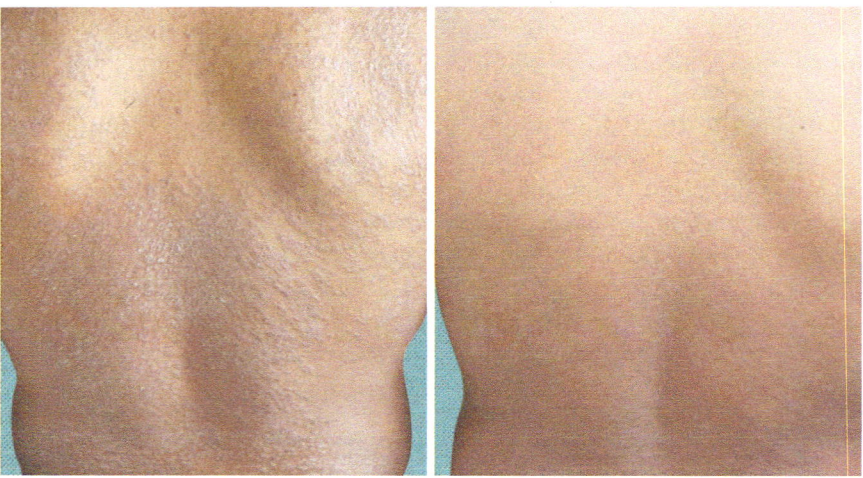

FIG. 5: Pre- and post-etanercept (8 weeks) in a case of psoriasis with hepatitis.

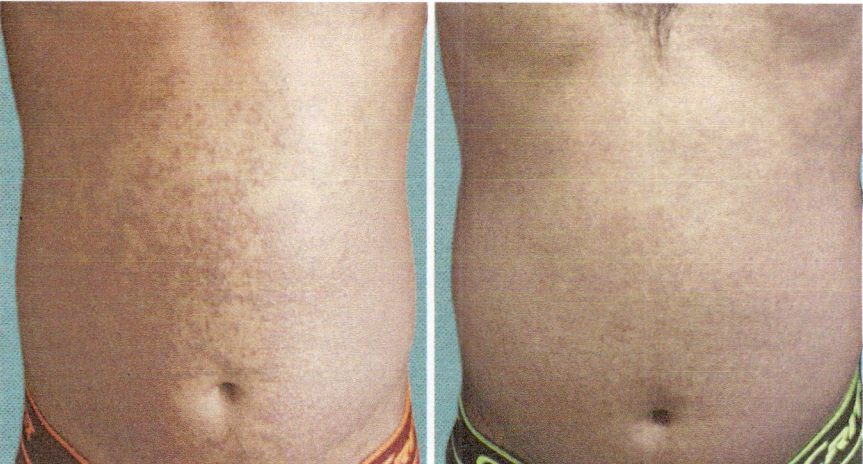

FIG. 6: Pre- and post-etanercept (8 weeks) in a case of psoriasis with hepatitis.

Management Pearl

Psoriasis presenting with hepatitis is not a common scenario, however, when it comes it possesses a lot of management dilemma. Usually, topical therapy is sufficient in most cases but psoriasis with high PASI scores or association with arthritis mandates use of some form of systemic or biologic therapy. Following points need to be kept in mind before starting therapy:

- In general, systemic antipsoriatic therapies should be postponed during active phases of HBV infection.[24] Treatment for psoriasis should commence only after effective control of the HBV infection is achieved using antiviral drugs. Active HBV infection can present in different phases, which are not necessarily sequential, such as (1) acute infection, characterized as a recent HBV infection that may be asymptomatic or symptomatic with jaundice; and (2) chronic infection, defined by the persistence of HBsAg for 6 months or more and comprising various phases, including immune-tolerant, HBeAg-positive immune-active, and HBeAg-negative immune reactivation phases.[25,26] Acitretin is the preferred drug that could be administered during the active phases of HBV infection. However, the administration of said drug should be reserved only for selected cases without a severe impairment of liver function.[27] Recently, apremilast has also been used in HBV infection without the risk of reactivation.[28]
- In clinical practice, it is common to encounter patients with serological markers that indicate prior exposure to HBV, showing low or undetectable viral loads. These patients may be in one of the following infectious phases: (1) inactive HBV infection [characterized by serum HBV DNA < 2,000 IU/mL, normal alanine aminotransferase (ALT) levels, presence of HBsAg and anti-HBe, minimal liver necroinflammation, and variable fibrosis]; (2) occult HBV infection (characterized by serum HBV DNA < 200 IU/mL or undetectable, HBsAg negative, anti-HBc positive, and anti-HBs negative); and (3) resolved HBV (rHBV) infection, indicated by positive anti-HBs with or without anti-HBc. Patients with inactive HBV infection, occult HBV, or rHBV are at risk of HBV reactivation (HBVr) (a sudden increase in HBV replication) after beginning

immunosuppressive therapy. The risk is significantly higher in inactive carriers than in those with occult HBV, and reactivation is even rarer in cases of rHBV.[29]

- Viral reactivation is characterized by two main aspects: (1) virologic (an increase in viral replication) and (2) biochemical [a rise in ALT and/or aspartate aminotransferase (AST) levels]. In patients who are HBsAg positive and anti-HBc positive, HBVr is defined as either: (1) an increase in HBV DNA by more than 2 logs (100-fold) from the baseline level, or (2) HBV DNA levels above 3 logs (1,000 IU/mL) in a patient with previously undetectable HBV DNA (recognizing that HBV DNA levels can fluctuate).

  For patients who are HBsAg negative and anti-HBc positive, both virologic and biochemical criteria are used to define reactivation. Virologic criteria include: (1) detectable HBV DNA or (2) reverse HBsAg seroconversion (reappearance of HBsAg). Biochemical criteria include: (1) a threefold increase in ALT above baseline or (2) an ALT level > 100 U/L, as used in some studies.[30]

- The risk of reactivation is broadly categorized based on the type of immunosuppressive therapy and the presence of HBV markers. It is defined as high risk (≥10% risk of HBVr), moderate risk (1–10% risk), or low risk (<1% risk), depending on the presence of HBsAg or the presence of anti-HBc with negative HBsAg.[31,32] While methotrexate, acitretin and apremilast are considered to be among low-risk group in HBsAg positive, caution needs to be exercised specially for first two drugs in view of their hepatotoxicity. Cyclosporine falls in moderate risk while TNF-α inhibitors come under high risk. In HBsAg-negative group, TNF-α inhibitors fall into moderate-risk group while other drugs mentioned above continue to be in the same group as HBsAg positive.

- While most reports focus on rheumatologic or gastroenterologic patients, TNF-α inhibitors have been associated with a 12–39% risk of HBVr in HBsAg-positive patients not receiving antiviral prophylaxis.[27] Studies suggest that the risk of HBVr is lower in HBsAg-positive patients treated with etanercept compared to those treated with infliximab. This difference may be due to variations in the drugs' administration methods or molecular structure. However, there is limited research on dermatologic patients. A recent systematic review found that five out of 14 psoriasis patients with chronic HBV, who were not on antiviral prophylaxis, experienced viral reactivation, with an adjusted yearly reactivation rate of 26.31%.[33] Among psoriasis and rheumatologic patients with chronic HBV who were treated with TNF-α inhibitors and given antiviral prophylaxis, the risk of reactivation ranges between 1 and 10%.[34]

  Current guidelines from the American Academy of Dermatology, the American Gastroenterological Association, the European Crohn's and Colitis Organization, and the American College of Rheumatology (ACR) recommend antiviral prophylaxis for patients with chronic HBV. This prophylaxis should begin simultaneously or 1–2 weeks before starting anti-TNF-α therapy.[35] Dermatologists should prescribe TNF-α inhibitors with caution to selected patients with severe psoriasis and chronic HBV infection for whom all other treatment options (such as topical treatment, phototherapy, acitretin, or apremilast) have been exhausted.

- *IL 17 inhibitors*: A prospective multicenter study involving 22 patients with chronic hepatitis B (CHB) who did not receive antiviral prophylaxis after starting secukinumab found that six patients (27.3%) developed HBVr.[36] Of these, three patients began antiviral treatment, resulting in a rapid decrease in viral load within 3 months. The other three patients with HBVr were monitored without antiviral drugs, and their viral loads remained low without acute hepatitis. Importantly, none of the three CHB patients who received antiviral prophylaxis developed HBVr. This study thus underscored the importance of antiviral prophylaxis in CHB patients starting with IL-17 inhibitors.

The study also included 24 patients with rHBV who did not receive antiviral prophylaxis, and one patient (4.2%) with a positive baseline viral load developed HBVr without acute hepatitis. These findings support the European Association for the Study of the Liver (EASL) and Asian Pacific Association for the Study of the Liver (APASL) guidelines, which recommend antiviral prophylaxis for patients with rHBV if they have a positive baseline viral load.

In a case report, a CHB patient treated with ixekizumab alongside entecavir did not experience HBVr after 18 months of treatment. Another report showed that a patient with rHBV did not experience HBVr during follow-up.[37] Given the limited data on HBVr risk in patients treated with ixekizumab or brodalumab, further studies with larger sample sizes are needed.

TAKE HOME MESSAGE

- Screening for LTBI is crucial before initiating systemic therapy in psoriasis patients, especially in high TB prevalence regions like India. IL-17/IL-23 inhibitors are preferred over TNF inhibitors due to lower TB reactivation risk.
- Managing psoriasis in pregnancy requires balancing disease control with fetal safety. TNF inhibitors (especially certolizumab) are safer options, and live vaccines should be deferred for infants exposed to biologics in utero.
- In psoriasis patients with hepatitis B, systemic therapy should be delayed until effective antiviral control is achieved. Biologic choice should consider reactivation risk, with TNF inhibitors requiring antiviral prophylaxis.
- For psoriasis patients with active hepatitis, apremilast and acitretin are preferred systemic options, while methotrexate and cyclosporine should be used cautiously due to hepatotoxicity.
- Real-world management of psoriasis in special populations often relies on expert consensus and evolving evidence. A multidisciplinary approach is key to optimizing treatment while minimizing risks.

REFERENCES

1. Henseler T, Christophers E. Psoriasis of early and late onset: characterization of two types of psoriasis vulgaris. J Am Acad Dermatol. 1985;13:450-6.
2. Dogra S, Yadav S. Psoriasis in India: prevalence and pattern. Indian J Dermatol Venereol Leprol. 2010;76:595-601.
3. Grimsrud KN, Sherwin CM, Constance JE, Tak C, Zuppa AF, Spigarelli MG, et al. Special population considerations and regulatory affairs for clinical research. Clin Res Regul Aff. 2015;32:47-56.
4. Salgame P, Geadas C, Collins L, Jones-López E, Ellner JJ. Latent tuberculosis infection--Revisiting and revising concepts. Tuberculosis (Edinb). 2015;95:373-84.
5. Neema S, Radhakrishnan S, Dabbas D, Vasudevan B. Latent tuberculosis in psoriasis patients planned for systemic therapy–A prospective observational study. Indian Dermatol Online J. 2021;12:429-32.
6. Neema S, Sandhu S, Mukherjee S, Vashisht D, Vendhan S, Sinha A, et al. Comparison of interferon gamma release assay and tuberculin skin test for diagnosis of latent tuberculosis in Psoriasis Patients Planned for Systemic Therapy. Indian J Dermatol. 2022;67:19-25.
7. Calzada-Hernández J, Anton J, Martín de Carpi J, et al. Dual latent tuberculosis screening with tuberculin skin tests and QuantiFERON-TB assays before TNF-α inhibitor initiation in children in Spain. Eur J Pediatr. 2023;182:307-17.

8. Askling J, Fored CM, Brandt L, Baecklund E, Bertilsson L, Cöster L, et al. Risk and case characteristics of tuberculosis in rheumatoid arthritis associated with tumor necrosis factor antagonists in Sweden. Arthritis Rheum. 2005;52:1986-92.
9. Wolfe F, Michaud K, Anderson J, Urbansky K. Tuberculosis infection in patients with rheumatoid arthritis and the effect of infliximab therapy. Arthritis Rheum. 2004;50:372-9.
10. Swoger JM, Regueiro M. Stopping, continuing, or restarting immunomodulators and biologics when an infection or malignancy develops. Inflamm Bowel Dis. 2014;20:926-35.
11. Solovic I, Sester M, Gomez-Reino JJ, Rieder HL, Ehlers S, Milburn HJ, et al. The risk of tuberculosis related to tumour necrosis factor antagonist therapies: a TBNET consensus statement. Eur Respir J. 2010;36:1185-206.
12. Torres T, Chiricozzi A, Puig L, Lé AM, Marzano AV, Dapavo P, et al. Treatment of psoriasis patients with latent tuberculosis using IL-17 and IL-23 inhibitors: a retrospective, multinational, multicentre study. Am J Clin Dermatol. 2024;25:333-42.
13. Murase JE, Chan KK, Garite TJ, Cooper DM, Weinstein GD. Hormonal effect on psoriasis in pregnancy and postpartum. Arch Dermatol. 2005;141:601-6.
14. Bobotsis R, Gulliver WP, Monaghan K, Lynde C, Fleming P. Psoriasis and adverse pregnancy outcomes: a systematic review of observational studies. Br J Dermatol. 2016;175:464-72.
15. Ben-David G, Sheiner E, Hallak M, Levy A. Pregnancy outcome in women with psoriasis. J Reprod Med. 2008;53:183-7.
16. Shavit E, Shear NH. An update on the safety of apremilast for the treatment of plaque psoriasis. Expert Opin Drug Saf. 2020;19:403-8.
17. Murase JE, Heller MM, Butler DC. Safety of dermatologic medications in pregnancy and lactation: Part I. Pregnancy. J Am Acad Dermatol. 2014;70:401.e1-14. quiz 415.
18. Trivedi MK, Vaughn AR, Murase JE. Pustular psoriasis of pregnancy: current perspectives. Int J Womens Health. 2018;10:109-15.
19. Sheth N, Greenblatt DT, Acland K, Barker J, Teixeira F. Generalized pustular psoriasis of pregnancy treated with infliximab. Clin Exp Dermatol. 2009;34:521-2.
20. Chhabra G, Chanana C, Verma P, Saxena A. Impetigo herpetiformis responsive to secukinumab. Dermatol Ther. 2019;32:e13040.
21. O'Byrne LJ, Alqatari SG, Maher GM, O'Sullivan AM, Khashan AS, Murphy GP, et al. Fetal and maternal outcomes after maternal biologic use during conception and pregnancy: A systematic review and meta-analysis. BJOG. 2022;129:1236-46.
22. Porter ML, Lockwood SJ, Kimball AB. Update on biologic safety for patients with psoriasis during pregnancy. Int J Womens Dermatol. 2017;3:21-5.
23. Strain J, Leis M, Lee KO, Fleming P. Certolizumab Pegol in Plaque Psoriasis: Considerations for Pregnancy. Skin Therapy Lett. 2021;26:1-5.
24. Nast A, Gisondi P, Ormerod AD, Saiag P, Smith C, Spuls PI, et al. European S3-Guidelines on the systemic treatment of psoriasis vulgaris--Update 2015--Short version--EDF in cooperation with EADV and IPC. J Eur Acad Dermatol Venereol. 2015;29:2277-94.
25. Ahn CS, Dothard EH, Garner ML, Feldman SR, Huang WW. To test or not to test? An updated evidence-based assessment of the value of screening and monitoring tests when using systemic biologic agents to treat psoriasis and psoriatic arthritis. J Am Acad Dermatol. 2015;73:420-8.e1.
26. Bojito-Marrero L, Pyrsopoulos N. Hepatitis B and Hepatitis C Reactivation in the Biologic Era. J Clin Transl Hepatol. 2014;2:240-6.
27. Pérez-Alvarez R, Díaz-Lagares C, García-Hernández F, Lopez-Roses L, Brito-Zerón P, Pérez-de-Lis M, et al. Hepatitis B virus (HBV) reactivation in patients receiving tumor necrosis factor (TNF)-targeted therapy: analysis of 257 cases. Medicine (Baltimore). 2011;90:359-71.
28. Tsentemeidou A, Sotiriou E, Sideris N, Bakirtzi K, Papadimitriou I, Lallas A, et al. Apremilast in Psoriasis Patients With Serious Comorbidities: a Case Series and Systematic Review of Literature. Dermatol Pract Concept. 2022;12:e2022179.
29. Terrault NA, Bzowej NH, Chang KM, Hwang JP, Jonas MM, Murad MH, et al. AASLD guidelines for treatment of chronic hepatitis B. Hepatology. 2016;63:261-83.
30. Visram A, Feld JJ. Defining and grading HBV reactivation. Clin Liver Dis. 2015;5:35–8.
31. Loomba R, Liang TJ. Hepatitis B Reactivation Associated With Immune Suppressive and Biological Modifier Therapies: Current Concepts, Management Strategies, and Future Directions. Gastroenterology. 2017;152:1297-309.
32. Perrillo RP, Gish R, Falck-Ytter YT. American Gastroenterological Association Institute technical review on prevention and treatment of hepatitis B virus reactivation during immunosuppressive drug therapy. Gastroenterology. 2015;148:221-44.e3.
33. Snast I, Atzmony L, Braun M, Hodak E, Pavlovsky L. Risk for hepatitis B and C virus reactivation in patients with psoriasis on biologic therapies: A retrospective cohort study and systematic review of the literature. J Am Acad Dermatol. 2017l;77:88-97.e5.

34. Piaserico S, Dapavo P, Conti A, Gisondi P, Russo FP. Adalimumab is a safe option for psoriasis patients with concomitant hepatitis B or C infection: a multicentre cohort study of 37 patients and review of the literature. J Eur Acad Dermatol Venereol. 2017;31:1853-9.
35. AlMutairi N, Abouzaid HA. Safety of biologic agents for psoriasis in patients with viral hepatitis. J Dermatolog Treat. 2018;29:553-6.
36. Chiu HY, Hui RC, Huang YH, Huang RY, Chen KL, Tsai YC, et al. Safety Profile of Secukinumab in Treatment of Patients with Psoriasis and Concurrent Hepatitis B or C: A Multicentric Prospective Cohort Study. Acta Derm Venereol. 2018;98:829-34.
37. Koike Y, Fujiki Y, Higuchi M, Fukuchi R, Kuwatsuka S, Murota H. An interleukin-17 inhibitor successfully treated a complicated psoriasis and psoriatic arthritis patient with hepatitis B virus infection and end-stage kidney disease on hemodialysis. JAAD Case Rep. 2019;5:150-2.

21. Novel Therapeutic Targets in Psoriasis: Biologics, Small Molecules, and Cell-based Therapies

Shraddha Madanagobalane

INTRODUCTION

There are a number of oral and topical therapies under development, such as oral interleukin 17 (IL-17) inhibitors, Janus kinase (JAK) inhibitors, and phosphodiesterase 4 (PDE4) inhibitors. Based on important developments in our knowledge of the immunopathogenesis of psoriasis, the creation of these more recent compounds is an excellent illustration of applied translational research, leading to a broad range of therapeutic options with various mechanisms of action. The newer treatments are:

- Newer biologics
- Oral small molecules
- Topicals
- *Newer biologics*:
  - IL-17 inhibitors: Bimekizumab
  - IL-23 inhibitors: Mirikizumab
  - IL-36 inhibitors for pustular psoriasis: Spesolimab, imsidolimab
- *Newer oral treatments*:
  - PDE4 inhibitors
  - JAK inhibitors
  - Oral tumor necrosis factor (TNF), IL-17, IL-23 inhibitors
  - Retinoic acid-related orphan receptors gamma T (RORγT) inhibitors
  - Sphingosine-1-phosphate receptor 1 (S1PR1) inhibitors
  - A3 adenosine receptor agonist (A3AR)
  - Heat shock protein 90 (HSP90) inhibitors
  - Rho associated protein kinase 2 (ROCK2) inhibitors
- *Emerging targets and treatments*:
  - Calcitonin gene-related peptide (CGRP) antagonist
  - Receptor interacting protein 1 (RIP1) kinase inhibitor
  - Bromodomain (BRD) and bromo-extraterminal (BET) inhibitor
  - Galectin 3 inhibitor
- *Newer topical treatments*:
  - Aryl hydrocarbon receptor (AhR) agonist
  - PDE4 inhibitors
  - JAK inhibitors
- *Emerging topical treatments*:
  - Topical RORγ agonists
  - IL-2 inhibitors
  - RNA modulation
  - Amygdalin analog
  - siRNA treatments

NEWER BIOLOGICS

Interleukin 17 Inhibitors

(Bimzelx) Bimekizumab:
- A humanized immunoglobulin G1 (IgG1) monoclonal antibody (mAb) called bimekizumab inhibits the cytokines IL-17A and IL-17F.
- In October 2023, the Food and Drug Administration (FDA) authorized it for the treatment of moderate-to-severe psoriasis.

- In the phase 3b BE RADIANT research, bimekizumab had a statistically significant better skin response than secukinumab. Bimekizumab's clinical effectiveness and tolerability in psoriasis patients were also demonstrated in the phase 3 BE SURE and BE VIVID trials.[1,2] Patients with moderate-to-severe psoriatic arthritis also reported positive results.[3,4]

Interleukin-23 Inhibitors

Mirikizumab:
- It is a humanized IgG4 mAb, which has demonstrated encouraging outcomes in clinical trials and particularly targets the p19 subunit of IL-23. Mirikizumab significantly reduces inflammation and improves psoriatic skin lesions by focusing on the IL-23/Th17 (T helper type 17) pathway.[5]
- In a more recent phase 3 multicenter, double-blinded study, mirikizumab at a dose of 250 mg was found to be more effective than secukinumab and placebo in treating plaque-type psoriasis while maintaining the safety profile of other IL-23 inhibitors. Up until week 16, there were four significant adverse cardiovascular events reported in the mirikizumab groups compared to none in the placebo and secukinumab groups.
- One patient receiving mirikizumab experienced a fatal myocardial infarction, which the researcher believed was caused by the study medication. Due to a refocused development strategy that prioritizes inflammatory bowel disease, Eli Lilly has chosen not to pursue licensing of mirikizumab in the psoriasis group.[6,7]

Biologics for Pustular Psoriasis

Interleukin-36 Inhibitors

Spesolimab:
- Spesolimab is an antagonistic IgG1 antibody with excellent affinity, specificity, and humanization that targets the interleukin-36 receptor (IL-36R) at a binding site.
- The effectiveness, safety, pharmacokinetics, and pharmacogenomics of spesolimab in individuals experiencing generalized pustular psoriasis (GPP) flares have been assessed in six investigations. When used to treat GPP flares, spesolimab produced quick and long-lasting improvements in skin clearance as well as symptoms and quality of life that were clinically significant. Additionally, spesolimab has a favorable safety profile and dramatically lowers the risk of GPP flares and flare occurrence.[8] For the treatment of GPP in adults and adolescents aged 12 years and up who weigh at least 40 kg, the recommended dosage of SPEVIGO SC (subcutaneous) is 600 mg (four 150-mg injections) given subcutaneously as a loading dose, followed by 300 mg (two 150-mg injections) given subcutaneously 4 weeks later and then every 4 weeks after that.[9]

Imsidolimab:
- Imsidolimab is a humanized IgG4 mAb with high affinity, which binds to IL-36R specifically and inhibits IL-36 signaling.
- In order to evaluate the clinical effectiveness, tolerability, and safety of several doses of imsidolimab in patients with active GPP, GALLOP was an open-label, single-arm, multiple-dose trial. In patients with GPP flares, imsidolimab showed a quick and long-lasting reduction in symptoms and pustular eruptions, and it seemed to be usually well tolerated. The doses used in this study were 750 mg intravenously on day 1 and three 100-mg SC doses of imsidolimab on days 29, 57, and 85. This dosage was accepted satisfactorily.
- No fatalities were reported, and most treatment-emergent adverse events (TEAEs) were mild to moderate in intensity. No patient dropped out of the study due to a TEAE.[10]

Others: Furthermore, recent research has indicated that the mast cell cytokines IL-37 and IL-38 may have a therapeutic use in the management of psoriasis.[11]

■ PHOSPHODIESTERASE 4 INHIBITORS

The development of *PDE4 inhibitors* has significantly advanced the treatment of psoriasis and other inflammatory conditions. Apremilast wase the first PDE4 inhibitor to be use in psoriasis.[12] Roflumilast, another PDE4 inhibitor, which was first approved for chronic obstructive pulmonary disease, has also shown promise in treating psoriasis in a clinical trial.[13] Other new oral PDE4 inhibitors are orismilast,[14] Hemay005 (mufemilast), and ME3183.[15]

Some key PDE4 inhibitors currently in development or approved for use are:

Apremilast (Otezla):
- Apremilast was the first PDE4 inhibitor approved for *psoriasis* in 2014.[12]
- *Mechanism*: It works by inhibiting the enzyme PDE4, which decreases the production of proinflammatory cytokines, thus reducing inflammation.
- *Efficacy*: Apremilast is used to treat moderate-to-severe *plaque psoriasis*, and has shown to be effective in improving symptoms in patients.

Orismilast:
- Orismilast is a novel PDE4 inhibitor with increased selectivity for the PDE4B and PDE4D subtypes, which are more directly involved in inflammation. This subtype selectivity may give orismilast an advantage over pan-PDE4 inhibitors like apremilast.[15]
- A phase IIb study (NCT05190419) included 202 patients with moderate-to-severe plaque psoriasis, who were randomized to receive either 20, 30, or 40 mg of orismilast twice a day, or a placebo.
  - Results: orismilast was more effective than apremilast at achieving a PASI 90 response (90% improvement in psoriasis severity), but the 40-mg group had higher discontinuation rates compared to apremilast. The 20-mg and 30-mg doses showed the best risk–benefit profile.
  - Side effects: Common adverse effects included nausea and diarrhea.[16]

Hemay005 (Mufemilast):
- Hemay005, also known as *mufemilast*, is another oral PDE4 inhibitor being investigated for the treatment of *psoriasis*.[17]
- *Clinical trials*:
  - In a *phase II trial* (NCT04102241), 216 patients with moderate-to-severe psoriasis were randomized into four groups: 15, 30, and 60 mg doses of Hemay005, plus a placebo.
  - Phase III study: A subsequent *phase III trial* (NCT04839328) will assess the 60 mg BID dose in comparison to a placebo.
  - Current status: The results of the phase II trial are not yet published, and patients are still being recruited for the phase III trial.[18]

ME3183:
- ME3183 is another oral PDE4 inhibitor designed to treat psoriasis and atopic dermatitis.[15,19]
- *Clinical trials*: Two phase I trials (ME3183-1 and ME3183-2) assessed the safety, tolerability, and pharmacokinetics of ME3183 in 126 healthy volunteers. Doses ranged up to 25 mg (single dose) and 10 mg twice a day.
  - Safety profile: ME3183 was generally well tolerated, with diarrhea and headache being the most common treatment-emergent side effects.
  - Potential: The drug showed safety and acceptability, suggesting it may have a favorable risk profile for patients with inflammatory diseases like psoriasis.

CHAPTER 21: Novel Therapeutic Targets in Psorias s: Biologics, Small Molecules...

JANUS KINASE INHIBITORS IN PSORIASIS TREATMENT

The JAK/signal transducer and activator of transcription (JAK/STAT) pathway plays a central role in the immune response and inflammation, including in diseases like psoriasis. JAK inhibitors have emerged as a promising class of oral therapies for managing moderate-to-severe psoriasis by targeting intracellular signaling of cytokines involved in inflammation.[20]

Janus Kinase Family and Mechanism of Action

- JAKs are intracellular enzymes that mediate the JAK/STAT signaling pathway, which is activated by cytokine binding to cell surface receptors.
- The JAK family consists of JAK1, JAK2, JAK3, and tyrosine kinase 2 (TYK2), each playing a role in specific immune responses.
- Upon activation by cytokines (e.g., IL-23, IL-12), JAK dimers phosphorylate the receptor, which recruits and activates STAT proteins. The activated STAT proteins then move to the nucleus to trigger the transcription of proinflammatory cytokines, promoting immune cell activation and inflammation.[20,21]
- By inhibiting specific JAK enzymes, JAK inhibitors block these pathways, reducing inflammation and cytokine production, which helps in treating diseases like psoriasis.

Approved and Emerging Janus Kinase Inhibitors for Psoriasis

- *Tofacitinib (Xeljanz)*: A pan Jak inhibitor did not get approval for the treatment of psoriasis due to safety issues;[22] however, it was the first JAK inhibitor approved for psoriatic arthritis in 2017.[23] Tofacitinib has shown efficacy in treating psoriasis as well.
- *Upadacitinib*: Approved for psoriatic arthritis and other indications;[24] it selectively inhibits JAK1 and has been shown to be effective in treating psoriasis.
- Other emerging JAK inhibitors for psoriasis treatment include baricitinib, peficitinib, brepocitinib, rospacitinib, and deucravacitinib (approved for psoriasis).[18]

Deucravacitinib
Mechanism of Action

Deucravacitinib is an allosteric inhibitor that specifically targets TYK2, one of the key enzymes in the JAK family. It works by binding to the regulatory domain of TYK2, which blocks the activation of downstream cytokines like IL-23, IL-12, and type I interferons.

Unlike other JAK inhibitors, which block the kinase's ATP-binding site, deucravacitinib's allosteric inhibition provides a more selective and potentially safer way to modulate immune responses.[25]

The *FDA* approved *deucravacitinib* (trade name *Sotyktu*) in *2022* for the treatment of moderate-to-severe psoriasis in adults.

The European Medicines Agency (EMA) followed with approval in 2023, and Japan approved it in the same year for more severe forms of psoriasis (erythrodermic and GPP).[26]

Efficacy of Deucravacitinib

- *Short-term efficacy (10–16 weeks)*:
  - PASI 75 (75% improvement in psoriasis severity) response rates for deucravacitinib were around 54.1% (compared to 39.7% for etanercept and 79.0% for infliximab)[27]
- *Long-term efficacy (44–60 weeks)*:
  - The PASI 75 response rate for deucravacitinib increased to 65.9%, showing sustained efficacy.
  - Deucravacitinib's long-term response was comparable to ustekinumab (68.0%) and adalimumab (62.8%), two established biologics.[28]

- A matching-adjusted indirect comparison (MAIC) suggested that deucravacitinib had greater long-term response rates at 2 years compared to adalimumab.[29]
- Other ongoing trials:
  - Deucravacitinib's efficacy in treating scalp psoriasis, nail psoriasis, and pediatric psoriasis is being evaluated in several phase III and phase IV trials.
  - Ongoing studies (e.g., NCT04036435) are assessing the drug's effectiveness and safety in various patient populations, including those with more complex forms of psoriasis.[18]

Safety Profile of Deucravacitinib
- *Safety*:
  - Deucravacitinib appears to have a better safety profile compared to other JAK inhibitors, with fewer serious side effects.
  - Herpesvirus reactivation has been observed as a mild side effect, which is a common concern with many immunomodulatory drugs.
  - Regular monitoring of triglyceride levels is recommended, particularly in high-risk patients.
  - Phase IV studies are ongoing, including a post-marketing surveillance study (NCT05633264) to further evaluate the drug's safety and effectiveness in the broader population.[18]
- *Common adverse events (AEs)*:
  - Mild increases in herpesvirus infections, with reactivation of herpes zoster or other viral infections reported
  - Elevated triglyceride levels may require monitoring, especially in patients at high risk.
- *Dosage*: It is administered orally (6 mg daily), offering an attractive alternative to injectable biologics for patients who prefer or require oral therapy.
- *Sustained responses*: Unlike some biologics, where response rates can decrease over time, deucravacitinib's efficacy appears to remain consistent, which is a key advantage in the long-term management of psoriasis.

ORAL TUMOR NECROSIS FACTOR INHIBITORS

- Sanofi is now developing an oral TNF inhibitor called SAR441566.[30,31] The effectiveness and safety of SAR441566 in patients with moderate-to-severe psoriasis were assessed in a randomized, double-blind, placebo-controlled phase I trial (NCT05453942), which included 38 patients. Although the trial is over, the results have not yet been made public.

ORAL INTERLEUKIN 17 INHIBITORS

- Lilly, Leo Pharma, and DICE Therapeutics have separately created at least three distinct compounds.
- Two phase I clinical trials using LY3509754 (Lilly) for psoriasis (NCT04152382, NCT04586920) were prematurely ended in 2019 because of liver function-related safety concerns.[32] Early-stage IL-17 inhibitors include DC-853 (Eli Lilly and Company), a quick follower of DC-806, and LEO 153339 (LEO Pharma, Ballerup, Denmark), which was recently studied in a phase I single ascending dose (SAD) and multiple ascending dose (MAD) trial in healthy subjects (NCT04883333). Lilly claims that DC-853 provides better metabolic stability and a greater affinity for the cytokine IL-17A.[33] Nevertheless, there are currently no published preclinical or clinical trial data on these medications.
- DICE Therapeutics developed the oral IL-17 inhibitor DC-806 and

studied its pharmacokinetic and safety characteristics.[34] The high-dose group that received 800 mg BD (43.7%) experienced a substantially greater ($p = 0.0008$) reduction in PASI at 4 weeks of treatment than the placebo group (13.3%). With its DELSCAPE DNA-encoded library-based platform to find small molecules targeting protein–protein interactions, DICE Therapeutics is reportedly creating a fast follower of DC-806 and DC-853 with enhanced potency and metabolic stability. Lilly recently completed the acquisition of DICE therapeutics.[35]

ORAL INTERLEUKIN 23 INHIBITORS

- A new oral IL-23R antagonist peptide called JNJ-77242113 (icotrokinra) specifically inhibits IL-23 signaling and the subsequent synthesis of cytokines.[36]
- JNJ-77242113 was administered at random to 225 patients with moderate-to-severe plaque psoriasis at doses of 25 mg once daily, 25 mg twice daily, 50 mg once daily, 100 mg once daily, or 100 mg twice daily for 16 weeks in a phase 2 dose-finding experiment. At week 16, the main outcome was a PASI 75 response. In individuals with moderate-to-severe plaque psoriasis, treatment with the IL-23 receptor antagonist peptide JNJ-77242113 was more effective than a placebo after 16 weeks of once- or twice-daily oral dosing.
- Two more trials of JNJ-77242113 are under underway: FRONTIER 2 (NCT05364554), a phase II trial designed to investigate the safety and efficacy of JNJ-77242113 at week 36, and a phase I trial involving a single dose to test the pharmacokinetics, safety, and tolerability (NCT05703841).[37]
- ICONIC-ADVANCE 1 and ICONIC-ADVANCE 2, two more studies in the phase 3 ICONIC clinical development program, are now underway and will assess the safety and effectiveness of icotrokinra in moderate-to-severe plaque psoriasis in comparison to both placebo and deucravacitinib.
- At the start of 2025, the phase 3 ICONIC-PsA program will begin to examine icotrokinra in psoriatic arthritis.[38,39]

RETINOIC ACID-RELATED ORPHAN RECEPTORS GAMMA T INHIBITOR

- It Is an essential transcription factor needed for Th17 cell development. RORγT controls the production of Th17 cytokines, such as IL-17A, IL-17F, IL-22, and IL-23 receptor.[40]
- Several RORγT inverse agonists, including VTP-43742, JTE-451, AUR101, ABBV-157, IMU-935, BMS-986251, AZD0284, SAR441169, ABBV-553, and BI 730357, have been studied in clinical studies for the treatment of moderate-to-severe psoriasis, with varying degrees of effectiveness thus far.
- The studies for AZD0284 and IMU-935 were discontinued because of their low efficacy, while the studies for VTP-43742, ABBV-553, and ABBV-157 were discontinued for safety reasons. BI 730357 studies were also discontinued.[41-43] Clinical studies for other developing compounds, such as VTP-45489, have not yet been conducted.

SPHINGOSINE-1-PHOSPHATE RECEPTOR AGONIST

Five G-protein-coupled receptors (GPCRs) are bound by the bioactive lipid sphingosine-1-phosphate (S1P), which controls vital cellular processes such as adhesion, migration, survival, and proliferation.[45,44] The skin, lymphoid tissue, and cardiovascular system all have notable expression of the S1P1 receptor (S1P1R).[46,47]

Ponesimod:
- It is an oral S1P1R selective modulator.
- In two phase II trials (NCT01208090 and NCT00852670), this medication was investigated for the treatment of moderate-to-severe psoriasis and showed effectiveness in reducing the numbers of circulating T and B lymphocytes, especially CD4+ cells, in healthy human subjects.[48,49] 326 patients participated in the multicenter, randomized, double-blind, placebo-controlled phase II trial NCT01208090. They were divided into three treatment groups: 20 mg QD, 40 mg BID, or placebo. 46%, 48.1%, and 13.4% of patients in each group, respectively, reached the primary objective of PASI 75 at 16 weeks of treatment.[50] During the maintenance phase, participants were then rerandomized to receive either a placebo, 20 mg, or 40 mg. A PASI 75 response was attained by the 28th week of the follow-up period in 71.4% of patients remaining on the 20 mg dosage and 77.4% of those continuing on the 40 mg dosage.
- However, there was a rapid decrease in effectiveness among those from the 20-mg and 40-mg groups who were rerandomized to the placebo. Dizziness, liver enzyme abnormalities, and dyspnea were the most commonly reported AEs.[50] NCT00852670's results are still pending publication. Ponesimod does not currently have a clinical trial under progress.

A3 AGONIST OF THE ADENOSINE RECEPTOR

- Adenosine signaling plays a crucial function in immune cell activation and proliferation.[51] By attaching to particular purinergic receptors (P2Y and P2X) linked to DAMP (damage-associated molecular pattern), elevated adenosine levels from ATP catabolism starts inflammation.
- Adenosine receptors are members of the GPCR class, which is responsible for a number of vital physiological functions, including metabolic management, vascular regulation, and immunological modulation.[52] Different types of adenosine receptors, including adenosine A1, A2A, A2B, and A3 receptors, may be involved in this process.

Peripheral blood mononuclear cells (PBMCs) with Gi proteins in individuals with psoriasis show elevated expression of A3AR.[53] As a result, allosteric modulators and highly selective A3AR agonists that produce anti-inflammatory effects have been developed.[54]

Namodenoson and Piclidenoson:
- Currently under investigation, Namodenoson and Piclidenoson are agonists that bind to this particular receptor found in inflammatory cells and inhibit immune-based cytokines.[55-57]
- Furthermore, A3AR signaling causes the nuclear factor kappa-B (NF-κB) and Wnt/β-catenin pathways to be downregulated, which causes inflammatory cells to undergo apoptosis. According to recent phase III clinical trials, Piclidenoson is a safe and efficient treatment for moderate to severe plaque-type psoriasis. Results compared to apremilast during this study indicated that a score of at least PASI 75 may be attained in 16 weeks. Piclidenoson has an outstanding safety/tolerability profile, outperforming apremilast. The dosage was 3 mg BD.[58]

HEAT SHOCK PROTEIN 90

Heat shock protein 90 is a chaperone protein, which plays a crucial role in the folding, stabilization, and activation of various intracellular proteins, including transcription factors and signaling molecules, which regulate inflammation.[59] As it is involved in the activation of proinflammatory pathways, HSP90 has become a target for therapeutic intervention in inflammatory diseases, including psoriasis.

Heat Shock Protein 90 and Psoriasis Pathophysiology

- In psoriasis, HSP90 is important in regulating the function of Act1, a key molecule in IL-17-dependent signaling, which is central to the development of the disease.
- Keratinocytes in psoriatic skin are characterized by overexpression of HSP90α, suggesting that HSP90 may contribute to the inflammatory processes seen in psoriasis by stabilizing and activating molecules involved in the immune response.[60]
- *RGN-305*: RGN-305 is an imidazopyridine derivative and a selective HSP90 inhibitor. The drug works by interfering with the function of HSP90, thereby destabilizing proteins involved in inflammatory pathways, including those regulated by IL-17 and TNF-α.

Clinical Trial Data

- *Phase Ib trial (NCT03675542)*:
  - Design: The trial was open-label and single-arm, testing RGN-305 in 11 patients with moderate-to-severe psoriasis. The doses tested were 250 mg and 500 mg of RGN-305 administered QD.[61]
  - Results:
    - Six patients (out of 11) showed a ≥50% improvement in PASI, with improvement ranging from 71 to 94% by week 12.
    - This demonstrates that RGN-305 has the potential to provide significant clinical benefit in treating psoriasis.
    - AEs: No significant adverse effects were noted in the study, although four of seven patients receiving the 500 mg dose developed an exanthematous skin reaction, which is a rash-like response.
    - A transcriptome analysis of psoriatic skin revealed that RGN-305 treatment resulted in a rapid and sustained reduction in inflammatory gene expression, particularly genes like *IL36G* and *CXCL8*, which are induced by TNF and IL-17.

Topical Application of Heat Shock Protein 90 Inhibitors

- Topical HSP90 inhibition could represent a novel therapeutic approach not only for psoriasis but also for a range of other immune-mediated skin diseases, where inflammation driven by immune signaling is a key factor.[62]

While further studies and clinical trials are needed to confirm long-term safety and efficacy, HSP90 inhibition represents a promising new approach in the treatment of psoriasis, especially for patients who have not responded to conventional therapies.

■ INHIBITORS OF ROCK 2

- The downstream mediators of Rho proteins, which belong to a family of guanosine triphosphate-binding proteins, are Rho associated protein kinase 1 and 2 (ROCK1 and 2).
- Kadmon Pharmaceuticals created the ROCK inhibitor belumosudil (KD025, Rezurock®). This drug has been approved by the FDA for graft versus host disease (GVHD). Belumosudil has a 100-fold higher selectivity for ROCK-2 than ROCK-

1. Additionally, belumosudil has a better safety profile than dual ROCK inhibitors.[63]
- Two phase 2 research studies (NCT02852967—in this study patients were divided into three cohorts of 400 mg once daily, 200 mg twice daily, and 400 mg twice daily for 12 weeks; and NCT02106195—this study was on the safety and tolerability at a dose of 200 mg once daily) on psoriasis have been finished.[64,65]

NEW APPROACHES AND THERAPIES

Antagonist of the Calcitonin Gene-related Peptide

- CGRP, a lengthy chain of sensory neuropeptides made up of 37 amino acids, is created by alternative splicing of the calcitonin gene. Both the peripheral and central nervous systems contain sensory nerves that contain CGRP, which is widely expressed in a variety of tissues and organs.
- These neuropeptides' endogenous roles include localized immune cell infiltration, which causes neurogenic inflammation, and vasodilator effects, which enhance blood flow.[66] Keratinocytes, Langerhans cells (LCs), mast cells, and fibroblasts all have high levels of CGRP expression in the skin, which can regulate the cells' rate of growth, differentiation, and activity.[67]

Rimegepant:
- An oral CGRP antagonist called rimegepant dramatically lowers the immune response and Th17 cell infiltration by directly blocking CGRP's ability to bind to its receptor.[68]
- The FDA has approved rimegepant, a drug used to treat acute migraines, under the brand name Nurtec™ ODT. CGRP is located close to LCs in psoriasis, which release IL-23 cytokines, which in turn stimulate $\gamma\delta$-T cells to produce IL-17A and IL-22 cytokines, hence activating keratinocyte proliferation. The neurogenic inflammation in psoriatic patients is caused by CGRP. For psoriasis, it is presently being evaluated in a phase 2 trial.[69]

Inhibitor of Receptor-interacting Protein 1 Kinase

- Receptor interacting protein kinase 1 (RIP 1): An essential enzyme for preserving tissue homeostasis and controlling innate and inflammatory reactions is kinase; even a small perturbation of the route might have serious repercussions.
- By inhibiting cellular apoptosis and necrosis pathways and influencing the differentiation and maturation of proinflammatory cytokines as well as inflammasome assembly, RIP1 kinase increases inflammation. Therefore, blocking this route has been essential in the treatment of inflammatory diseases.[70,71]

GSK2982772—benzoxazepinone:
- Benzoxazepinone (GSK2982772) was the first synthetic RIP1 kinase inhibitor. It reduces inflammation by downregulating several TNF-α-dependent cellular responses.[72]
- The first RIPK1 inhibitor to enroll in a clinical phase Ia trial for psoriasis was GSK772. In psoriasis, phase Ib/IIa clinical trials (NCT02776033 and NCT04316585) have been conducted. In phase IIa clinical studies, GSK'772 has shown satisfactory safety against mild-to-moderate plaque psoriasis; nonetheless, further data is needed to explain the drug's effectiveness.[73]

Inhibitors of Bromodomain and Bromoextraterminal

- Proteins called BRD and BET decipher the epigenetic code in cells to regulate gene development and expression.

- These proteins are essential for preserving both healthy physiological states and diseased ones, including inflammatory and metabolic diseases. According to studies, it can inhibit the synthesis of IL-17, IL-23, and IL-36, among other proinflammatory cytokines.[74]
- 46 proteins with 61 bromodomains encoded by the human genome perform a wide range of biological tasks, including chromatin-based gene transcription.

BD2-selective BET inhibitor (GSK620):
- *Efficacy*: The effectiveness of GSK620 was assessed in an in vivo model of psoriasis-induced NF-κB mice. Comparing GSK620 to apremilast, the PASI was considerably lower. In the case of GSK620, the reduction of the clinical score for erythema, plaque development, and epidermal hyperplasia was determined to be more significant. Additionally, GSK620 suppresses the expression of genes for proinflammatory cytokines including IL-17 and IL-22.[75]
- *AEs*: There may be difficulties, particularly with on-target dose-limiting toxicity, which includes thrombocytopenia, fatigue, hypertension, and gastrointestinal bleeding, even though many BET BrD inhibitors have entered clinical trials and significantly contributed to the development of this novel class of epigenetic medications.[74]

Inhibitor of Galectin 3

- A biological regulator of several physiological processes linked to immune-related disorders is galectin-3. Additionally, it controls immune cell proliferation and differentiation, including keratinocyte differentiation.
- Galectin-3 is in charge of angiogenesis and cell fibrosis in psoriasis.[76] According to studies, psoriatic individuals have higher serum levels of galectin, and the epidermis of psoriatic patches exhibits higher expression of the protein.[77,78]
- *Belapectin*: A new galectin-3 antagonist called belapectin is presently being developed. It has not yet been used clinically to treat psoriasis, although it has been utilized as a clinical candidate to treat patients with head and neck squamous cell carcinoma and metastatic melanoma.[79]

■ TOPICAL THERAPIES

Newer treatments have been developed as a result of recent discoveries about the pathophysiology of psoriasis, as **Table 2**[18] illustrates, attention is increasingly being paid to topical treatments that target novel therapeutic pathways. The latest topical therapies include:
- Modulators of the AhR
- Inhibitors of PDE4
- JAK inhibitors

New topical therapies:
- Topical RORγ agonists
- IL-2 inhibitors
- RNA modulation
- Amygdalin analog

Aryl Hydrocarbon Receptor Agonist

- Both endogenous and exogenous stimuli have the ability to activate the ligand-mediated transcription factor known as AhR.
- It is a receptor that controls the genes in charge of regular physiological function and is found in a variety of tissues and cells, such as the skin, lungs, intestine, etc. Through balancing between the upregulation and downregulation barriers, it preserves skin homeostasis.
- The AhR–ARNT complex preserves the epidermal barrier and promotes the production of the proteins loricrin and filaggrin in the upregulated barrier. The

cytokines IL-13 and IL-14 decrease the expression of loricrin and filaggrin in the downregulated barrier.
- Therefore, AhR's role in immune system activation may be a significant pathogenic factor in inflammatory conditions like psoriasis.[80]

Tapinarof:
- A new AhR agonist with anti-inflammatory properties, tapinarof 1%/benvitimod cream inhibits T cell activation (Th17 and Th22) and suppresses proinflammatory cytokines (IL-17 and IL-22).
- It controls the expression of the skin barrier proteins filaggrin and loricrin, which are in charge of preserving skin homeostasis. By acting on fibroblasts and keratinocytes, tapinarof AhR agonist has contributed to the reduction of inflammation.[81]
- The AhR-ARNT complex increases the Nrf2 transcription factor pathway, which results in the expression of genes for antioxidant enzymes (quinone oxidoreductase 1 and heme oxygenase-1). This lowers the levels of reactive oxygen species (ROS), which causes cellular damage in psoriatic skin, and lessens the oxidative stress of epidermal cells.[82]

Phosphodiesterase 4 Inhibitors

Topical roflumilast (Zoryve®):
- *Approved*: July, 2022 for plaque psoriasis;[83] FDA approval for children (ages 6-11) in October, 2023[84]
- *Formulation*: Available as 0.3% cream
- *Efficacy*: Demonstrated long-term effectiveness in a 52-week study, improving itch and skin lesions; effective in flexural psoriasis
- *Safety*: Profile similar to the vehicle; few application site reactions reported, with no new AEs in long-term use[85]

Topical crisaborole:
- Approved for atopic dermatitis (2% ointment)[86]
- *Efficacy*: Effective in treating flexural, anogenital, and facial psoriasis[86]
- *Usage*: Off-label use observed for psoriasis, despite lack of regulatory approval for this indication[87,88]

Janus Kinase Inhibitors

Topical ruxolitinib:
- Targets JAK1 and JAK2
- *Efficacy*: Phase II study showed significant improvements in plaque psoriasis (lesion thickness, erythema, scaling) compared to placebo, with a reduction in lesion severity score over 50%.[89] The 1.5% formulation was slightly more effective than calcipotriene.
- *Safety*: Mild side effects such as stinging and itching noted at the application site

Brepocitinib cream:
- An inhibitor of TYK2/JAK1 indicated for psoriasis and atopic eczema.
- *Pharmacokinetics*: Systemic concentration in psoriasis patients is 45% lower than in atopic dermatitis patients. Therefore, in individuals with <50% BSA, 3% topical treatment twice daily was deemed safe.[90]
- *Efficacy*: A phase IIb study with 344 participants showed no significant improvement in psoriasis lesions across various dosage groups at 12 weeks compared to vehicle controls.[91]
- *Safety*: Well tolerated with AEs occurring at comparable rates across groups

■ NEWER THERAPIES

Topical Inverse Agonists for RORγ

The expression of the proinflammatory cytokine IL-17 is significantly influenced by the transcription factor RORγ.[92] Numerous research teams have discovered artificial substances that target RORγ via distinct mechanisms. Either they (1) decrease the recruitment of coactivator proteins (inverse agonists), (2) increase the recruitment of coactivator proteins (agonists), or (3) have no effect on basal transcriptional activity (silent ligands/neutral antagonists).

A strong inverse agonist that targets RORγ is GSK2981278.[93]

Mechanism of action:
- GSK2981278 regulates the main transcription pathways associated with Th17 cell production and differentiation by acting on this receptor. Preclinical research has shown that GSK2981278 significantly reduces Th17 cytokine production in human tissue-based systems as well as in vitro trials.[93,94]

Safety, tolerability, and effectiveness:
- This was assessed in a phase I randomized, double-blind clinical trial. The product was applied repeatedly over the course of 19 days to six different test regions (each measuring roughly 1.1 cm^2) inside the psoriatic plaques of 15 participants.[95]
- A vehicle, betamethasone valerate 0.1% cream as a positive control, and six topical formulations of GSK2981278 ointment at different concentrations (0.03%, 0.1%, 0.8%, or 4%) was assessed. Only the positive control showed a decrease in infiltrate thickness by the end of the 19-day period, indicating that the other treatment groups did not experience improvement.
- The short treatment duration, a small region of application, or the potential that targeting RORγ is not a practical strategy topically for psoriasis could be reasons for the lack of benefit in this study.

Inhibitors of Interleukin 2

- IL-2 contributes to the upregulation of T-cell activation and proliferation. BMS-509744, which is a small molecule, prevents IL-2-inducible T-cell kinase. Using an imiquimod-induced lesion mouse model, preclinical research has investigated the effects of topically applied BMS-509744. This has shown encouraging results, such as decreased lesion thickness, decreased inflammatory cell infiltration, and decreased messenger RNA levels of Th17-related cytokines (IL-17A, IL-17F, and IL-22).[96]

Modulation of RNA

- MicroRNAs, which are short, noncoding RNA sequences, are crucial for regulating gene expression and keratinocyte and T-cell proliferation and differentiation.[97] When comparing psoriasis patients to healthy persons, differences in miRNA expression levels have been reported. These variations include both overexpression and downregulation of distinct miRNA subtypes.[97-99]
- Gaining insight into miRNA behavior may open the door to possible modulation. The viability of topical distribution using various carriers has been demonstrated by research. For example, psoriasis patients and mice models that resemble psoriasis showed increased expression of microRNA-210.[100] Using this information, a study has looked into using a nanocarrier gel carrying miRNA-210 antisense topically in a mouse model. Erythema, scaling, acanthosis, and inflammatory infiltrates improved as a result of the intervention's reduction of miRNA-210 expression in skin lesions and T cells. It appears that more research in this area is necessary.[101]

Analog of Amygdalin

- Analogs of amygdalin are derived from a naturally occurring cyanogenic glycoside, which is present in the seeds and kernels of

Prunus trees (as well as other food plants) and is known to have anti-inflammatory qualities.
- Although there was no scientific proof to back its usage, laetrile, a synthetic version of amygdalin, gained popularity in the 1970s as an alternative cancer treatment.[102] Amygdalin analogs are believed to have an anti-inflammatory impact via reducing the expression of the thymic stromal lymphopoietin (*TSLP*) gene. TSLP, an inflammatory cytokine, is widely distributed in psoriasis sufferers' epidermis.
- It stimulates dendritic cells and promotes the generation of IL-23 by working with the CD40 ligand, which is produced from T cells. FIB-116 has shown the ability to reduce certain cytokines associated with psoriasis both systemically in mice serum (IL-17α, IL-6) and locally in the skin (IL-17α, TNF-α, and IFN-γ).[103]
- The possible clinical use of FIB-116 is not currently being investigated by any clinical trials.

RNA Interference

RNA interference (RNAi) has the ability to suppress the expression of molecules implicated in the pathogenesis of psoriasis. The field of RNAi therapies has seen significant advancements. To improve the formulation and administration of RNAi therapies, more studies are necessary.

Targeted siRNA Treatment for Psoriasis

One promising approach to treating psoriasis is to use small interfering RNA (siRNA) therapy to target harmful genes.

Compared to current systemic treatments for psoriasis, this may provide clear benefits. By preventing DNA from being translated into proteins, siRNAs—small double-stranded RNA molecules—silence genes and specifically disrupt the expression of particular genes.

The critical function that siRNA plays in modifying the pathophysiology of psoriasis has been clarified by recent research. The use of siRNA can block a variety of mediators that contribute to the development of psoriasis, such as differentiation regulators, inflammatory cytokines, proliferative agents, and cellular signaling molecules.[104]

Targeting Keratinocytes

Mediating keratinocyte proliferation and apoptosis: By focusing on keratinocyte proliferation, differentiation, apoptosis, and migration, siRNA technology can slow the development of psoriasis.[105]

Fibroblast growth factor receptor 2 (FGFR2): The inhibition of keratinocyte growth is achieved through the siRNA silencing of FGFR2.[106]

Nuclear factor of activated T cells 2 (NFAT2): NFAT2 knockdown diminishes epidermal thickness and keratinocyte proliferation.[107]

TRAF3 interacting protein 2 (TRAF3IP2): By increasing apoptotic signaling and preventing the G2/M cell cycle phase, TRAF3IP2 knockdown reduces the proliferation of keratinocytes and endothelial cells.[108]

WT1 transcription factor (WT1) and WT1-associated protein (WTAP):
- In addition to siRNA silencing individual genes, some studies indicate that certain genes have inter-regulatory interactions. For instance, WT1 is connected to WTAP.
- Both exhibit strong functional and expressive connections. WT1 overexpression has the opposite consequences from low expression, which suppresses keratinocyte growth and promotes apoptosis.[109] In a similar vein, keratinocyte proliferation is increased by overexpressing WTAP and decreased by inhibiting it.[110]

- Consequently, there may be an upstream–downstream regulatory link between WTAP and WT1, indicating the need for additional collaborative research.

Signal transducer and activator of transcription 3 (STAT3) and STAT1:
- The signaling system known as JAK/STAT is linked to numerous important pathogenic mediators of psoriasis.[111]
- The transmission of cytokine and growth factor signals, which controls inflammatory reactions, immune cell activation, keratinocyte proliferation, and aberrant differentiation, is largely dependent on the JAK/STAT signaling system.[112]

STAT3:
- In psoriatic keratinocytes, STAT3 is abundantly expressed and active. The degree of psoriasis is positively correlated with its activity. When psoriatic keratinocytes' *STAT3* gene is silenced utilizing siRNA, ultrasonic irradiation, and microbubble technology, keratinocyte development is inhibited and apoptosis is induced.[113]
- Inhibiting casein kinase 2 (CK2) in human keratinocytes decreases the inflammatory response, aberrant differentiation, and epidermal hyperplasia via suppressing the STAT3 and threonine kinase (AKT) signaling pathways.[114]
- Bcl-2 and STAT3 have been found to interact strongly in protein interaction networks. Keratinocytes exhibit growth inhibition, apoptosis, and enhanced UVB sensitivity when Bcl2L1 and IGF1R are silenced using siRNA.[115]

Signal transducer and activator of transcription 1 (STAT 1):
- It was established that avidin controls the proliferation of psoriatic keratinocytes through the STAT signaling pathway when keratinocytes, whether or not they were treated with avidin, were transfected with siRNA that targets STAT1 and STAT3.[116]

Mediating keratinocyte differentiation:
- Research has shown that the keratinocyte phenotype can change from psoriatic to normal by blocking genes that control differentiation.
- *Grainyhead-like transcription factor 2 (GRHL2)*: GRHL2 is promoted to normal differentiation in keratinocytes through siRNA-mediated knockdown.[117]
- *Sphingosine-1-phosphate lyase 1 (SGPL1)*: SGPL1 inhibition reduces cell proliferation and promotes proper differentiation by blocking S1P cleavage enzymes in keratinocytes.
- *Cathepsin B (CTSB)*: The inflammatory reactions and increased proliferation brought on by IL-17A[118] are both reversed by silencing CTSB.
- *Vascular endothelial growth factor (VEGF) secretion inhibition, angiogenesis inhibition*: By producing substances like VEGF, inflammatory cells encourage the migration, proliferation, and survival of endothelial cells. This action exacerbates the illness by inducing angiogenesis, which in turn causes vascular erythematous plaques to form.[119]
- *Aquaporin-1 (AQP1)*: A protein called AQP1 is involved in the membrane of water channels. Antiangiogenic treatments may target AQP1's function in maintaining endothelial cell activity during angiogenesis.[120]
- *TRAF3 interacting protein 2 (TRAF3IP2)*: In keratinocytes and endothelial cells, downregulation of TRAF3IP2 modifies VEGF production and secretion.[108]

Therefore research in targeted siRNA therapy for psoriasis could lead to future clinical treatment options.[105]

CONCLUSION

Some of the molecules mentioned in this chapter may never reach clinical use, while others may emerge as widely adopted and successful treatments for psoriasis. However, it is crucial to continue advancing our understanding of the disease pathogenesis. As our knowledge of psoriasis expands, we can anticipate the discovery of new treatment targets, leading to the development of highly specific, individualized therapies.

TAKE HOME MESSAGE

- Newer biologics like Bimekizumab (IL-17 blocker) has been approved by USFDA in October 2023 and has shown to be effective in psoriasis and psoriatic arthritis.
- Spesolimab an IL-36 receptor blocker has proven efficacy in generalized pustular psoriasis.
- Imsidolimab showed a quick and long lasting reduction in generalized pustular psoriasis.
- Orismilast a novel PDE4 inhibitor has been found to be more effective than apremilast in phase II studies.
- Deucravacitinib a specific Tyk 2 inhibitor has been approved for plaque psoriasis in 2022.
- One can expect oral IL-17 and oral IL-23 inhibitors in the near future.
- Tapinarof a new aryl hydrocarbon receptor agonist has emerged as a promising topical therapy in psoriasis.
- Topical roflumilast has been approved in plaque psoriasis in July 2022. It is also used in the pediatric age group (6–11 years).
- Small interfering RNA therapy will probably be the future of psoriasis management where the harmful genes are targeted.

REFERENCES

1. Reich K, Warren RB, Lebwohl M, Gooderham M, Strober B, Langley RG, et al. Bimekizumab versus secukinumab in plaque psoriasis. N Engl J Med. 2021;385:142-52.
2. Reich K, Papp KA, Blauvelt A, Langley RG, Armstrong A, Warren RB, et al. Bimekizumab versus ustekinumab for the treatment of moderate to severe plaque psoriasis (BE VIVID): efficacy and safety from a 52-week, multicentre, double-blind, active comparator and placebo controlled phase 3 trial. Lancet. 2021;397:487-98.
3. Coates LC, McInnes IB Merola JF, Warren RB, Kavanaugh A, Gottlieb AB, et al. Safety and efficacy of bimekizumab in patients with active psoriatic arthritis: Three-year results from a phase IIb randomized controlled trial and its open-label extension study. Arthritis Rheumatol. 2022;74(12):1959-70.
4. McInnes IB, Asahina A, Coates LC, Landewé R, Merola JF, Ritchlin CT, et al. Coarse J, Mease PJ. Bimekizumab in patients with psoriatic arthritis, naive to biologic treatment: a randomised, double-blind, placebo-controlled, phase 3 trial (BE OPTIMAL). Lancet. 2023;401(10370):25-37.
5. Blauvelt A, Kimball AB, Augustin M, Okubo Y, Witte MM, Capriles CR, et al. Efficacy and safety of mirikizumab in psoriasis: Results from a 52-week, double-blind, placebo-controlled, randomized withdrawal, phase III trial (OASIS-1). Br J Dermatol. 2022;187:866-77.
6. Papp K, Warren RB, Green L, Reich K, Langley RG, Paul C, et al. Safety and efficacy of mirikizumab versus secukinumab and placebo in the treatment of moderate-to-severe plaque psoriasis (OASIS-2): a phase 3, multicentre, randomised, double-blind study. Lancet Rheumatol. 2023;5:e542-52.
7. Taylor NP. (2021). Lilly scraps IL-23 psoriasis program despite phase 3 success, focuses on IBD race against AbbVie, J&J. [online] Available from https://www.fiercebiotech.com/biotech/lilly-scraps-il-23-psoriasis-program-despite-phase-3-success-focuses-ibd-race-against [Last accessed January 2025].
8. Morita A, Okubo Y, Imafuku S, Terui T. Spesolimab, the first-in-class anti-IL-36R antibody: From bench to clinic. J Dermatol. 2024;51(11):1379-91.
9. SPEVIGO® [package insert]. Ridgefield: Boehringer Ingelheim Pharmaceuticals, Inc; 2024.
10. Warren RB, Reich A, Kaszuba A, Placek W, Griffiths CEM, Zhou J, et al. Imsidolimab, an anti-interleukin-36 receptor monoclonal antibody, for the treatment of generalized pustular psoriasis: results from the phase II GALLOP trial. Br J Dermatol. 2023;189(2):161-9.
11. Conti P, Pregliasco FE, Bellomo RG, Gallenga CE, Caraffa A, Kritas SK, et al. Mast Cell Cytokines IL-1, IL-33, and IL-36 Mediate Skin Inflammation in Psoriasis: A Novel Therapeutic Approach with the Anti-Inflammatory Cytokines IL-37, IL-38, and IL-1Ra. Int J Mol Sci. 2021;22:8076.

12. Fala L. Otezla (Apremilast), an Oral PDE-4 Inhibitor, Receives FDA Approval for the Treatment of Patients with Active Psoriatic Arthritis and Plaque Psoriasis. Am Health Drug Benefits. 2015;8(Spec Feature):105-10.
13. Gyldenløve M, Meteran H, Zachariae C, Egeberg A. Long-term clearance of severe plaque psoriasis with oral roflumilast. J Eur Acad Dermatol Venereol. 2023;37:e429-30.
14. Warren RB, Strober B, Silverberg JI, Guttman E, Andres P, Felding J, et al. Oral orismilast: Efficacy and safety in moderate-to-severe psoriasis and development of modified release tablets. J Eur Acad Dermatol Venereol. 2023;37:711-20.
15. Kubota-Ishida N, Kaji C, Matsumoto S, Wakabayashi T, Matsuhira T, Okura I, et al. ME3183, a novel phosphodiesterase-4 inhibitor, exhibits potent anti-inflammatory effects and is well tolerated in a non-clinical study. Eur J Pharmacol. 2024;962:176202.
16. Warren RB, French LE, Blauvelt A, Langley RG, Egeberg A, Mrowietz U, et al. Orismilast in moderate-to-severe psoriasis: Efficacy and safety from a 16-week, randomized, double-blinded, placebo-controlled, dose-finding, and phase 2b trial (IASOS). J Am Acad Dermatol. 2024;90(3):494-503.
17. Liu X, Chen R, Zeng G, Gao Y, Liu X, Zhang D, et al. Determination of a PDE4 inhibitor Hemay005 in human plasma and urine by UPLC-MS/MS and its application to a PK study. Bioanalysis. 2018;10(11):863-75.
18. Carmona-Rocha E, Rusiñol L, Puig L. New and Emerging Oral/Topical Small-Molecule Treatments for Psoriasis. Pharmaceutics. 2024;16(2):239.
19. Kato S, Cho N, Koresawa T, Otake K, Kano A. Safety, Tolerability, and Pharmacokinetics of a Novel Oral Phosphodiesterase 4 Inhibitor, ME3183: First-in-Human Phase 1 Study. Clin Pharmacol Drug Dev. 2023;13(4):341-8.
20. Villarino AV, Kanno Y, Ferdinand JR, O'Shea JJ. Mechanisms of Jak/STAT signaling in immunity and disease. J Immunol. 2015;194:21-7.
21. O'Shea JJ, Schwartz DM, Villarino AV, Gadina M, McInnes IB, Laurence A. The JAK-STAT pathway: Impact on human disease and therapeutic intervention. Annu Rev Med. 2015;66:311-28.
22. Helfand C. (2015). FDA Swats down Pfizer's Xeljanz in Plaque Psoriasis. Fierce Pharma. 2015. [online] Available from https://www.fiercepharma.com/regulatory/fda-swats-down-pfizer-s-xeljanz-plaque-psoriasis [Last accessed January 2025].
23. Tian F, Chen Z, Xu T. Efficacy and safety of tofacitinib for the treatment of chronic plaque psoriasis: A systematic review and meta-analysis. J Int Med Res. 2019;47:2342-50.
24. Abbvie. (2021). RINVOQ® (Upadacitinib) Receives U.S. FDA Approval for Active Psoriatic Arthritis. Abbvie. 2021. [online] Available from https://news.abbvie.com/2021-12-14-RINVOQ-R-upadacitinib-Receives-U-S-FDA-Approval-for-Active-Psoriatic-Arthritis [Last accessed January 2025].
25. Kaur M, Misra S. Deucravacitinib: moderate-to-severe plaque psoriasis preventable? J Basic Clin Physiol Pharmacol. 2024;35(4-5):225-30.
26. Hoy SM. Deucravacitinib: First Approval. Drugs. 2022;82:1671-9.
27. Sbidian E, Chaimani A, Garcia-Doval I, Doney L, Dressler C, Hua C, et al. Systemic pharmacological treatments for chronic plaque psoriasis: A network meta-analysis. Cochrane Database Syst Rev. 2022;5:CD011535.
28. Armstrong AW, Warren RB, Zhong Y, Zhuo J, Cichewicz A, Kadambi A, et al. Short-, Mid-, and Long-Term Efficacy of Deucravacitinib Versus Biologics and Nonbiologics for Plaque Psoriasis: A Network Meta-Analysis. Dermatol Ther. 2023;13:2839-57.
29. Armstrong AW, Park SH, Patel V, Hogan M, Wang WJ, Davidson D, et al. Matching-Adjusted Indirect Comparison of the Long-Term Efficacy of Deucravacitinib Versus Adalimumab for Moderate to Severe Plaque Psoriasis. Dermatol Ther. 2023;13:2589-603.
30. Vugler A, O'Connell J, Nguyen MA, Weitz D, Leeuw T, Hickford E, et al. An orally available small molecule that targets soluble TNF to deliver anti-TNF biologic-like efficacy in rheumatoid arthritis. Front Pharmacol. 2022;13:1037983.
31. Pharmaceutical Technology. SAR-441566 by Sanofi for Psoriasis: Likelihood of Approval; Pharm Technol. 2023.
32. Datta-Mannan A, Regev A, Coutant DE, Dropsey AJ, Foster J, Jones S, et al. Safety, Tolerability, and Pharmacokinetics of an Oral Small Molecule Inhibitor of IL-17A (LY3509754): A Phase I Randomized Placebo-Controlled Study. Clin Pharmacol Ther. 2024;115(5):1152-61.
33. DICE Therapeutics. (2025). Unlocking the Potential of Oral Medicines. [online] Available from https://www.dicetherapeutics.com/pipeline [Last accessed January 2025].
34. Budwick D. (2022). DICE Therapeutics Announces Positive Topline Data from Phase 1 Clinical Trial of Lead Oral IL-17 Antagonist, DC-806, for Psoriasis. [online] Available from https://www.globenewswire.com/news-release/2022/10/11/2531642/0/en/DICE-Therapeutics-Announces-Positive-Topline-Data-from-Phase-1-Clinical-Trial-of-Lead-Oral-IL-17-Antagonist-DC-806-for-Psoriasis.html [Last accessed January 2025].

35. Lilly Investors. (2023). Lilly Completes Acquisition of DICE Therapeutics. [online] Available from https://investor.lilly.com/news-releases/news-release-details/lilly-completes-acquisition-dice-therapeutics [Last accessed January 2025].
36. Bissonnette R, Pinter A, Ferris LK, Gerdes S, Rich P, Vender R, et al. An Oral Interleukin-23-Receptor Antagonist Peptide for Plaque Psoriasis. N Engl J Med. 2024;390(6):510-21.
37. Bader K. (2023). New Positive Results of Oral IL-23 Receptor Antagonist for Psoriasis. Dermatology Times. 2023. [online] Available from https://www.dermatologytimes.com/view/new-positive-results-of-oral-il-23-receptor-antagonist-for-psoriasis [Last accessed January 2025].
38. Janssen Research & Development, LLC. (2025). A Study of JNJ-77242113 for the Treatment of Participants With Moderate to Severe Plaque Psoriasis. [online] Available from https://clinicaltrials.gov/study/NCT06143878?term=jnj-77242113&rank=10 [Last accessed January 2025].
39. Janssen Research & Development, LLC. (2025). A Study of JNJ-77242113 for the Treatment of Participants With Moderate to Severe Plaque Psoriasis (ICONIC-ADVANCE 2). [online] Available from https://clinicaltrials.gov/study/NCT06220604?tab=results [Last accessed January 2025].
40. Tang L, Yang X, Liang Y, Xie H, Dai Z, Zheng G. Transcription factor retinoid-related orphan receptor γt: a promising target for the treatment of psoriasis. Front Immunol. 2018;9:1210.
41. Gege C. RORγt inhibitors as potential back-ups for the phase II candidate VTP-43742 from Vitae Pharmaceuticals: Patent evaluation of WO2016061160 and US20160122345. Expert Opin Ther Pat. 2017;27:1-8.
42. Pandya VB, Kumar S, Sachchidanand S, Sharma R, Desai RC. Combating Autoimmune Diseases with Retinoic Acid Receptor-Related Orphan Receptor-γ (RORγ or RORc) Inhibitors: Hits and Misses. J Med Chem. 2018;61:10976-95.
43. Capone A, Volpe E. Transcriptional Regulators of T Helper 17 Cell Differentiation in Health and Autoimmune Diseases. Front Immunol. 2020;11:348.
44. Blankenbach KV, Schwalm S, Pfeilschifter J, Meyer Zu Heringdorf D. Sphingosine-1-Phosphate Receptor-2 Antagonists: Therapeutic Potential and Potential Risks. Front Pharmacol. 2016;7:167.
45. Obinata H, Hla T. Sphingosine 1-phosphate and inflammation. Int Immunol. 2019;31:617-25.
46. Herzinger T, Kleuser B, Schäfer-Korting M, Korting HC. Sphingosine-1-phosphate signaling and the skin. Am J Clin Dermatol. 2007;8:329-36.
47. Schaper K, Kietzmann M, Bäumer W. Sphingosine-1-phosphate differently regulates the cytokine production of IL-12, IL-23 and IL-27 in activated murine bone marrow derived dendritic cells. Mol Immunol. 2014;59:10-8.
48. Yiu ZZN, Warren RB. Novel Oral Therapies for Psoriasis and Psoriatic Arthritis. Am J Clin Dermatol. 2016;17:191-200.
49. D'Ambrosio D, Steinmann J, Brossard P, Dingemanse J. Differential effects of ponesimod, a selective S1P1 receptor modulator, on blood-circulating human T cell subpopulations. Immunopharmacol Immunotoxicol. 2015;37:103-9.
50. Vaclavkova A, Chimenti S, Arenberger P, Holló P, Sator PG, Burcklen M, et al. Oral ponesimod in patients with chronic plaque psoriasis: A randomised, double-blind, placebo-controlled phase 2 trial. Lancet. 2014;384:2036-45.
51. Magni G, Ceruti S. Adenosine signaling in autoimmune disorders. Pharmaceuticals. 2020;13(9):1-22.
52. Cheng Y, Man N, Xu T, Fu R, Wang X, Wang X, et al. Transdermal delivery of nonsteroidal anti-inflammatory drugs mediated by polyamidoamine (PAMAM) dendrimers. J Pharm Sci. 2007;96(3):595-602.
53. Cohen S, Barer F, Itzhak I, Silverman MH, Fishman P. Inhibition of IL-17 and IL-23 in human keratinocytes by the A3 adenosine receptor agonist piclidenoson. J Immunol Res. 2018;2018:2310970.
54. Koscsó B, Csóka B, Pacher P, Haskó G. Investigational A3 adenosine receptor targeting agents. Expert Opin Investig Drugs. 2011;20(6):757-68.
55. Cohen S, Fishman P. Targeting the A3 adenosine receptor to treat cytokine release syndrome in cancer immunotherapy. Drug Des Devel Ther. 2019;13:491-7.
56. Lee JY, Jhun BS, Oh YT, Lee JH, Choe W, Baik HH, et al. Activation of adenosine A3 receptor suppresses lipopolysaccharide-induced TNF-alpha production through inhibition of PI 3-kinase/Akt and NF-kappaB activation in murine BV2 microglial cells. Neurosci Lett. 2006;396(1):1-6.
57. Haskó G, Németh ZH, Vizi ES, Salzman AL, Szabó C. An agonist of adenosine A3 receptors decreases interleukin-12 and interferon-gamma production and prevents lethality in endotoxemic mice. Eur J Pharmacol. 1998;358 (3):261-8.
58. Papp KA, Beyska-Rizova S, Gantcheva ML, Slavcheva Simeonova E, Brezoev P, Celic M, et al.; COMFORT-1 Study Investigators. Efficacy and safety of piclidenoson in plaque psoriasis: Results from a randomized phase 3 clinical trial

59. Ben Abdallah H, Johansen C, Iversen L. Key Signaling Pathways in Psoriasis: Recent Insights from Antipsoriatic Therapeutics. Psoriasis Targets Ther. 2021;11:83-97.
60. Wang WM, Jin HZ. Heat shock proteins and psoriasis. Eur J Dermatol. 2019;29(2):121-5.
61. Bregnhøj A, Thuesen KKH, Emmanuel T, Litman T, Grek CL, Ghatnekar GS, et al. HSP90 inhibitor RGRN-305 for oral treatment of plaque-type psoriasis: Efficacy, safety and biomarker results in an open-label proof-of-concept study. Br J Dermatol. 2022;186:861-74.
62. BenAbdallah H, Seeler S, Bregnhøj A, Ghatnekar G, Kristensen LS, Iversen L, et al. Heat shock protein 90 inhibitor RGRN-305 potently attenuates skin inflammation. Front. Immunol. 2023;14:1128897.
63. Yoon JH, Nguyen TT, Duong VA, Chun KH, Maeng HJ. Determination of KD025(SLx-2119), a Selective ROCK2 Inhibitor, in Rat Plasma by High-Performance Liquid Chromatography-Tandem Mass Spectrometry and its Pharmacokinetic application. Molecules. 2020;25:1369.
64. Kadmon Corporation, LLC. (2022). Phase 2, Open-label, Study of KD025 in Subjects With Psoriasis Vulgaris Who Failed First-line Therapy. [online] Available from https://clinicaltrials.gov/study/NCT02317627 [Last accessed January 2025].
65. Kadmon Corporation, LLC. (2022). A Safety and Tolerability Study of Belumosudil (KD025) Treatment in Subjects With Moderately Severe Psoriasis Vulgaris. [online] Available from https://clinicaltrials.gov/study/NCT02106195 [Last accessed January 2025].
66. Zhang X, He Y. The role of nociceptive neurons in the pathogenesis of psoriasis. Front Immunol. 2020;11.
67. Innani S, Tomar Y, Rana V, Singhvi G. Navigating the landscape of psoriasis therapy: novel targeted pathways and emerging trends. Expert Opin Ther Targets. 2023;27(12):1247-56.
68. Lipton RB, Croop R, Stock EG, Stock DA, Morris BA, Frost M, et al. Rimegepant, an oral calcitonin gene–related peptide receptor antagonist, for Migraine. N Engl J Med. 2019;381(2):142-9.
69. Weill Cornell Medicine. Rimegepant Clinical Trial A Pilot Study of Rimegepant in Moderate Plaque-type Psoriasis. [online] Available from https://jcto.weill.cornell.edu/rimegepant#:~:text=What%20is%20Rimegepant%20normally%20used,for%20the%20treatment%20of%20migraines [Last accessed January 2025].
70. Christofferson DE, Li Y, Hitomi J, Zhou W, Upperman C, Zhu H, et al. A novel role for RIP1 kinase in mediating TNFα production. Cell Death Dis. 2012;3(6):e320.
71. Dannappel M, Vlantis K, Kumari S, Polykratis A, Kim C, Wachsmuth L, et al. RIPK1 maintains epithelial homeostasis by inhibiting apoptosis and necroptosis. Nature. 2014;513(7516):90-4.
72. Harris PA, Berger SB, Jeong JU, Nagilla R, Bandyopadhyay D, Campobasso N, et al. Discovery of a first-in-class receptor interacting protein 1 (RIP1) kinase specific clinical candidate (GSK2982772) for the treatment of inflammatory diseases. J Med Chem. 2017;60(4):1247-61.
73. Xin Y, Dai P, Shao H, Zhuang C, Li J. Discovery of novel biaryl benzoxazepinones as dual-mode receptor-interacting protein kinase-1 (RIPK1) inhibitors. Bioorg Med Chem. 2024;100:117611.
74. Gajjela BK, Zhou MM. Bromodomain inhibitors and therapeutic applications. Curr Opin Chem Biol. 2023;75:102323.
75. Gilan O, Rioja I, Knezevic K, Bell MJ, Yeung MM, Harker NR, et al. Selective targeting of BD1 and BD2 of the BET proteins in cancer and immunoinflammation. Science. 2020;368(6489):387-94.
76. Pasmatzi E, Papadionysiou C, Monastirli A, Badavanis G, Tsambaos D. Galectin 3: an extraordinary multifunctional protein in dermatology. Current knowledge and perspectives. An Bras Dermatol. 2019;94(3):348-54.
77. Hayran Y, Allı N, Akpınar Ü, Öktem A, Yücel Ç, Fırat Oguz E, et al. Serum galectin-3 levels in patients with psoriasis. Int J Clin Pract. 2021;75(10):e14545.
78. Zhou X, Su J, Zhang CL, Dai H, Wang WH. Decreased expression of galectin-3 in the epidermis of psoriasis patients. Eur J Dermatol. 2024;34(4):371-7.
79. Curti BD, Koguchi Y, Leidner RS, Rolig AS, Sturgill ER, Sun Z, et al. Enhancing clinical and immunological effects of anti-PD-1 with belapectin, a galectin-3 inhibitor. J Immunother Cancer. 2021;9(4):e002371.
80. Furue M, Tsuji G, Mitoma C, Nakahara T, Chiba T, Morino-Koga S, et al. Gene regulation of filaggrin and other skin barrier proteins via aryl hydrocarbon receptor. J Dermatol Sci. 2015;80(2):83-8.
81. Smith SH, Jayawickreme C, Rickard DJ, Nicodeme E, Bui T, Simmons C, et al. Tapinarof is a natural AhR agonist that resolves skin inflammation in mice and humans. J Invest Dermatol. 2017;137(10):2110-9.
82. Bissonnette R, Stein Gold L, Rubenstein DS, Tallman AM, Armstrong A. Tapinarof in the treatment of psoriasis: A review of the unique mechanism of action of a novel therapeutic aryl hydrocarbon receptor-modulating agent. J Am Acad Dermatol. 2021;84(4):1059-67.

83. Nicolas SE, Bear MD, Kanaan AO, Coman OA, Dima L. Roflumilast 0.3% Cream:A Phosphodiesterase 4 Inhibitor for the Treatment of Chronic Plaque Psoriasis. Am J Ther. 2023;30:e535-e542.
84. Sheldon A. FDA Approves Arcutis'ZORYVE® (roflumilast) Cream 0.3% for Treatment of Psoriasis in Children Ages 6 to 11. Westlake Village: Arcutis Biotherapeutics; 2023.
85. Lebwohl MG, Kircik LH, Moore AY, Stein Gold L, Draelos ZD, Gooderham MJ, et al. Effect of Roflumilast Cream vs Vehicle Cream on Chronic Plaque Psoriasis: The DERMIS-1 and DERMIS-2 Randomized Clinical Trials. JAMA. 2022;328: 1073-84.
86. Hashim PW, Chima M, Kim HJ, Bares J, Yao CJ, Singer G, et al. Crisaborole 2% ointment for the treatment of intertriginous, anogenital, and facial psoriasis: A double-blind, randomized, vehicle-controlled trial. J Am Acad Dermatol. 2020;82(2): 360-5.
87. Liu Y, Li W. Successful treatment with crisaborole for facial lesions refractory to adalimumab in a man with psoriasis: A case report. Dermatol Ther. 2022;35:e15424.
88. Robbins AB, Gor A, Bui MR. Topical Crisaborole-A Potential Treatment for Recalcitrant Palmoplantar Psoriasis. JAMA Dermatol. 2018;154:1096-7.
89. Punwani N, Scherle P, Flores R, Shi J, Liang J, Yeleswaram S, et al. Preliminary clinical activity of a topical JAK1/2 inhibitor in the treatment of psoriasis. J Am Acad Dermatol. 2012;67:658-64.
90. Maleki F, Chang C, Purohit VS, Nicholas T. Pharmacokinetic Profile of Brepocitinib with Topical Administration in Atopic Dermatitis and Psoriasis Populations: Strategy to Inform Clinical Trial Design in Adult and Pediatric Populations. Pharm Res. 2024;41(4):623-36.
91. Landis MN, Smith SR, Berstein G, Fetterly G, Ghosh P, Feng G, et al. Efficacy and safety of topical brepocitinib cream for mild-to-moderate chronic plaque psoriasis: A phase IIb randomized double-blind vehicle-controlled parallel-group study. Br J Dermatol. 2023;189:33-41.
92. Bronner SM, Zbieg JR, Crawford JJ. RORγ antagonists and inverse agonists: a patent review. Expert Opin Ther Pat. 2016;27(1):101-12.
93. Smith SH, Peredo CE, Takeda Y, Bui T, Neil J, Rickard D, et al. Development of a Topical Treatment for Psoriasis Targeting RORγ: From Bench to Skin. PLoS ONE. 2016;11:e0147979.
94. Ecoeur F, Weiss J, Kaupmann K, Hintermann S, Orain D, Guntermann C. Antagonizing Retinoic Acid-Related-Orphan Receptor Gamma Activity Blocks the T Helper 17/Interleukin-17 Pathway Leading to Attenuated Pro-inflammatory Human Keratinocyte and Skin Responses. Front Immunol. 2019;10:577.
95. Kang EG, Wu S, Gupta A, vonMackensen YL, Siemetzki H, Freudenberg JM, et al. A phase I randomized controlled trial to evaluate safety and clinical effect of topically applied GSK2981278 ointment in a psoriasis plaque test. Br J Dermatol. 2018;178:1427-9.
96. Otake S, Otsubaki T, Uesato N, Ueda Y, Murayama T, Hayashi M. Topical Application of BMS-509744, a Selective Inhibitor of Interleukin-2-Inducible T Cell Kinase, Ameliorates Imiquimod-Induced Skin Inflammation in Mice. Biol Pharm Bull. 2021;44(4):528-34.
97. Pradyuth S, Rapalli VK, Gorantla S, Waghule T, Dubey SK, Singhvi G. Insightful exploring of microRNAs in psoriasis and its targeted topical delivery. Dermatol Ther. 2020;33:e14221.
98. Guo S, Zhang W, Wei C, Wang L, Zhu G, Shi Q, et al. Serum and skin levels of miR-369-3p in patients with psoriasis and their correlation with disease severity. Eur J Dermatol. 2013;23:608-13.
99. Zhang W, Yi X, An Y, Guo S, Li S, Song P, et al. MicroRNA-17-92 cluster promotes the proliferation and the chemokine production of keratinocytes: Implication for the pathogenesis of psoriasis. Cell Death Dis. 2018;9:567.
100. Wu R, Zeng J, Yuan J, Deng X, Huang Y, Chen L, et al. MicroRNA-210 overexpression promotes psoriasis-like inflammation by inducing Th1 and Th17 cell differentiation. J Clin Invest. 2018;128(6):2551-68.
101. Feng H, Wu R, Zhang S, Kong Y, Liu Z, Wu H, et al. Topical administration of nanocarrier miRNA-210 antisense ameliorates imiquimod-induced psoriasis-like dermatitis in mice. J Dermatol. 2020;47(2):147-54.
102. Milazzo S, Horneber M. Laetrile treatment for cancer. Cochrane Database Syst Rev. 2015;2015: CD005476.
103. Gago-López N, Lagunas Arnal C, Perez JJ, Wagner EF. Topical application of an amygdalin analogue reduces inflammation and keratinocyte proliferation in a psoriasis mouse model. Exp Dermatol. 2021;30(11):1662-74.
104. Purewal JS, Doshi GM. RNAi in psoriasis: A melodic exploration of miRNA, shRNA, and amiRNA with a spotlight on siRNA. Eur J Pharmacol. 2024;985: 177083.
105. Zhao F, Zhao J, Wei K, Jiang P, Shi Y, Chang C, et al. Targeted siRNA Therapy for Psoriasis: Translating Preclinical Potential into Clinical Treatments. Immunotargets Ther. 2024;13:259-71.
106. Xu N, Brodin P, Wei T, Meisgen F, Eidsmo L, Nagy N, et al. MiR-125b, a microRNA downregulated in psoriasis, modulates keratinocyte proliferation by

targeting FGFR2. J Invest Dermatol. 2011;131(7):1521-9.
107. Hampton PJ, Jans R, Flockhart RJ, Parker G, Reynolds NJ. Lithium regulates keratinocyte proliferation via glycogen synthase kinase 3 and NFAT2 (Nuclear Factor of Activated T Cells 2). J Cell Physiol. 2012;227(4):1529-37.
108. Song Y, Chen L, Li Y, Lin Q, Liu W, Zhang L. Knockdown of TRAF3IP2 suppresses the expression of VEGFA and the proliferation of keratinocytes and vascular endothelial cells. Heliyon. 2019;5(5):e01642.
109. Liao Y, Su Y, Wu R, Zhang P, Feng C. Overexpression of Wilms tumor 1 promotes IL-1β expression by upregulating histone acetylation in keratinocytes. Int Immunopharmacol 2021;96:107793.
110. Kong Y, Wu R, Zhang S, Zhao M, Wu H, Lu Q, et al. Wilms' tumor 1-associating protein contributes to psoriasis by promoting keratinocytes proliferation via regulating cyclinA2 and CDK2. Int Immunopharmacol. 2020;88:106918.
111. Yu J, Zhao Q, Wang X, Zhou H, Hu J, Gu L, et al. Pathogenesis, multi-omics research, and clinical treatment of psoriasis. J Autoimmun. 2022;133:102916.
112. Zhou X, Chen Y, Cui L, Shi Y, Guo C. Advances in the pathogenesis of psoriasis: from keratinocyte perspective. Cell Death Dis. 2022;13(1):81.
113. Ran LW, Wang H, Lan D, Jia HX, Yu SS. Effect of RNA interference targeting STAT3 gene combined with ultrasonic irradiation and SonoVue microbubbles on proliferation and apoptosis in keratinocytes of psoriatic lesions. Chin Med J (Engl). 2018;131(17):2097-104.
114. Huang W, Zheng X, Huang Q, Weng D, Yao S, Zhou C, et al. Protein Kinase CK2 promotes proliferation, abnormal differentiation, and proinflammatory cytokine production of keratinocytes via regulation of STAT3 and Akt pathways in psoriasis. Am J Pathol. 2023;193(5):567-78.
115. Lerman G, Volman E, Sidi Y, Avni D. Small-interfering RNA targeted at antiapoptotic mRNA increases keratinocyte sensitivity to apoptosis. Br J Dermatol. 2011;164(5):947-56.
116. Qin X, Chen C, Zhang Y, Zhang L, Mei Y, Long X, et al. Acitretin modulates HaCaT cells proliferation through STAT1- and STAT3-dependent signalling. Saudi Pharm J. 2017;25(4):620-4.
117. Zhu H, Hou L, Liu J, Li Z. MiR-217 is down-regulated in psoriasis and promotes keratinocyte differentiation via targeting GRHL2. Biochem Biophys Res Commun. 2016;471(1):169-76.
118. Jeon S, Song J, Lee D, Kim GT, Park SH, Shin DY, et al. Inhibition of sphingosine 1-phosphate lyase activates human keratinocyte differentiation and attenuates psoriasis in mice. J Lipid Res. 2020;61(1):20-32.
119. Xu D, Wang J. Downregulation of cathepsin B reduces proliferation and inflammatory response and facilitates differentiation in human HaCaT keratinocytes, ameliorating IL-17A and SAA-induced psoriasis-like lesion. Inflammation. 2021;44(5):2006-17.
120. Nicchia GP, Stigliano C, Sparaneo A, Rossi A, Frigeri A, Svelto M. Inhibition of aquaporin-1 dependent angiogenesis impairs tumour growth in a mouse model of melanoma. J Mol Med (Berl). 2013;91(5):613-23.

22
Overview of Psoriasis Research Trends

Shraddha Madanagobalane

■ INTRODUCTION

Psoriasis is a multifactorial, heterogeneous inflammatory skin disease. Unravelling genetic predispositions, newer immunological pathways, and microbiome insights have paved the way for newer therapeutic targets. Extensive research over the last decade in psoriasis has changed the scope of its treatment. The future holds promise for more treatments improving outcome and quality of life for individuals living with psoriasis.

Management of psoriasis has come a long way from conventional treatments to molecular targeted therapy and toward genetic modulations. The administration of these have also evolved from subcutaneous delivery to include more convenient oral and topical medications.

Recent research in psoriasis has been predominantly focused on keratinocytes which forms the basis of newer therapeutic targets. In this chapter, we will discuss the following areas of keratinocyte research:
- Genetics
- Noncoding ribonucleic acid (RNA)
- Antimicrobial peptides (AMPs)
- Cytokines and receptors
- Keratinocytes interaction
- Metabolism

■ GENETICS

Numerous genetic risk factors have been identified, such as genes related to cytokine signaling (*IL12B* and *IL23R*), interferon signaling, nuclear factor-κB (NF-κB) signaling (*TNFAIP3*, *NFKBIA*, *NFKBIZ*, *TNIP1*, and *RELA*), antigen presentation (HLA-Cw6), and cytokine signaling.[1-3]

In psoriatic lesions, activation of keratinocytes and skin infiltration by T lymphocytes and macrophages are linked to >80% of elevated genes.[4]

The psoriasis associated susceptibility locus 1 (PSORS1) was the most potent of the >80 psoriasis susceptible loci that have been found. At least 100 psoriasis susceptibility genes have been discovered over time, the majority of which are connected to skin barrier function, innate immunity, and adaptive immunity.

At least 100 psoriasis susceptibility genes have been discovered over time, the majority of which are connected to skin barrier function, innate immunity, and adaptive immunity.[3,5]

CARD14 and NF-κB Pathway Activation in Psoriasis

- *CARD14* encodes for CARMA2 (CARD-containing MAGUK protein 2) is a key

player in activating the NF-κB signaling pathway. This pathway is central to inflammation and immune responses, and its dysregulation is involved in the pathogenesis of psoriasis.[1]
- *Mutations in CARD14* lead to a *gain-of-function* effect, where the protein's altered function results in *increased NF-κB* and mitogen-activated protein kinase (MAPK) signaling pathways. This promotes the expression of inflammatory cytokines, chemokines such as *CCL20* and AMPs, all of which contribute to psoriasis.[6,7]
- *PSORS2* is the psoriasis susceptibility locus associated with *CARD14 mutations*, further emphasizing its role in the disease's pathogenesis.[1]

TNFAIP3/A20 and TNIP1: Negative Regulation of TNF Signaling

- TNFAIP3 (encoding A20) and TNIP1 (encoding ABIN1) are key negative regulators of the tumor necrosis factor (TNF) receptor signaling pathway, which is implicated in psoriasis.
- A20 functions as a feedback inhibitor of TNF signaling, preventing excessive inflammation. However, in psoriasis patients, there are lower levels of A20 in the epidermis, contributing to increased inflammation.
- The deletion of TNFAIP3/A20 results in upregulation of proinflammatory genes in keratinocytes, reinforcing the importance of this pathway in the pathophysiology of psoriasis.[8]

VEGFA/Flt1/Nrp1 Axis in Psoriasis

- VEGFA is a vascular endothelial growth factor that plays a critical role in angiogenesis and is often elevated in inflammatory conditions, including psoriasis.
- It signals through receptors such as Flt1 (VEGFR1) and Flk1 (VEGFR2), as well as the coreceptor neuropilin-1 (Nrp1). In psoriasis, VEGFA expression is elevated in keratinocytes, contributing to both inflammation and tissue remodeling.
- Studies have shown that keratinocyte-specific deletion of Flt1 or Nrp1 reduces VEGFA-induced psoriasis, indicating that the VEGF-Flt1-Nrp1 axis is a key mediator in psoriasis pathogenesis and a potential target for therapeutic intervention.[9]

TRAF3IP2 (ACT1) in IL-17A Signaling

- TRAF3IP2 encodes ACT1, an adapter protein crucial for interleukin-17A (IL-17A) receptor signaling. IL-17A is a central cytokine in psoriasis, promoting inflammation and the expression of proinflammatory genes in keratinocytes.
- TRAF3IP2 mutations can alter the IL-17A response, and knockdown of TRAF3IP2 in keratinocytes leads to suppressed IL-17A signaling and enhanced cell differentiation, suggesting that modulating this pathway could have therapeutic potential for controlling the disease.[10,11]

Implications for Treatment

The identification of genetic variants and molecular mechanisms involved in psoriasis opens the door for targeted therapies. For instance:
- Inhibiting NF-κB (e.g., through targeting CARD14 or other downstream mediators) could reduce the inflammatory responses characteristic of psoriasis.
- Modulating VEGFA signaling may help to address vascular changes and keratinocyte hyperproliferation in psoriasis.
- Targeting IL-17A and its downstream signaling pathways (including TRAF3IP2) could offer specific therapeutic strategies aimed at reducing the chronic inflammation and skin lesions in psoriasis.

Overall, the complex interplay between these genetic variants and molecular pathways underscores the multifactorial nature of psoriasis and highlights potential avenues

CHAPTER 22: Overview of Psoriasis Research Trends

for precision medicine and more effective treatments.

■ NONCODING RIBONUCLEIC ACID

Noncoding RNA mediates cellular processes such as chromatin remodeling, transcription, post-transcriptional modification, and signal transduction. Psoriasis is also influenced by epigenetic regulation. One of the epigenetic controls which is crucial to the etiology of disease is noncoding RNA regulation. Psoriasis is associated with the malfunctioning of microRNAs, which are small noncoding RNAs that suppress the expression of protein-coding genes at the posttranscriptional stage.[12] The expression of genes linked to cell division, proliferation, and apoptosis is significantly and widely impacted by sRNA.

The types of ncRNAs include microRNA (miRNA), long noncoding RNA (lncRNA), and circular RNA (circRNA).

MicroRNA

MicroRNAs are short ncRNAs that regulate gene expression at the posttranscriptional level by binding to the target messenger RNAs (mRNAs), leading to their degradation or translational repression. Dysregulation of miRNAs has been implicated in various aspects of psoriasis, particularly in regulating immune cell differentiation, keratinocyte proliferation, and inflammation. In psoriasis, several miRNAs are abnormally expressed, contributing to the disease's pathophysiology.[13]

- *miR-210*: Upregulated in psoriasis, miR-210 promotes Th17 and Th1 cell differentiation through the STAT6 signaling pathway, both of which are involved in driving inflammation in psoriasis.
- *miR-155*: Upregulated in psoriasis, miR-155 plays a critical role in regulating cytokine production in keratinocytes, particularly IL-6 and CXCL8, via the GATA3/IL-37 regulatory axis. This enhances the inflammatory response in psoriatic lesions.
- *miR-125a*: Downregulated in psoriasis, miR-125a normally suppresses keratinocyte proliferation and promotes apoptosis by inhibiting the IL-23R/JAK2/STAT3 signaling pathway. Its downregulation in psoriasis leads to unchecked keratinocyte proliferation and survival, contributing to disease pathology.
- *Other miRNAs*: Over 250 miRNAs have been found to be differentially expressed in psoriatic skin lesions, peripheral blood mononuclear cells, and plasma, highlighting the extensive role of miRNAs in the disease.

Long Noncoding RNA

Long noncoding RNAs are RNA molecules longer than 200 nucleotides and play roles in chromatin remodeling, gene expression regulation, and cellular differentiation. In psoriasis, lncRNAs are involved in controlling the immune response and keratinocyte behavior.

Studies have shown that patients with psoriasis who were treated with adalimumab and have reduced expression of specific lncRNAs compared to untreated patients, suggesting that lncRNAs may be involved in the inflammatory and immune responses associated with psoriasis.

Circular RNA

Circular RNAs are a class of noncoding RNAs that form covalently closed loops and are involved in regulating gene expression through sponging miRNAs. By binding to specific miRNAs, circRNAs prevent miRNAs from repressing their target genes, thus modulating the expression of genes involved in cell proliferation and inflammation. In psoriasis, circRNAs have been shown to regulate these processes, contributing to the excessive cell turnover and inflammation seen in psoriatic lesions.[14]

Role of Noncoding RNAs in Psoriasis Pathogenesis

Noncoding RNAs influence several aspects of psoriasis pathogenesis, including:

- *Immune cell differentiation and inflammation*: miRNAs such as miR-210 and miR-155 regulate the differentiation of immune cells such as Th1 and Th17 cells, which are key drivers of inflammation in psoriasis. Elevated levels of these miRNAs contribute to the chronic inflammatory response.
- *Keratinocyte proliferation and apoptosis*: miRNAs such as miR-125a modulate keratinocyte behavior by regulating signaling pathways that control cell division, survival, and apoptosis. In psoriasis, the dysregulation of these miRNAs results in excessive keratinocyte proliferation and abnormal differentiation.
- *Gene expression regulation*: lncRNAs and circRNAs act as regulators of gene expression by interacting with miRNAs, transcription factors, and chromatin remodeling complexes. Their dysregulation in psoriasis exacerbates the disease by maintaining an environment of chronic inflammation and hyperproliferation.[15]
- Noncoding RNAs, including miRNAs, lncRNAs, and circRNAs, play crucial roles in the regulation of immune responses, cell proliferation, apoptosis, and inflammation in psoriasis. The dysregulation of these ncRNAs contributes significantly to the pathogenesis of psoriasis, making them potential therapeutic targets for novel treatments. RNA interference (RNAi) and the modulation of specific miRNAs and ncRNAs offer a promising avenue for targeted therapies in psoriasis management. Understanding the complex network of ncRNA interactions will be key to developing effective treatments for this chronic inflammatory skin disease.[14]

RNA Interference and Potential Psoriasis Treatment

RNA interference is a mechanism that can specifically target and degrade mRNAs, resulting in sequence-specific suppression of gene expression. Given the involvement of miRNAs and other ncRNAs in psoriasis, RNAi-based therapies have emerged as a promising potential treatment. By manipulating miRNA expression or using RNAi to block specific ncRNAs involved in the disease, it may be possible to reduce inflammation, control keratinocyte proliferation, and improve clinical outcomes in patients with psoriasis.[16,17]

ANTIMICROBIAL PEPTIDES

Antimicrobial peptides play an important role in innate immunity due to their ability to disrupt microbial membranes, leading to the death of bacteria, fungi, and some viruses.[18] Their amphipathic nature and positive charge allow them to interact effectively with the lipid bilayers of microbial cells, resulting in membrane disruption.[19]

Different types of AMPs, such as cathelicidins and defensins, possess additional functions beyond their antimicrobial activity. They can modulate immune responses, facilitating a broader role in inflammation and tissue repair, which is especially relevant in conditions such as psoriasis.[20]

Cathelicidins

Cathelicidins, in particular, are produced as inactive precursors (propeptides) and are converted into active forms [cathelicidin antimicrobial peptides (CAMPs)] through the action of serine proteases. LL-37 (cathelicidin) is the most studied cathelicidin related to psoriasis, where its expression is increased in response to inflammation. This heightened expression in keratinocytes and deposition by neutrophils may contribute to both antimicrobial defense and modulation of the inflammatory response in psoriatic lesions.[21]

Understanding the functions and mechanisms of AMPs in skin conditions can lead to new therapeutic strategies aimed at harnessing their properties for treating infections and inflammatory skin diseases.

Defensins

The cationic microbial peptides known as defensins have three pairs of intramolecular disulfide bonds formed by six conserved cysteine residues. Humans have several defensin genes that constitute multiple gene clusters, as opposed to the one human cathelicidin gene CAMP. Similar to LL-37, β-defensins and lysosomes have been shown to activate plasmacytoid dendritic cells (pDCs) by improving self-DNA or self-RNA recognition. Both CD4+ T cells and neutrophils are susceptible to the chemotactic action of S100A7.[21]

S100 Proteins

S100 proteins, a family of low molecular weight (13 kDa) proteins distinguished by the presence of two calcium-binding helix-loop-helix motifs, are another class of AMPs implicated with psoriasis. There are 21 known S100 proteins, including S100A7 (psoriasin), S100A8 (calgranulin A), S100A9 (calgranulin B), S100A12 (calgranulin C), and S100A15 (psoriasin).[22] These proteins have antimicrobial properties and are expressed at higher levels in psoriasis patients' serum and lesional skin.[23]

■ CYTOKINES AND RECEPTORS

Cytokines and their receptors facilitate communication between immune cells and keratinocytes, which is essential to the pathophysiology of psoriasis. Since treatments that target TNF-α, IL-17A, and IL-23 are the most effective in treating people with psoriasis, it is already recognized that these three factors are crucial. Researchers have recently focused more on cytokines produced by or receptors expressed on keratinocytes. One of the main causes of psoriasis is thought to be the cytokine axis between IL-23 and IL-17. The maintenance and growth of immune cells that produce IL-17 depend on the expression of IL-23 by immune cells. The primary downstream cytokine of IL-23 and IL-17A is most closely linked to and well researched in the pathophysiology of psoriasis.[24] IL-17A uses a variety of cell signaling pathways to attach to its receptors on keratinocytes. In order to activate innate immunity, it triggers the production of keratinocyte-derived AMPs (e.g., S100A7, LL37, and DEFB4A); chemokines (e.g., CXCL1, CXCL8, and CCL20) that attract leukocytes, including neutrophils, Th17 cells, mDCs, and macrophages; and several proinflammatory genes (e.g., IL-1β, IL-6, IL-8, and TNF-α). These actions amplify the IL-23/IL-17A axis and create "feed forward" inflammatory circuits. However, through keratinocytes' increased expression of IL-19 and IL-36, IL-17A may indirectly cause epidermal hyperplasia.

What needs further understanding?

It is the involvement of keratinocyte-produced IL-23 in psoriasis, despite the fact that keratinocytes also produce this substance. Li and colleagues recently shown, using a transgenic mouse model, that keratinocyte-derived IL-23 was adequate to trigger the release of IL-17 by immune cells that produce it, resulting in a persistent inflammatory response of the skin. Subsequent research revealed that psoriasis may be exacerbated by epigenetic regulation by H3K9 dimethylation, which regulated IL-23 production in keratinocytes.[25] Although other IL-17s are upregulated in psoriatic lesions, their function is yet unclear. IL-17A, also known as IL-17, IL-17B, IL-17C, IL-17D, IL-17E (IL-25), and IL-17F, which functions via an IL-17 receptor heterodimer, are the six members of the IL-17 family of cytokines. Similar to IL-23, IL-17E (IL-25), which is produced by keratinocytes and immune cells, was shown to be strongly expressed in the epidermal layer of psoriatic patients' lesional skin. Mouse skin developed psoriasis-like pathology after receiving an injection of IL-17E. In psoriasis, IL-17A mechanically increases the expression of epidermal IL-17E. It also activates STAT3 to stimulate keratinocyte proliferation and the generation of inflammatory cytokines and chemokines through its receptor, IL-17RB, on keratinocytes.[26] Another member of the IL-17 family, IL-17C, has been found to be an epithelial cytokine that is mostly generated by keratinocytes in the skin. In some inflammatory skin conditions, including psoriasis and atopic dermatitis (AD), keratinocytes have been shown to have elevated levels of IL-17C.[27] Up until now, biologics have mostly targeted IL-17A blockage; more recently, bimekizumab has been used to block 17A and 17F.

Crosstalk Between Keratinocytes

In both the onset and maintenance stages of psoriasis, keratinocytes are crucial. Keratinocytes, which are a component of the innate immune system, are able to react to many stimuli. Self-nucleotides and AMPs are released by stressed keratinocytes, which encourage pDC activation. Interferon-α (IFN-α), IFN-γ, TNF-α, and IL-1β are then produced by mDCs, activating and maturing them. Keratinocytes not only contribute to the initiation phase but also intensify psoriatic inflammation in the maintenance phase.[28] When keratinocytes are synergistically activated by proinflammatory cytokines, they can produce a large number of chemokines (e.g., CXCL1/2/3, CXCL8, CXCL9/10/11, CCL2, and CCL20) to attract leukocytes (e.g., neutrophils, Th17 cells, dendritic cells, and macrophages), AMPs (e.g., S100A7/8/9/12, hBD2, and LL37) to trigger innate immunity, and other inflammatory mediators to intensify inflammation. Keratinocytes are immune cells as well. Keratinocyte-secreted cytokines, such as IL-17C and IL-36, have an autocrine effect on keratinocytes.[29] Its importance during the early phases of psoriatic inflammation, or the "priming" for plaque development, is suggested by the identification of IL-17C as a functional regulator of the initial psoriatic cytokine network.[30] The primary skin cells that create (and react to) IL-17C, which fuels psoriatic inflammation, are keratinocytes.[31] TNF-α, IL-17A, IL-22, and IL-1β stimulate keratinocytes to generate IL-36 cytokines, including IL-36α/β/γ. Keratinocytes are stimulated by IL-36 to generate TNF-α and IL-17C.[32] According to emerging data, psoriasis involves a crosstalk between keratinocytes, TH17 cells, and dendritic cells.[33]

Importance of Keratinocytes' DDX5-sIL-36R Axis

The defective DDX5-sIL-36R axis in keratinocytes, which contributes to the pathophysiology of both psoriasis and AD, is another current focus on keratinocytes in psoriasis. The phenotypic transition between AD and psoriasis is a frequent side effect of biological therapies. The importance of the DDX5-sIL-36R axis in keratinocytes for the pathophysiology of AD and psoriasis has been revealed by recent studies.[34] By activating the CD93–p38 MAPK–AKT–SMAD2/3 signaling pathway, IL-17D caused DDX5 to be inhibited in keratinocytes. Because of the pre-mRNA splicing events caused by the decrease in DDX5, keratinocytes produced more IL-36 receptor (IL-36R) at the expense of soluble IL-36R (sIL-36R). This led to the selective amplification of IL-36R-mediated inflammatory responses in the skin. Both psoriasis and AD experienced cutaneous inflammation as a result of this augmentation of IL-36R-mediated inflammatory responses. The idea that AD and psoriasis evolve through a similar molecular pathway is supported by recent research. As a result, keratinocytes play a crucial role in regulating the phenotypic shift in people who have a DDX5 keratinocyte deficiency. This has sparked conjecture that if psoriasis is initially developed in people with a DDX5 deficiency in keratinocytes and then treated with IL-17A/IL-17RA neutralizing antibodies, the psoriasis pathogenesis may be alleviated, but the skin phenotype of AD may manifest. People with an AD phenotype may have a similar phenotypic shift after receiving IL-4Rα neutralizing antibodies. Clinical data are needed to further validate this idea.[34]

Keratinocytes in Psoriasis Recurrence

The skin's resident memory T cells [tissue-resident memory T cells (TRM)] are currently thought to have a significant role in psoriasis recurrence. Basal keratinocytes can create a long-lasting memory of inflammation, according to recent studies.[35] Basal keratinocytes can react to a variety of stimuli, including infections and traumas, thanks to their inflammatory memory. Following an inflammatory episode, the persistence of cellular and molecular alterations in basal keratinocytes might influence skin inflammatory responses and lead to the recurrence or modified presentation of inflammatory diseases. Therefore, the ability of basal keratinocytes to develop inflammatory memory in the setting of psoriasis implies that they may play a role in the recurrence of the illness.[36] Furthermore, Wang X et al. found that inflammatory memory-producing keratinocytes generate a lot of IL-15 (unpublished). In other inflammatory circumstances, the activation of CD8+ TRM cells depends on 38IL-15, which is produced by keratinocytes in the hair follicle.[37] To ascertain if basal keratinocytes with inflammatory memory control TRM cell activation by releasing IL-15, therefore encouraging psoriasis recurrence, more research is necessary.

Keratinocytes in Immunometabolism

The entire body's metabolism is impacted by the inflammatory cascade that occurs in psoriasis, and the long-term consequences of inflammation may lead to significant metabolic alterations. Metabolic abnormalities can impact the occurrence, development, efficacy, and prognosis of diseases. The mechanisms through which metabolic dysregulation impacts psoriasis offer significant promise for the development of efficient clinical diagnostics, treatment monitoring, and the further identification of novel metabolic-based therapeutic targets. The fundamental processes of psoriasis remain unclear, despite the fact that metabolomic alterations are well documented. In psoriatic skin, metabolic and nutritional sensing mechanisms can synchronize the activation and differentiation of keratinocytes and immune cells. An important mediator of inflammation and a master indicator of intracellular metabolic state is the phosphoinositide 3-kinase (PI3K)/Akt/mTOR cascade.[38] The encouragement of cell differentiation and proliferation and the extracellular nutritional status triggers are closely related to mechanistic Target of rapamycin (mTOR), the master sensor of nutrients and growth factors. Depending on the metabolic requirements and available "food," this serine/threonine kinase forms the mTORC1 and mTORC2, which control the anabolic and catabolic cellular processes. In summary, when mTORC1 is blocked, cell growth mechanisms such as protein synthesis, lipid and nucleotide synthesis, and glycolysis are downregulated, but survival and maintenance mechanisms such as autophagy and protein degradation [ubiquitin–proteasome system (UPS)] are increased. However, mTORC1 inhibits the growth, migration, and proliferation of cells.[38] mTORC1 is inhibited in the keratinocytes of the epidermis, but it is active in the cells of the basal layer in healthy skin, increasing their differentiation and decreasing their proliferative capacity.[39] Keratinocytes have been demonstrated to proliferate and differentiate when exposed to IL-1β, IL-17A, IL-22, and TNF-α, which activates mTORC1 and its downstream pathways.[40]

CONCLUSION

- T cells and keratinocytes experience metabolic abnormalities
- A key player in cell differentiation and proliferation, the PI3K/Akt/mTOR cascade is a crucial mediator of inflammation.
- mTORC1 inhibits the growth, migration, and proliferation of cells
- When differentiation begins, healthy keratinocytes immediately turn off Akt/mTORC1 signaling. Since Ki-67-positive cells in the basal layer of healthy skin also had mTOR activity, this seems to be related to proliferation regulation.
- Keratinocytes appear to need mTOR inactivation in order to begin terminal differentiation
- In contrast, the mTORC1 cascade is abnormally active in all levels of the epidermis in an inflammatory environment, such as psoriasis.

Gut microbiota: Recent research has shown that changes in the gut and skin microbiota affect immune response and host homeostasis, especially Th17 cell growth. The IL-23R/IL-22 pathway controls the intestinal barrier's function and the number of segmented filamentous bacteria (SFB). When the gut barrier is compromised and bacteria or their components spread throughout the body, the IL-23 pathway is triggered, which starts the barrier's repair process and triggers Th17 reactions to destroy the invasive microorganisms.[41] Therefore, nutritional approaches that modulate gut microbiota may have a role in the future management of psoriasis. Studies investigating the function of the gut microbiota in autoimmune illnesses, and specifically psoriasis, have proliferated in recent years.

TAKE HOME MESSAGE

- Recent research has focussed on keratinocytes.
- CARD 14 gene, a key gene in the activation of NFκB pathway is dysregulated in psoriasis.
- TNFAIP3 and TNIP1, negative regulators in TNF receptor signaling pathway has been implicated in psoriasis.
- Dysregulation of micro RNAs has been proven in various aspects of psoriasis.
- Antimicrobial peptides play an important role in innate immunity and can modulate immune response in psoriasis.
- Defective DDX5-sIL-36R axis in keratinocytes contribute to the pathophysiology of both psoriasis and atopic dermatitis. The phenotypic transition between atopic dermatitis and psoriasis is a frequent side effect of biologic therapies.
- Apart from tissue resident memory T cells, keratinocytes are also involved in the recurrences of psoriasis.
- Recent research has shown that an imbalance in gut microbiome can lead to the induction of IL-23 pathway. Therefore modulation of gut microbiome may have a role in the future management of psoriasis.

REFERENCES

1. Greb JE, Goldminz AM, Elder JT, Lebwohl MG, Gladman DD, Wu JJ, et al. Psoriasis. Nat Rev Dis Primers. 2016;2:16082.
2. Harden JL, Krueger JG, Bowcock AM. The immunogenetics of Psoriasis: A comprehensive review. J Autoimmun. 2015;64:66-73.
3. Tsoi LC, Stuart PE, Tian C, Gudjonsson JE, Das S, Zawistowski M, et al. Large scale meta-analysis characterizes genetic architecture for common psoriasis associated variants. Nat Commun. 2017; 8:15382.
4. Swindell WR, Johnston A, Voorhees JJ, Elder JT, Gudjonsson JE. Dissecting the psoriasis transcriptome: inflammatory- and cytokine-driven gene expression in lesions from 163 patients. BMC Genomics. 2013;14:527.
5. Mahil SK, Capon F, Barker JN. Genetics of psoriasis. Dermatol Clin. 2015;33:1-11.
6. Mellett M, Meier B, Mohanan D, Schairer R, Cheng P, Satoh TK, et al. CARD14 gain-of-function mutation alone is sufficient to drive IL-23/IL-17-mediated psoriasiform skin inflammation in vivo. J Invest Dermatol. 2018;138:2010-23.
7. Afonina IS, Van Nuffel E, Baudelet G, Driege Y, Kreike M, Staal J, et al. The paracaspase MALT1 mediates CARD14-induced signaling in keratinocytes. EMBO Rep. 2016;17:914-27.
8. Devos M, Mogilenko DA, Fleury S, Gilbert B, Becquart C, Quemener S, et al. Keratinocyte expression of A20/TNFAIP3 controls skin inflammation associated with atopic dermatitis and psoriasis. J Invest Dermatol. 2019;139:135-45.
9. Benhadou F, Glitzner E, Brisebarre A, Swedlund B, Song Y, Dubois C, et al. Epidermal autonomous VEGFA/Flt1/Nrp1 functions mediate psoriasis-like disease. Sci Adv. 2020;6:eaax5849.
10. Lambert S, Swindell WR, Tsoi LC, Stoll SW, Elder JT. Dual role of Act1 in keratinocyte differentiation and host defense: TRAF3IP2 silencing alters keratinocyte differentiation and inhibits IL-17 responses. J Invest Dermatol. 2017;137:1501-11.
11. Zhou X, Chen Y, Cui L, Shi Y, Guo C. Advances in the pathogenesis of psoriasis: from keratinocyte perspective. Cell Death Dis. 2022;13(1):81.
12. Bartel DP. MicroRNAs: target recognition and regulatory functions. Cell 2009;136:215-33.
13. Srivastava A, Nikamo P, Lohcharoenkal W, Li D, Meisgen F, Xu Landén N, et al. MicroRNA-146a suppresses IL-17-mediated skin inflammation and is genetically associated with psoriasis. J Allergy Clin Immunol. 2017;139(2):550-61.
14. Guo J, Zhang H, Lin W, Lu L, Su J, Chen X. Signaling pathways and targeted therapies for psoriasis. Signal Transduct Target Ther. 2023;8(1):437. Erratum in: Signal Transduct Target Ther. 2024; 9(1):25.
15. Hawkes JE, Nguyen GH, Fujita M, Florell SR, Callis Duffin K, Krueger GG, et al. microRNAs in Psoriasis. J Invest Dermatol. 2016;136(2):365-71.
16. Jiang X, Shi R, Ma R, Tang X, Gong Y, Yu Z, et al. The role of microRNA in psoriasis: A review. Exp Dermatol. 2023;32(10):1598-612.
17. Timis TL, Orasan RI. Understanding psoriasis: Role of miRNAs. Biomed Rep. 2018;9(5):367-74.
18. Lai Y, Gallo RL. AMPed up immunity: how antimicrobial peptides have multiple roles in immune defense. Trends Immunol. 2009;30(3):131-41.
19. Wimley WC. Describing the mechanism of antimicrobial peptide action with the interfacial activity model. ACS Chem Biol. 2010;5(10):905-17.
20. Mukherjee S, Vaishnava S, Hooper LV. Multi-layered regulation of intestinal antimicrobial defense. Cell Mol Life Sci. 2008;65(19):3019-27.
21. Takahashi T, Yamasaki K. Psoriasis and Antimicrobial Peptides. Int J Mol Sci. 2020;21(18):6791.
22. Eckert RL, Broome AM, Ruse M, Robinson N, Ryan D, Lee K. S100 proteins in the epidermis. J Invest Dermatol. 2004;123(1):23-33.
23. Büchau AS, Gallo RL. Innate immunity and antimicrobial defense systems in psoriasis. Clin Dermatol. 2007;25(6):616-24.
24. Sieminska I, Pieniawska M, Grzywa TM. The Immunology of Psoriasis-Current Concepts in Pathogenesis. Clin Rev Allergy Immunol. 2024; 66(2):164-91.
25. Li H, Yao Q, Mariscal AG, Wu X, Hülse J, Pedersen E, et al. Epigenetic control of IL-23 expression in keratinocytes is important for chronic skin inflammation. Nat Commun. 2018;9(1):1420.
26. Xu M, Lu H, Lee YH, Wu Y, Liu K, Shi Y, et al. An interleukin-25-mediated autoregulatory circuit in keratinocytes plays a pivotal role in psoriatic skin inflammation. Immunity. 2018;48:787-98.e4.
27. Lauffer F, Jargosch M, Baghin V, Krause L, Kempf W, Absmaier-Kijak M, et al. IL-17C amplifies epithelial inflammation in human psoriasis and atopic eczema. J Eur Acad Dermatol Venereol. 2020;34:800-9.
28. Lowes MA, Russell CB, Martin DA, Towne JE, Krueger JG. The IL-23/T17 pathogenic axis in psoriasis is amplified by keratinocyte responses. Trends Immunol. 2013;34:174-81.
29. Sachen KL, Arnold Greving CN, Towne JE. Role of IL-36 cytokines in psoriasis and other inflammatory skin conditions. Cytokine. 2022;156:155897.
30. Boonpethkaew S, Meephansan J, Jumlongpim O, Tangtanatakul P, Soonthornchai W, Wongpiyabovorn J, et al. Transcriptomic profiling

of peripheral edge of lesions to elucidate the pathogenesis of psoriasis vulgaris. Int J Mol Sci. 2022;23(9):4983.
31. Vandeghinste N, Klattig J, Jagerschmidt C, Lavazais S, Marsais F, Haas JD, et al. Neutralization of IL-17C reduces skin inflammation in mouse models of psoriasis and atopic dermatitis. J Invest Dermatol. 2018;138:1555-63.
32. Miura S, Garcet S, Li X, Cueto I, Salud-Gnilo C, Kunjravia N, et al. Cathelicidin antimicrobial peptide LL37 induces toll-like receptor 8 and amplifies IL-36γ and IL-17C in human keratinocytes. J Invest Dermatol. 2023;143:832-41.e4.
33. Kamata M, Tada Y. Crosstalk: keratinocytes and immune cells in psoriasis. Front Immunol. 2023;14:1286344.
34. Ni X, Xu Y, Wang W, Kong B, Ouyang J, Chen J, et al. IL-17D-induced inhibition of DDX5 expression in keratinocytes amplifies IL-36R-mediated skin inflammation. Nat Immunol. 2022;23(11):1577-87.
35. Seok J, Cho SD, Lee J, Choi Y, Kim SY, Lee SM, et al. A virtual memory CD8+ T cell-originated subset causes alopecia areata through innate-like cytotoxicity. Nat Immunol. 2023;24(8):1308-17.
36. Wang X, Lai Y. Keratinocytes in the pathogenesis, phenotypic switch, and relapse of psoriasis. Eur J Immunol. 2024;54(5):e2250279.
37. Larsen SB, Cowley CJ, Sajjath SM, Barrows D, Yang Y, Carroll TS, et al. Establishment, maintenance, and recall of inflammatory memory. Cell Stem Cell. 2021;28(10):1758-74.e8.
38. Sarandi E, Krueger-Krasagakis S, Tsoukalas D, Sidiropoulou P, Evangelou G, Sifaki M, et al. Psoriasis immunometabolism: progress on metabolic biomarkers and targeted therapy. Front Mol Biosci. 2023;10:1201912.
39. Buerger C. Epidermal mTORC1 Signaling Contributes to the Pathogenesis of Psoriasis and Could Serve as a Therapeutic Target. Front Immunol. 2018;9:2786.
40. Buerger C, Shirsath N, Lang V, Berard A, Diehl S, Kaufmann R, et al. Inflammation dependent mTORC1 signaling interferes with the switch from keratinocyte proliferation to differentiation. PLoS One. 2017;12(7):e0180853.
41. Martin AM, Sun EW, Rogers GB, Keating DJ. The Influence of the Gut Microbiome on Host Metabolism Through the Regulation of Gut Hormone Release. Front Physiol. 2019;10:428.

23. Personalized Medicine in Psoriasis

Shraddha Madanagobalane

■ INTRODUCTION

The concept of personalized or precision medicine emphasizes the customization of medical treatment to the individual patient's characteristics. These terms are often used interchangeably, though there is a subtle difference in their focus. Personalized medicine centers around tailoring treatment to the individual, while precision medicine generally involves grouping patients based on shared characteristics (such as genetic makeup or specific biomarkers) to identify the most effective treatment strategies for those groups. In psoriasis treatment, this approach is particularly relevant as it could enable more effective and individualized care.

As of now, psoriasis treatment is primarily based on clinical factors rather than genetic markers. These clinical factors include:
- Age
- Sex
- Comorbidities
- Disease severity (measured through scales such as DLQI—Dermatology Life Quality Index)
- Psoriasis type (plaque, guttate, inverse, etc.)
- Site and extent of involvement (e.g., scalp, nails, and body surface area affected)
- Symptoms (such as itching, pain, or scaling)

However, with advancements in the understanding of psoriasis' underlying mechanisms—particularly the genetic, epigenetic, and inflammatory pathways—the potential for more targeted therapies has expanded significantly. The goal is not just to clear the skin, but to achieve long-term remission, minimize side effects, and ultimately improve quality of life.

■ RESPONSE VARIABILITY IN PSORIASIS TREATMENT

A key point is the variability in treatment response among psoriasis patients. Some individuals are super responders, experiencing near-complete clearance of symptoms with targeted therapies, while others may be super nonresponders, showing little to no improvement despite similar treatments.[1,2] This variability may be due to a combination of genomic, epigenetic, and exposomic factors:
- *Genomic factors*: Specific gene variants may influence the way a patient responds to certain drugs, especially biologics targeting immune pathways such as tumor necrosis factor-α (TNF-α), interleukin-17 (IL-17), or IL-23.
- *Epigenetic factors*: Changes in gene expression caused by environmental exposures (such as UV light, stress, diet,

etc.) may also contribute to psoriasis pathogenesis and treatment outcomes.
- *Exposomic factors*: These are the environmental, behavioral, and lifestyle factors that influence disease progression, including smoking, alcohol consumption, diet, and other external triggers.

ROLE OF BIOMARKERS

The identification of *biomarkers*—whether *genetic, inflammatory, or epigenetic*—is essential for *patient stratification*. These biomarkers can help predict which treatment is likely to work best for a patient, guiding decisions on whether they would benefit from biologics, small molecules, phototherapy, or topical treatments. Biomarkers can also assist in:
- *Predicting treatment response*: For instance, certain genetic or inflammatory biomarkers might indicate that a patient will respond well to an IL-23 inhibitor but not to an IL-17 inhibitor.
- *Minimizing side effects*: By identifying those at risk for adverse reactions, healthcare providers can select therapies with the least potential for harm.
- *Ensuring long-term remission*: By monitoring how a patient's biomarkers change over time, clinicians can adjust treatment plans to sustain disease control.
- *Cost-effectiveness*: Choosing the right treatment for the right patient not only improves outcomes but can also save costs by avoiding ineffective treatments.

CURRENT RESEARCH AND FUTURE DIRECTIONS

Ongoing research in *genetic, epigenetic, and immune system* biomarkers is steadily providing new insights. For example, genetic studies have identified specific *single nucleotide polymorphisms (SNPs)* linked to psoriasis, which may help to identify individuals at higher risk for severe disease or poor treatment response. Additionally, *gene expression profiles* in skin biopsies are being explored to help to stratify patients based on disease subtype.

In the future, we may see more *precision-based approaches* in psoriasis treatment that incorporate *genomic testing, serum biomarkers, and patient lifestyle assessments*. As this research progresses, it will likely lead to more *personalized treatment plans* that not only target the disease more effectively but also take into account the patient's unique genetic and environmental factors.

By combining clinical judgment with advanced genetic and biomarker testing, the future of psoriasis treatment will be more personalized, cost-effective, and potentially more successful at providing *long-term remission* while improving *quality of life* for patients.

Genetic Biomarkers

The exploration of *genetic biomarkers* in psoriasis treatment continues to evolve, especially as more targeted biologic therapies such as *anti-TNF, anti-IL-12/23, anti-IL-17, and anti-IL-23* are increasingly used to manage the disease. Understanding the genetic underpinnings of how patients respond to these treatments can potentially guide more personalized and effective care. Below are the key findings for each class of biologics.

Biomarkers Predictive of Response to TNF-α Inhibitors

Tumor necrosis factor-α inhibitors (such as *etanercept, infliximab, and adalimumab*) are among the first biologic therapies used in psoriasis. Genetic biomarkers predictive of response to TNF-α inhibitors include:
- *HLA-C*06:02*: Some studies have shown a *favorable association* between the

HLA-C*06:02 allele and a better response to *anti-TNF therapies*. However, recent studies have *questioned this association*, indicating that it may not be a robust predictive marker across all patient populations.[3]

- *Single nucleotide polymorphisms in the TNF gene*: SNPs in the *TNF gene*, such as *rs1800629, rs1799964, rs1799724, and rs361520*, have shown *varied results* in predicting response to anti-TNF therapy. These SNPs can potentially help to tailor therapy, but more research is needed to establish clear, consistent predictive value.
- *TNF receptor superfamily member 1B (TNFRSF1B)*:
  - *TNFRSF1B rs1061622-TT* has been associated with a *better response* to all *anti-TNF* therapies, and particularly etanercept.
  - The *rs1061622-G polymorphism* has been associated with *poorer outcomes* in patients receiving anti-TNF treatments.
  - These findings suggest that genetic variations in the TNF receptor pathway may affect both the *efficacy* and *tolerability* of TNF-α inhibitors.[3]

Biomarkers Predictive of Response to IL-12/IL-23 Inhibitors

Ustekinumab (an anti-IL-12/IL-23 monoclonal antibody) is an important drug in the treatment of psoriasis, and research into genetic biomarkers predictive of its response has yielded several insights:

- *HLA-C*06:02*: The *HLA-C*06:02 allele* has been shown to be *positively associated with a better clinical and faster response to ustekinumab*. However, a *recent meta-analysis* raised questions about the significance of this allele alone in predicting treatment response. It is now suggested that a *panel of biomarkers*, rather than a single allele, would be more reliable in predicting outcomes.[4]
- *Polymorphisms in IL-17, IL-12, and IL-23R genes*: Studies on *polymorphisms* in the *IL-17, IL-12, and IL-23R genes* have not shown *statistically significant* results in predicting response to *IL-12/IL-23 inhibitors* such as ustekinumab. This suggests that while these pathways are central to psoriasis pathogenesis, specific gene variations within these loci may not be strong enough predictors for treatment response.[5]

Biomarkers Predictive of Response to Anti-IL-17 Inhibitors

Secukinumab and *ixekizumab*, which target *IL-17*, are often used for patients who do not respond to other biologics. The genetic markers associated with response to *anti-IL-17 therapies* are less well-established:

- *HLA-C*06:02*: There have been studies on the *HLA-C*06:02 allele*, but they have shown *no statistically significant differences* in the efficacy of *secukinumab* in patients who carry this polymorphism versus those who do not. This suggests that *HLA-C*06:02* may not be a strong predictor for response to *anti-IL-17 therapies*.[6]
- *Polymorphisms in IL-17*: Research on *polymorphisms in the IL-17 gene* has also shown *no significant results* in predicting response to *anti-IL-17 therapies*, further complicating the use of genetic markers to guide therapy for IL-17 inhibitors.[7]

Biomarkers Predictive of Response to Anti-IL-23 Inhibitors

For anti-IL-23 therapies (e.g., *guselkumab, tildrakizumab, and risankizumab*), there is *currently no data* from *pharmacogenetic studies* that suggest specific biomarkers predictive of response. This may be due to the relatively newer introduction of these therapies, and the need for further research to identify relevant genetic markers in the IL-23 pathway.

Inflammatory Biomarkers

Inflammatory biomarkers are crucial in understanding the pathophysiology of psoriasis and guiding its management.[8] The summary of key inflammatory molecules and their relevance to the disease are:

- *Adiponectin*:
  - Levels are lower in patients with psoriasis
  - This adipokine has anti-inflammatory properties, and its reduction may contribute to systemic inflammation observed in psoriasis.
- *Th1 cytokines*:
  - Elevated levels of IL-2, IL-12, and IFN-γ are noted in psoriasis.
  - These cytokines are associated with the activation and maintenance of the inflammatory response.
- *Macrophagic M1 cytokines*:
  - IL-1, IL-6, and TNF-α are elevated in psoriasis.
  - These proinflammatory molecules play a pivotal role in the development and progression of psoriatic lesions.
- *Th17 cytokines*:
  - Elevated IL-6 and IL-17 are characteristics of psoriasis.
  - These cytokines drive the pathogenic inflammation in psoriatic plaques
- *Transforming growth factor-β (TGF-β)*: Its role is controversial in psoriasis. While it has both proinflammatory and anti-inflammatory effects depending on the context, its precise function in psoriasis remains debated.[9]
- *Th2/Treg cytokines*:
  - IL-4 and TGF-β levels are decreased in psoriasis.[10]
  - The reduction in these cytokines suggests an imbalance favoring pro-inflammatory responses
- *YKL-40*:
  - This mammalian chitinase-3-like protein is associated with inflammatory diseases.
  - It correlates with higher Psoriasis Area and Severity Index (PASI) scores, indicating its potential as a marker of disease severity.[11]
- *Profilin-1 (PFN1)*:
  - Identified as a disease biomarker for psoriasis
  - PFN1, a protein involved in cytoskeletal structure, may play a role in the inflammatory or structural changes associated with psoriasis.[12]

Epigenetic Biomarkers in Psoriasis

Epigenetic regulation plays a significant role in psoriasis pathogenesis, with *microRNAs (miRNAs)* and *long noncoding RNAs (lncRNAs)* emerging as critical components.[13,14] These molecules influence gene expression without altering the DNA sequence, making them valuable for diagnostics, prognostics, and therapeutic interventions.

MicroRNAs

- MicroRNAs are small noncoding RNA molecules (~22 nucleotides) involved in RNA silencing and posttranscriptional regulation of gene expression.[13]
- *Role in psoriasis*:
  - miRNAs show promise as biomarkers for diagnosis, prognosis, and treatment response
  - Dysregulated miRNA expression can contribute to immune dysregulation and keratinocyte hyperproliferation in psoriasis.

- *Notable miRNAs in psoriasis*:
  - *miR-155*:
    - Overexpressed in psoriatic patients
    - Linked to proinflammatory pathways
  - *miR-210*:
    - Positively correlated with serum IL-17/IL-17A levels[15]
    - Therapeutic potential: In a mouse model, miR-210 ablation mitigated immune imbalances and blocked psoriasis-like inflammation induced by imiquimod or IL-23.[16]
  - *Differential expression*: A study identified 246 differentially expressed miRNAs in psoriasis (80 downregulated and 146 upregulated) when comparing psoriatic patients to healthy controls.[17]

Long Noncoding RNAs

- Long noncoding RNAs are nonprotein-coding RNA molecules (≥200 nucleotides) that are the most numerous group of noncoding RNAs.[14]
- *Role in psoriasis*: lncRNAs regulate gene expression via chromatin remodeling, transcriptional control, and post-transcriptional mechanisms.
- *Notable lncRNAs in psoriasis*:
  - PRINS (*psoriasis-susceptibility-related RNA gene induced by stress*):
    - Reduced levels in psoriatic patients
    - Study findings:
      - Correlated with upregulated miRNAs (miR-124-3p, miR-203a-5p, miR-129-5p, miR-146a-5p, and miR-9-5p) in psoriasis compared to healthy controls.[18]
      - An inverse relationship between PRINS and miRNA expression suggests the potential of the PRINS-miRNA-mRNA axis as a *personalized medicine target*.[18]
  - lncRNA-MSX2P1:
    - Promotes IL-22-stimulated keratinocyte growth by inhibiting miR-6731-5p and activating S100A7.[19]
    - The positive correlation between MSX2P1 and S100A7 highlights the *MSX2P1-miR-6731-5p-S100A7 complex* as a potential *innovative therapeutic target*.

IMPLICATIONS FOR PSORIASIS MANAGEMENT

- The discovery of epigenetic biomarkers such as miRNAs and lncRNAs opens avenues for:
  - *Noninvasive diagnostics*: Blood or tissue-based assays for miRNA/lncRNA profiles.
  - *Therapeutic interventions*: Targeting specific miRNAs or lncRNA pathways to restore immune balance.
  - *Personalized medicine*: Leveraging PRINS-miRNA-mRNA or MSX2P1-mediated pathways for tailored treatments.

Further studies are needed to validate these findings and fully elucidate the mechanisms by which miRNAs and lncRNAs regulate psoriasis pathogenesis.[14]

COMMERCIAL DIAGNOSTICS AND EMERGING PRECISION MEDICINE TECHNOLOGIES IN PSORIASIS

Advancements in precision medicine have driven the development of innovative diagnostic tools and technologies for psoriasis, aimed at improving treatment outcomes and reducing the trial-and-error approach in therapy selection. Two notable companies leading this charge are Mindera Health and Castle Biosciences, Inc.

Mindera Health

Mindera Health focuses on precision medicine for inflammatory skin diseases, including psoriasis. Their proprietary technologies—*SkinAtlas* and *Mind.Px*™—utilize cutting-edge tools such as artificial intelligence (AI) and next-generation sequencing (NGS) for comprehensive analytics and personalized treatment approaches.[20]

SkinAtlas

- A database integrating patient images, health data, and skin samples
- Utilizes AI and machine learning for analytics on therapy response, helping refine clinical decision making[20]

Mind.Px™ Dermal Diagnostic Patch

- A patented dermal patch with microneedles that collects RNA from the skin[21]
- *Analysis*:
  - Employs NGS and machine learning to identify biomarkers predictive of therapeutic response to biologics targeting *TNF-α, IL-17,* or *IL-23*.[1,20]
  - Patients are categorized as *responders* or *nonresponders,* guiding treatment selection to minimize trial-and-error.[1,2]

Clinical Studies

- *STAMP (STAMP-1 and STAMP-2)*:
  - *Focus*: Validation of baseline dermal biomarkers as response classifiers for achieving *PASI75* at week 12.
  - *Findings*:
    - Classifiers derived for IL-23 inhibitors, IL-17 inhibitors, and TNF-α inhibitors showed *positive predictive values* of 93.1, 92.3, and 85.7%, respectively.
    - Across the cohort, *99.5% of patients* were predicted to respond to at least one drug class.
  - *Significance*: Demonstrated the power of dermal biomarkers combined with machine learning in predicting biologic response before drug exposure.[1]
- *MATCH study*:
  - *Focus*: Validated a physician questionnaire alongside biomarker-guided therapy.
  - *Findings*:
    - In the informed group (where physicians received Mind.Px™ results), *84.4%* of therapeutic decisions aligned with Mind.Px™ predictions, compared to *53.8%* in the uninformed group.
    - Informed patients achieved *PASI75* sooner than uninformed patients ($p = 0.004$).
    - Barriers to using Mind.Px™ outcomes included payer formulary constraints.[2]
  - *Clinical significance*: Highlights the importance of integrating biomarker data into clinical decision making to enhance treatment outcomes.

Significance of Mindera Health's Technologies

- *Personalized medicine*: Mind.Px™ facilitates the selection of the most effective biologic therapy for individual patients, avoiding unnecessary exposure to ineffective treatments.
- *Reduced trial-and-error*: Predictive algorithms streamline treatment decisions, reducing time, and costs associated with therapeutic mismatches.
- *Data-driven decision making*: AI and machine learning models provide objective and evidence-based support for clinicians.

TABLE 1: Comparison between Mindera Health versus Castle Biosciences		
Aspect	**Mindera Health**	**Castle Biosciences**
Core technology	Mind.Px™ dermal patch with RNA sampling via microneedles	Skin scraping technology for RNA collection
Focus	Predictive response to biologic therapies (anti-TNF-α, IL-17, and IL-23)	Identifying diagnostic and treatment-response gene expression profiles
Analytical approach	RNA sequencing + machine learning for therapeutic predictions	RT-PCR-based analysis of lesional versus nonlesional gene expression
Current utility	Biomarker-driven categorization of responders and nonresponders	Gene expression profiling to guide therapy selection
Clinical studies	STAMP, MATCH (evaluating predictive power of Mind.Px™)	Multisite longitudinal study for inflammatory dermatoses

(anti-TNF-α: anti-tumor necrosis factor-α; IL-17: interleukin-17; RT-PCR: real-time polymerase chain reaction)

Castle Biosciences

Castle Biosciences is a diagnostic company aiming to leverage insights from a patient's unique biology to guide clinical decision making and optimize health outcomes. Their work focuses on developing technologies to improve therapy selection for inflammatory dermatoses, including psoriasis.

Clinical Study and Approach

- *Objective*: Evaluate the utility of *skin scrapings* in inflammatory dermatoses, particularly psoriasis, to develop gene expression profiles for guiding systemic therapy selection.
- *Methodology*:
  - Multisite longitudinal clinical study
  - Gene expression analysis conducted using *real-time polymerase chain reaction (RT-PCR)* on RNA extracted from lesional skin samples.
- *Findings*:
  - Analysis of *28 genes* showed *seven genes* were increased, and *one gene* was decreased in lesional skin compared to nonlesional skin in psoriasis.
  - These differential expression patterns may form the basis for diagnostic and therapeutic biomarkers.[22]

A comparison of the two available commercial diagnostics is given in **Table 1**.[23]

Significance of Castle Biosciences' Work

- *Noninvasive diagnostics*: Skin scraping is a minimally invasive technique, making it patient-friendly.
- *Gene expression profiling*: Identifying gene sets associated with psoriatic lesions offers insights into disease mechanisms and treatment responses.
- *Precision medicine*: Focused on creating multialgorithmic profiles to tailor systemic therapy to individual patient biology.[23]

■ CONCLUSION

While both Mindera Health and Castle Biosciences aim to revolutionize psoriasis management through precision medicine, their approaches diverge in methodology. Mindera Health's *Mind.Px™* dermal patch focuses on predictive treatment response using advanced machine learning, while Castle Biosciences leverages *skin scraping* to identify diagnostic and therapeutic gene profiles. Together, these innovations hold promise for a future where psoriasis treatment is personalized and highly effective.

TAKE HOME MESSAGE

Genetic biomarkers and biologic therapy response
- TNF-alpha inhibitors (Etanercept, Infliximab, Adalimumab):
  - HLA-C*06:02 and TNFRSF1B polymorphisms may influence treatment response.
- IL-12/23 inhibitors (ustekinumab):
  - HLA-C*06:02 may be linked to a faster and better response, but not a definitive predictor.
- IL-17 inhibitors (secukinumab, ixekizumab):
  - No strong genetic markers identified for predicting response.
- IL-23 inhibitors (guselkumab, tildrakizumab, risankizumab):
  - Limited genetic data available; more research needed.

Inflammatory biomarkers in psoriasis
- Key molecules include:
  - Th1 cytokines (IL-2, IL-12, IFN-γ) → Maintain inflammation.
  - Th17 cytokines (IL-6, IL-17) → Drive psoriatic plaque formation.
  - Macrophagic M1 cytokines (IL-1, IL-6, TNF-α) → Contribute to psoriatic lesions.
  - YKL-40 → Associated with disease severity.
  - Adiponectin → Lower levels linked to systemic inflammation.

Epigenetic biomarkers
- MicroRNAs (miRNAs) regulate immune responses:
  - miR-155 → Overexpressed in psoriasis, linked to inflammation.
  - miR-210 → Correlates with IL-17 levels, potential therapeutic target.
- Long Non-coding RNAs (lncRNAs) regulate gene expression:
  - PRINS → Reduced in psoriasis, interacts with miRNAs.
  - lncRNA-MSX2P1 → Linked to keratinocyte proliferation.

Commercial precision medicine technologies like Mindera Health and castle biosciences are already in use.

REFERENCES

1. Bagel J, Wang Y, Montgomery P, Abaya C, Andrade E, Boyce C, et al. A machine learning-based test for predicting response to psoriasis biologics. SKIN J Cutan Med. 2021;5(6):621-8.
2. Strober B, Bukhalo M, Armstrong A, Pariser D, Kircik L, Parhami S, et al. Interim clinical utility findings of a transcriptomic psoriasis biologic test demonstrate altered physician prescribing behaviour and improved patient outcomes. SKIN J Cutan Med. 2022;6(6):458-62.
3. Membrive Jiménez C, Pérez Ramírez C, Sánchez Martín A, Vieira Maroun S, Arias Santiago SA, Ramírez Tortosa MDC, et al. Influence of genetic polymorphisms on response to biologics in moderate-to-severe Psoriasis. J Pers Med. 2021; 11:293.
4. van Vugt LJ, van den Reek JMPA, Hannink G, Coenen MJH, de Jong EMGJ. Association of HLA-C*06:02 status with differential response to ustekinumab in patients with Psoriasis: a systematic review and meta-analysis. JAMA Dermatol. 2019;155:708-15.
5. Ovejero-Benito MC, Muñoz-Aceituno E, Reolid A, Saiz-Rodríguez M, Abad-Santos F, Daudén E. Pharmacogenetics and pharmacogenomics in moderate-to-severe Psoriasis. Am J Clin Dermatol. 2018;19:209-22.
6. Costanzo A, Bianchi L, Flori ML, Malara G, Stingeni L, Bartezaghi M, et al. Secukinumab shows high efficacy irrespective of HLA-Cw6 status in patients with moderate-to-severe plaque-type psoriasis: SUPREME study. Br J Dermatol. 2018;179:1072-80.
7. Muñoz-Aceituno E, Martos-Cabrera L, Ovejero-Benito MC, Reolid A, Abad-Santos F, Daudén E. Pharmacogenetics update on biologic therapy in Psoriasis. Medicina (Kaunas). 2020;56(12):719.
8. Camela E, Potestio L, Fabbrocini G, Ruggiero A, Megna M. New frontiers in personalized medicine in psoriasis. Expert Opin Biol Ther. 2022;22(12):1431-3.
9. Cataldi C, Mari NL, Lozovoy MAB, Martins LMM, Reiche EMV, Maes M, et al. Proinflammatory and anti-inflammatory cytokine profiles in psoriasis: use as laboratory biomarkers and disease predictors. Inflamm Res. 2019;68:557-67.

10. Divyapriya D, Priyadarssini M, Indhumathi S, Rajappa M, Chandrashekar L, Mohanraj PS. Evaluation of cytokine gene expression in psoriasis. Postepy Dermatol Alergol. 2021;38(5):858-65.
11. Khashaba SA, Attwa E, Said N, Ahmed S, Khattab F. Serum YKL-40 and IL 17 in Psoriasis: reliability as prognostic markers for disease severity and responsiveness to treatment. Dermatol Ther. 2021;34:e14606.
12. Xu M, Deng J, Xu K, Zhu T, Han L, Yan Y, et al. In-depth serum proteomics reveals biomarkers of psoriasis severity and response to traditional Chinese medicine. Theranostics. 2019;9(9):2475-88.
13. Timis TL, Orasan RI. Understanding psoriasis: role of miRNAs. Biomed Rep. 2018;9(5):367-74.
14. Aydin B, Arga KY, Karadag AS. Omics-driven biomarkers of psoriasis: recent insights, current challenges, and future prospects. Clin Cosmet Investig Dermatol. 2020;13:611-25.
15. El-Komy M, Amin I, El-Hawary MS, Saadi D, Shaker O. Upregulation of the miRNA-155, miRNA-210, and miRNA-20b in psoriasis patients and their relation to IL-17. Int J Immunopathol Pharmacol. 2020;34:2058738420933742.
16. Wu R, Zeng J, Yuan J, Deng X, Huang Y, Chen L, et al. MicroRNA-210 overexpression promotes psoriasis-like inflammation by inducing Th1 and Th17 cell differentiation. J Clin Invest. 2018;128(6):2551-68.
17. Chen XM, Yao DN, Wang MJ, Wu XD, Deng JW, Deng H, et al. Deep Sequencing of serum exosomal microRNA level in psoriasis vulgaris patients. Front Med. 2022;9:895564.
18. Abdallah HY, Tawfik NZ, Soliman NH, Eldeen LAT. The lncRNA PRINS-miRNA-mRNA axis gene expression profile as a circulating biomarker panel in psoriasis. Mol Diagn Ther. 2022;26(4):451-65.
19. Qiao M, Li R, Zhao X, Yan J, Sun Q. Up-regulated lncRNA-MSX2P1 promotes the growth of IL-22-stimulated keratinocytes by inhibiting miR-6731-5p and activating S100A7. Exp Cell Res. 2018; 363(2):243-54.
20. Mindera Health. (2020). Mindera Health SkinAtlas™: The Dataset for Dermal Intelligence™. [online] Available from https://minderahealth.com/platform [Last accessed January, 2025].
21. Dickerson T, Taft B, Lee BI. MiNDERA Corporation. Microneedle Devices and Methods, And Skin Condition Assays. US 2023/0383352;2023.
22. Quick AP, Farberg AS, Goldberg MS, Wilkinson J, Silverberg JI. Feasibility of a novel, non-invasive sample collection technique to develop a molecular test guiding therapeutic selection for patients with atopic dermatitis and psoriasis. Poster presented at: Revolutionizing Atopic Dermatitis. virtual; 2022.
23. Haran K, Kranyak A, Johnson CE, Smith P, Farberg AS, Bhutani T, et al. Commercial Diagnostics and Emerging Precision Medicine Technologies in Psoriasis and Atopic Dermatitis. Psoriasis (Auckl). 2024;14:87-92.

24

Advances in Psoriasis Research: Genomics, Proteomics, and Bioinformatics

Shraddha Madanagobalane, Madhumitha Venugopal

GENOMICS

■ INTRODUCTION

The genomics of psoriasis has undergone significant advancements over the years, shedding light on the complex interplay of genetic factors underlying its pathogenesis. Advanced genomics in psoriasis has significantly enhanced our understanding of the disease's complex genetic architecture, providing insights into its pathogenesis, heterogeneity, and potential therapeutic targets.

■ EARLY DISCOVERIES AND FAMILIAL AGGREGATION

Early observations of familial aggregation provided initial evidence for the genetic basis of psoriasis. Studies in the mid-20th century identified a higher prevalence of psoriasis among relatives of affected individuals, suggesting a hereditary component to the disease. These findings spurred further investigations into specific genetic markers and susceptibility loci associated with psoriasis.

■ GENOME-WIDE ASSOCIATION STUDIES

The advent of genome-wide association studies (GWAS) in the 2000s revolutionized the field of psoriasis genetics. GWAS are hypothesis-free approaches that scan the entire genome for genetic variations [single nucleotide polymorphisms (SNPs)] associated with a particular disease.[1] In psoriasis, GWAS identified numerous susceptibility loci across different populations, highlighting the polygenic nature of the disease.

Key Findings from Genome-wide Association Studies

- *Human leukocyte antigen-C (HLA-C) and major histocompatibility complex (MHC) region*: The most significant genetic association in psoriasis is with the MHC region on chromosome 6p21. The HLA-Cw6 allele has consistently shown the strongest association with psoriasis susceptibility. Other HLA alleles (e.g., HLA-B27 and HLA-B57) and non-HLA genes within the MHC region (e.g., TNFAIP3 and LCE3C_LCE3B-del) have also been implicated.
- *Non-MHC loci*: Beyond the MHC region, GWAS have identified additional susceptibility loci involved in immune regulation, skin barrier function, and inflammatory responses. Examples include genes encoding interleukins (IL-23R, IL-12B, and IL-13), TNF receptor-associated factor (TRAF3IP2), and proteins involved in nuclear factor κB (NF-κB) signaling pathways.

- *Genetic heterogeneity*: GWAS have revealed genetic heterogeneity in psoriasis, with differences in susceptibility loci observed between populations of different ancestry. This underscores the importance of conducting diverse population studies to capture the full spectrum of genetic variants associated with psoriasis.

NEXT-GENERATION SEQUENCING TECHNOLOGIES

Next-generation sequencing (NSG) has revolutionized genomic research in psoriasis by enabling comprehensive profiling of the entire genome, transcriptome, and epigenome.[1] Key applications include:
- *Whole-genome sequencing (WGS)*: WGS allows for the identification of rare variants, structural variations, and novel genetic loci associated with psoriasis susceptibility. It provides a comprehensive view of genetic variations across the genome, offering insights into both coding and noncoding regions that may influence disease risk.
- *Whole-exome sequencing (WES)*: WES focuses on sequencing the protein-coding regions (exons) of the genome, identifying rare variants and mutations within genes implicated in immune dysregulation, skin barrier function, and inflammatory responses in psoriasis.

TRANSCRIPTOMICS AND GENE EXPRESSION PROFILING

Transcriptomic studies using RNA sequencing (RNA-seq) have uncovered dysregulated gene expression patterns in psoriatic skin lesions compared to normal skin. These studies have elucidated key molecular pathways involved in psoriasis pathogenesis, such as:
- *IL-23/Th17 pathway*: Increased expression of genes encoding interleukin-23 (IL-23), IL-17A, and IL-17F cytokines, highlighting the pivotal role of Th17 cell-mediated immune responses in driving chronic inflammation and keratinocyte proliferation in psoriasis.
- *NF-κB signaling*: Activation of NF-κB signaling pathway genes, which regulate inflammatory responses and contribute to the perpetuation of psoriatic lesions.

EPIGENOMICS AND REGULATORY ELEMENTS

Epigenetic modifications, such as DNA methylation and histone modifications, play critical roles in gene regulation and disease pathogenesis.[1] Advanced genomic techniques in psoriasis have revealed:
- *Epigenetic alterations*: Differential DNA methylation patterns in psoriatic versus healthy skin, influencing gene expression and contributing to disease heterogeneity and severity.
- *Enhancer landscapes*: Mapping of enhancer elements and chromatin accessibility profiles in psoriatic skin, identifying regulatory regions that control gene expression in response to environmental stimuli and immune activation.

INTEGRATIVE MULTIOMICS APPROACHES

Integrating genomic, transcriptomic, epigenomic, and proteomic data using advanced bioinformatics tools allows for a comprehensive understanding of psoriasis pathophysiology:
- *Network analysis*: Constructing gene regulatory networks and protein interaction networks to identify key molecular hubs and pathways driving psoriasis pathogenesis.
- *Machine learning and predictive modeling*: Utilizing machine learning algorithms to predict disease outcomes, treatment responses, and identify biomarkers for

personalized medicine approaches in psoriasis management.

THERAPEUTIC IMPLICATIONS AND PRECISION MEDICINE

Genomic discoveries in psoriasis have translated into clinical applications, particularly in the realm of personalized medicine and targeted therapies. Biomarker discovery and genetic profiling have facilitated:

- *Risk prediction*: Genetic profiling can help to stratify patients based on disease severity and risk of developing psoriatic arthritis or other comorbidities.
- *Treatment response prediction*: Identification of genetic variants associated with treatment response to biologic therapies [e.g., tumor necrosis factor (TNF) inhibitors, interleukin-17 (IL-17) inhibitors] allows for more personalized treatment decisions.
- *Biologic therapies*: Biologics targeting specific cytokines (e.g., TNF-α, IL-17, and IL-23) identified through genomic insights have revolutionized psoriasis treatment, offering improved efficacy and safety profiles compared to traditional systemic therapies.
- *Precision medicine*: Genetic profiling and biomarker discovery enable stratification of patients based on disease subtype, severity, and treatment response, guiding personalized therapeutic strategies tailored to individual genetic profiles.

CHALLENGES AND FUTURE DIRECTIONS

Despite significant progress, challenges remain in fully understanding the genetic architecture of psoriasis and translating genomic insights into clinical practice. Key challenges include:

- *Polygenic nature*: Psoriasis is influenced by multiple genetic variants, each contributing modestly to disease risk. Integrative approaches combining genomics with other omics data (proteomics and metabolomics) are needed to decipher complex gene-environment interactions.
- *Environmental factors*: The role of environmental triggers (e.g., stress, infections) in modulating genetic susceptibility requires further investigation to fully understand disease onset and exacerbation
- *Data integration and interpretation*: Integrating multiomics data and translating findings into clinically relevant insights require sophisticated computational tools and collaborative efforts across disciplines.
- *Precision medicine implementation*: Overcoming barriers to widespread adoption of personalized medicine approaches in clinical practice, including cost-effectiveness, accessibility to advanced genomic testing, and validation of biomarkers.

CONCLUSION

The genomics of psoriasis has made remarkable strides, from identifying susceptibility loci through GWAS to elucidating molecular pathways via NGS and functional genomics. These discoveries have not only enhanced our understanding of psoriasis pathogenesis but also paved the way for personalized medicine approaches that promise to improve patient outcomes. Continued interdisciplinary research and technological advancements will be critical in harnessing the full potential of genomics for precision medicine in psoriasis management.

PROTEOMICS

INTRODUCTION

Proteomics, the comprehensive study of proteins expressed in biological systems, has provided valuable insights into the pathogenesis, biomarkers, and potential therapeutic targets in psoriasis. This detailed discussion will cover the applications, methodologies, key findings, and implications of proteomics in understanding psoriasis.

APPLICATIONS OF PROTEOMICS IN PSORIASIS

Proteomics in psoriasis focuses on characterizing:
- *Protein expression profiles*: Differences in protein abundance and post-translational modifications (PTMs) between psoriatic lesional and nonlesional skin.
- *Identification of biomarkers*: Discovery of protein biomarkers for disease diagnosis, prognosis, and treatment response.
- *Elucidation of pathophysiological pathways*: Mapping protein-protein interactions (PPIs) and signaling pathways implicated in psoriasis pathogenesis.

METHODOLOGIES IN PROTEOMICS

Mass Spectrometry

Mass spectrometry (MS) is a cornerstone technique in proteomics, enabling high-throughput identification and quantification of proteins.[2] Key MS-based approaches include:
- *Shotgun proteomics*: Comprehensive analysis of all proteins in a sample by digesting proteins into peptides and analyzing them using liquid chromatography-tandem mass spectrometry (LC-MS/MS).
- *Quantitative proteomics*: Relative or absolute quantification of proteins to compare protein expression levels between samples (e.g., psoriatic lesional vs. nonlesional skin).

Two-dimensional Gel Electrophoresis and Protein Microarrays

- *Two-dimensional (2D) gel electrophoresis*: Separation of proteins based on their isoelectric point (pI) and molecular weight, followed by protein identification using MS.[2]
- *Protein microarrays*: High-throughput screening of protein interactions, protein expression, and antibody profiling in psoriasis samples.

KEY FINDINGS FROM PROTEOMICS STUDIES IN PSORIASIS

- *Differential protein expression profiles*: Proteomics studies have identified proteins differentially expressed in psoriatic lesional skin compared to nonlesional or healthy skin. Examples include:
  - *Keratins and filaggrin*: Abnormal expression of keratins (e.g., K16 and K17) and filaggrin-related proteins, contributing to abnormal keratinocyte differentiation and hyperproliferation.[3,4]
  - *S100 proteins*: Elevated levels of S100A7, S100A8, and S100A9 proteins, which are involved in inflammatory responses and contribute to chronic inflammation in psoriatic lesions.[3,4]
- *Signaling pathways and immune activation*: Proteomics has elucidated dysregulated signaling pathways in psoriasis, such as:
  - *NF-κB pathway*: Activation of NF-κB signaling, promoting proinflammatory cytokine production and perpetuating inflammation in psoriatic skin.[2]
  - *Interleukin pathways*: Increased expression of IL-17 and IL-23 pathway proteins, driving Th17 cell-mediated immune responses and keratinocyte hyperproliferation.
- *Post-translational modifications*: PTMs play a crucial role in regulating protein function and stability in psoriasis. Proteomics has identified PTMs such as phosphorylation, acetylation, and ubiquitination that

modulate protein activity and contribute to disease pathogenesis.[4]

■ IMPLICATIONS FOR DIAGNOSIS AND THERAPY

Proteomics research in psoriasis has several clinical implications:
- *Biomarker discovery*: Identification of protein biomarkers for early diagnosis, disease prognosis, and prediction of treatment response in psoriasis.
- *Therapeutic targets*: Discovery of proteins and pathways amenable to targeted therapies, including biologics targeting cytokines (e.g., IL-17 and IL-23) identified through proteomic studies.
- *Personalized medicine*: Integration of proteomic data with genomic and clinical information to tailor therapeutic strategies based on individual patient profiles.

■ CHALLENGES AND FUTURE DIRECTIONS

Challenges in proteomics research in psoriasis include:
- *Sample complexity and variability*: Variations in protein expression and PTMs across different psoriasis subtypes and disease stages.
- *Data integration*: Integrating proteomic data with genomic, transcriptomic, and clinical data to gain a comprehensive understanding of psoriasis pathophysiology.
- *Validation and translation*: Validating proteomic findings in larger patient cohorts and translating discoveries into clinically relevant biomarkers and therapeutic targets.

■ CONCLUSION

Proteomics has emerged as a powerful tool in unravelling the molecular mechanisms underlying psoriasis, from identifying differential protein expression profiles to elucidating dysregulated signaling pathways. Advances in proteomic technologies offer promising avenues for biomarker discovery, personalized medicine approaches, and the development of targeted therapies aimed at improving outcomes for patients with psoriasis. Continued research and technological innovations will further enhance our understanding of psoriasis pathogenesis and facilitate the translation of proteomic discoveries into clinical practice.

BIOINFORMATICS

■ INTRODUCTION

Bioinformatics plays a crucial role in advancing our understanding of psoriasis by integrating and analyzing vast amounts of biological data, including genomic, transcriptomic, proteomic, and clinical information.[5]

■ APPLICATIONS OF BIOINFORMATICS IN PSORIASIS

- *Genomic analysis*:
  - *Genome-wide association studies*: Bioinformatics tools are used to analyze large-scale genomic data to identify genetic variants associated with psoriasis susceptibility and severity. GWAS have identified numerous loci, including HLA-C and IL-23R, highlighting the genetic basis of psoriasis.
  - *Variant annotation and prioritization*: Bioinformatics pipelines annotate genetic variants and prioritize those most likely to contribute to disease pathogenesis, aiding in the identification of potential therapeutic targets.
- *Transcriptomic profiling*:
  - *RNA sequencing*: Bioinformatics tools quantify gene expression levels and identify differentially expressed

genes (DEGs) between psoriatic and healthy skin. This approach reveals dysregulated pathways, such as the IL-23/Th17 axis, providing insights into disease mechanisms.
  - *Gene ontology (GO) enrichment analysis*: Bioinformatics tools categorize DEGs based on their biological functions, cellular components, and molecular processes, elucidating functional changes in psoriasis.
- *Proteomics and metabolomics*:
  - *Protein-protein interaction networks*: Bioinformatics methods construct PPI networks to elucidate protein interactions and pathways dysregulated in psoriasis. This approach identifies key proteins (e.g., cytokines and signaling molecules) and potential therapeutic targets.
  - *Metabolic pathway analysis*: Bioinformatics tools analyze metabolomic data to identify altered metabolic pathways in psoriatic skin, linking metabolite profiles to disease progression and severity.
- *Systems biology approaches*:
  - *Network analysis*: Integration of multiomics data using network-based approaches (e.g., pathway analysis and coexpression networks) identifies interconnected molecular networks driving psoriasis pathophysiology. This holistic view enhances our understanding of complex disease mechanisms.
  - *Machine learning and predictive modeling*: Bioinformatics employs machine learning algorithms to predict disease outcomes, treatment responses, and patient stratification based on multiomics data integration.

This approach supports personalized medicine in psoriasis management.

■ CONTRIBUTIONS TO PSORIASIS RESEARCH

- *Biomarker discovery and validation*: Bioinformatics identifies and validates biomarkers (e.g., genetic variants, DEGs, and protein signatures) associated with psoriasis diagnosis, prognosis, and treatment response. These biomarkers aid in clinical decision-making and personalized therapy.[5]
- *Drug target identification*: Bioinformatics identifies druggable targets (e.g., cytokines and enzymes) within dysregulated pathways implicated in psoriasis. This knowledge accelerates the development of targeted therapies (e.g., biologics and small molecules) aimed at modulating disease mechanisms.
- *Clinical applications and precision medicine*: Bioinformatics integrates multiomics data to stratify psoriasis patients based on molecular subtypes, disease severity, and response to therapies.[5] This personalized approach optimizes treatment strategies and improves patient outcomes.

■ CHALLENGES AND FUTURE DIRECTIONS

- *Data integration and standardization*: Addressing challenges in integrating and harmonizing multiomics data across different platforms and studies to ensure data quality, reproducibility, and robustness in bioinformatics analyses.
- *Clinical translation*: Validating bioinformatics findings in large, diverse patient cohorts and translating discoveries into

CHAPTER 24: Advances in Psoriasis Research: Genomics, Proteomics, and Bioinformatics

clinical practice for improved diagnosis, treatment, and management of psoriasis.
- *Precision medicine approaches*: Further refining personalized medicine strategies based on individual molecular profiles (genetic, transcriptomic, and proteomic) to optimize therapeutic outcomes and minimize adverse effects in psoriasis patients.[5]

In conclusion, bioinformatics plays a pivotal role in advancing our understanding of psoriasis by integrating multiomics data, identifying biomarkers, elucidating disease mechanisms, and facilitating personalized medicine approaches. Further innovation in bioinformatics methodologies and collaborative research efforts will further enhance our ability to unravel the complexities of psoriasis and improve patient care.

■ CONCLUSION

Bioinformatics has revolutionized psoriasis research by integrating multiomics data to uncover genetic, transcriptomic, proteomic, and metabolic factors contributing to disease pathogenesis. It plays a crucial role in biomarker discovery, drug target identification, and personalized medicine, enhancing diagnosis and treatment strategies. Advanced computational tools, including machine learning and network analysis, enable precise patient stratification and predictive modeling. However, challenges such as data integration, standardization, and clinical translation remain. Continued advancements in bioinformatics methodologies and collaborative research efforts will be essential for translating genomic insights into improved patient care and precision medicine approaches in psoriasis management.

TAKE HOME MESSAGE

Genetic basis of psoriasis
- Psoriasis has a strong genetic component, with early studies highlighting familial aggregation.
- Genome-wide association studies (GWAS) have identified multiple susceptibility loci, including the HLA-Cw6 allele, which has the strongest association with psoriasis.

Advancements in genomic technologies
- *Next-generation sequencing (NGS)* has enabled detailed profiling of rare variants and novel loci.
- Transcriptomic studies using RNA sequencing have uncovered key dysregulated pathways like IL-23/Th17 and NF-κB signaling.
- Epigenomic research has revealed DNA methylation and histone modifications influencing psoriasis pathogenesis.

Integrative multiomics approaches
- Combining genomic, transcriptomic, epigenomic, and proteomic data provides a comprehensive understanding of psoriasis.
- Machine learning and network analysis help predict disease outcomes and treatment responses.

Clinical and therapeutic implications
- Genetic profiling aids in risk prediction and stratifying patients for personalized treatment.
- Biologic therapies targeting cytokines (e.g., IL-17, IL-23 inhibitors) have revolutionized treatment.

REFERENCES

1. Jiang S, Hinchliffe TE, Wu T. Biomarkers of An Autoimmune Skin Disease--Psoriasis. Genomics Proteomics Bioinformatics. 2015;13(4):224-33.
2. Chularojanamontri L, Charoenpipatsin N, Silpa-Archa N, Wongpraparut C, Thongboonkerd V. Proteomics in Psoriasis. Int J Mol Sci. 2019;20(5):1141.
3. Lundberg KC, Fritz Y, Johnston A, Foster AM, Baliwag J, Gudjonsson JE, et al. Proteomics of skin proteins in psoriasis: from discovery and verification in a mouse model to confirmation in humans. Mol Cell Proteomics. 2015;14(1):109-19.
4. Kromann B, Olsson A, Zhang YM, Løvendorf MB, Skov L, Dyring-Andersen B. Proteins in the Skin and Blood in Patients with Psoriasis: A Systematic Review of Proteomic Studies. Dermatology. 2024;240(2):317-28.
5. Li AH, Li WW, Yu XQ, Zhang DM, Liu YR, Li D. Bioinformatic Analysis and Translational Validation of Psoriasis Candidate Genes for Precision Medicine. Clin Cosmet Investig Dermatol. 2022;15:1447-58.

Index

Page numbers followed by *b* refer to box, *f* refer to figure, *fc* refer to flowchart, and *t* refer to table.

A

Abramowitz sign 17
Abrocitinib 115
Acitretin 104-106, 108, 141, 142, 144, 145, 147, 148, 177, 179
   metabolism 107
   therapy, monitoring during 107
Acquired immunodeficiency syndrome 50
Acrodermatitis continua 14
   of Hallopeau 170
Acute cutaneous lupus 171
Adalimumab 115, 123, 126, 128, 177, 179
Adenosine receptor 220
Adiponectin 247
Adjunctive treatments 158
Aggregatibacter actinomycetemcomitans 25
Akkermansia muciniphila 52
Alanine aminotransferase 105
Alcohol 27
   consumption 3
Amino-terminal type III procollagen peptide 105
Amygdalin, analog of 225
Angiotensin-converting enzyme 50
Antimicrobial peptides 234, 237
Antirheumatic drugs
   biologic disease-modifying 159
   disease-modifying 142
Anxiety 58
   disorder, generalized 58
Apoptosis 237
Apremilast 116, 142, 144, 145, 216
Aquaporin-1 227
Arthritis, peripheral 159
Artificial intelligence 67
Aryl hydrocarbon receptor

   agonist 223
   modulators 78
Aspartate aminotransferase 105
Atherosclerosis 55*fc*, 62
Auspitz sign 9, 9*f*, 10*fc*
Autoimmune 195
   t-cell, chronic 51
   thyroid disease 58
Axial disease 159

B

Bacillus species 52
Baricitinib 115
Bifidobacterium species 51
Bimekizumab 123, 127, 214
Biomarker discovery 257
   and validation 258
Biopsy 36
Bipolar disorder 58
Blood lipids 56
Body
   area 68
   mass index 54
   surface area 68, 184
Brepocitinib 116
Brepocitinib cream 224
Brodalumab 123
Bromodomain, inhibitors of 222
Bulkeley's membrane 9*f*, 10*f*

C

Calcipotriene 140, 141
   cream 73
Calcipotriol 73, 74, 140, 141
Calcitonin gene-related peptide, antagonist of 222
Calcitriol 144
Candida albicans 26
Cardiometabolic disease 57
Cardiovascular disease 54, 154, 164
   reduction of 57

Castle biosciences 250, 250*t*
   work, significance of 250
Cathelicidins 237
Cathepsin B 227
Certolizumab 125
Certolizumab pegol 123, 129, 177
Cesarean delivery 60
Chikungunya 26
Childhood psoriasis 54
Chlamydophila psittaci 25
Chromosome 29
Chronic kidney disease 58
Coal tar products 75
Combination therapy 92, 139, 143, 148
Complete blood count 179
Contact dermatitis 73
Coronavirus disease-2019 26, 50, 59
Corticosteroids, withdrawal of 170
Counseling patients 186
Coxsackie B 26
C-reactive protein 69
Crisaborole 117
Crohn's disease 59
Cyclosporine 107-109, 111, 141, 143, 147, 159, 178, 179
Cytochrome P450 107
Cytokine 238
   and receptors 234
   in depression, emerging role of 183
   ligand 31
Cytomegalovirus 25

D

Dactylitis 155, 156*f*, 159-163
Deep Koebner phenomenon 11
Defensins 238
Dendritic cells 32, 84
Depression 54, 58

Index

treatment of 186
Dermatitis herpetiformis 171
Dermatology life quality index 52, 65, 115, 186, 198
  score 193
Dermatology practice 189
Dermatology specific 65
Dermoscopy 16, 36
  Auspitz sign 9, 10f
Deucravacitinib 114, 217
Diabetes
  mellitus 61
  screening of 194
  type 2 56
Discoid dermatitis 37
Disease distribution factors 199
Dithranol 140, 141
  inhibits 74
Drug
  class of 62
  eruption reaction 171
  name of 125-128, 179
  target identification 258
Dual biologic therapy 146
Dynamic hepatic scintigraphy 105
Dysbiosis 51
Dyshidrotic eczema 171

E

Eczema, infected 171
Elective surgery 130
Emollients 72, 176
Enhancer landscapes 254
Enthesitis 159-163
  validated scoring systems for 155f
Environmental factors 255
Environmental triggers 3
Epidermal proliferation 55fc
Epigenetic alterations 254
Epstein–Barr virus 25
Erythema
  lasting 87
  moderate 92
  persistent 87
  severe 92
Erythroderma 171
  dermoscopy of 12f
  secondary to psoriasis 12f
    complications of 13t

Erythrodermic psoriasis 11
Etanercept 123, 125, 177, 179
Ethanol consumption 108
Ethnic and racial differences 2
Etretinate 141
Exanthematous pustulosis, acute generalized 171
Excimer laser 93
Excimer light
  therapy 91
  use of 91

F

Faecalibacterium prausnitzii 51
Familial aggregation 253
Fatigue 58
Fecal microbiota transplantation 51
Fertility, male 103
Fetal exposure 207
Filaggrin 256
Filgotinib 115
Fitzpatrick skin 92
  type 92
Flexural lesions 16
Flexural psoriasis 16, 17f
  dermoscopy of 18f
Folic acid supplementation 102
Follicular psoriasis 19, 20f
  dermoscopy of 20f
Fracture 60
Fumaric acid esters 110, 117, 142, 144
Fungi 26

G

Galectin, inhibitor of 223
Gene
  expression regulation 237
  in pustular psoriasis 30, 30t
  ontology enrichment analysis 258
Genetic 28, 234
  and environmental factors, interaction between 4
  biomarkers 245
  factors 2
Genital psoriasis 17, 18f
Genome-wide association studies 253, 257

Genomic loci 29, 29t
Gestational diabetes 60
Gestational hypertension 60
Glycoprotein 105
Goeckerman regimen 75
Golimumab 126, 129
Gout 58
Grainyhead-like transcription factor 2 227
Guselkumab 123, 128, 129, 246
Gut
  dysbiosis 51
  microbiome 51
  microbiota 27, 241
Guttate psoriasis 11, 11f

H

Hailey–Hailey disease 44
Heat shock protein 220, 221
Helicobacter pylori 25
Hepatitis 130
  B 59
    virus 104
  C 59
    virus 25, 104
Hepatotoxic drugs, use of 104
Heritability, missing 30
Herpes zoster 59, 115
High-pressure mercury lamps 83
Human endogenous retrovirus 26
Human immunodeficiency virus 25, 50, 59, 72, 104, 143, 148, 164
Human leukocyte antigen 2, 26, 253
Human papillomavirus 25
Hyperkeratosis 68
Hyperkeratotic variants 8t
Hyperlipidemia 107
Hypertension 56
Hypopigmentation, zone of 7

I

Immune
  activation 256
  cell differentiation and inflammation 237
  system dysfunction 23
Immunity locale, zone of 8

Index

Immunoglobulin G1 123, 126, 127
Immunological factors 2
Immunometabolism 240
Impetigo 171
  herpetiformis 170
Infection 3, 23, 59
  route of 24-26
Inflammatory biomarkers 247
Inflammatory bowel disease 61, 59, 154
Inflammatory diseases 51
Inflammatory multisystem disorder, chronic 82
Inflammatory papulosquamous lesions 36
Infliximab 123, 125, 177
Infrared rays 83
Inhibit inflammatory cytokines 114
Intense pulsed light therapy 84
Interferon gamma 26, 32
Interleukin 124, 164
  blockers 127t, 128t
  inhibitors of 215, 225
  pathways 256
Intestinal inflammation 51
Intralesional corticosteroids 73
Iodine 170
Itacitinib 115
Itch, chronic 60
Ixekizumab 123, 127, 177, 179, 180

J

Janus kinase 143, 146
  family 217
  inhibitor 77, 114, 115, 164, 214, 217, 224
JDA-GPPSI scoring system 69t

K

Keratinocyte 239, 240
  apoptosis of 84
  appear 241
  danger signal from 33
  in psoriasis recurrence 240
  interaction 234
  proliferation 237
  targeting 226
Keratins 256

Koebner phenomenon 3, 10
  negative 11

L

Lactobacillus 51
Langerhans cell 84
  histiocytosis 45
Latent tuberculosis infection, testing for 204
Leflunomide 159, 164
Leukonychia 68
Lichen
  planopilaris 41
  planus 39
  simplex chronicus 43
Lifestyle 26
  factors 3
Light source, classification of 84
Light-emitting device 84
Linear psoriasis 21
Lipid
  chromatography-tandem mass spectrometry 256
  metabolism 55fc
    dysregulated 28
  profiles 107
Lithium 170
Liver
  enzymes 107, 110
  function tests 126, 127
Low PASI score 66t
Low-density lipoprotein 52
Lunula, red spots in 68
Lupus erythematosus 48

M

Machine learning 258
Macrolide antibiotic 77
Macrophagic M1 cytokines 247
Maintenance therapy 87
Maintenance treatment 90
Malassezia 26
Malignancy 58, 130
Mapping protein-protein interactions 256
Mass spectrometry 256
Matrix metalloproteinase 105
Medication adherence 198
Mediterranean diet 51
Mental disorders 28
Mental health diseases 58

Metabolic dysfunction 164
Metabolic parameters, dysfunction in 56fc
Metabolic pathway analysis 258
Metabolic syndrome 54, 55fc, 62t, 154
  adverse effects on 62
  leads 54
Metabolism 234
Metabolomics 258
Metalloproteinase, tissue inhibitor of 105
Methotrexate 100, 101, 141-144, 158, 164, 177-179
  hepatotoxic risks of 102
  hepatotoxicity, monitoring 105t
  monitoring for 104t
Methoxypsoralen 82, 90
Micro ribonucleic acid 236, 247
Microbial imbalance 51
Microbiome factors 4
Microorganisms 24-26
Mind.Px™ dermal diagnostic patch 249
Mindera health 249, 250, 250t
  technologies, significance of 249
Minimal erythema dose 87
Minimum phototoxic dose 89
  testing 90
Mirikizumab 214
Miscellaneous systemic combination therapies 143t
Mitogen-activated protein 50
Mitogen-stimulated mononuclear cell proliferation 74
Mitotic activity, reducing 75
Moisturizers 176
Molluscum contagiosum 8
Monochromatic excimer light laser 91
Monoclonal antibody, type of 125-128
Musculoskeletal system 59
Mutation 30
Mycobacterium 59
Mycophenolate mofetil 143
Mycoplasma faucium 25
Mycosis fungoides 47

N

Nail 244
  affected area 19
  bed and matrix 68*t*
  bed hyperkeratosis 68
  changes 19, 19*t*
  matrix disease 68
  plate crumbling 68
Nail psoriasis 18, 19*f*, 65, 68
  dermoscopy of 19*f*
  scores, severity of 69
  severity index 68
    modified 68
    targeted 68
Namodenoson 220
Narrowband ultraviolet B 85, 93
  treatment methodology of 85
Nasopharyngitis 115
Nephrotoxicity 109
Neuropeptide-degrading enzymes, activity of 4
Next-generation sequencing technologies 254
Nonalcoholic fatty liver disease 57
Nonbiologic pharmaceuticals 114
Nonmelanoma skin cancer 126, 143
Nonsteroidal anti-inflammatory drugs 50, 148
Novel therapeutic targets 214
Nuclear factor-kappa 30
Nutrients, metabolism of 51

O

Obesity 55, 62
Onycholysis 68
Open body language, use 190
Oral comorbidities 60
Oral interleukin inhibitors 214, 218, 219
Oral mucosa 18
Oral psoralen plus ultraviolet A 89*t*
Oral sphingosine-1-phosphate receptor 1 118
Oral tumor necrosis factor inhibitors 218
Orismilast 216
Orphan receptor gamma T inhibitors 118, 219
Osteoporosis 60

P

Palmar psoriasis 15*f*
Palmoplantar psoriasis 15, 170
Papulosquamous disorder 7
Parakeratosis 9, 49
Parvovirus B19 25
Pediatric psoriasis, biologic treatments for 179*t*
Peficitinib 115
Perceived stress scale 185
Perifollicular scaling 21
Periodontitis 60
Personality disorders 58
Personalized medicine 244, 249, 257
Personalized medicine target 248
Phosphodiesterase 4 inhibitor 77, 116, 164, 214, 216, 224
Photochemotherapy depending 89
Photodynamic therapy 84
Phototherapy 148
  mechanisms of action of 83
  safety measures during 95
  systemic medications with 144
  targeted 91
Phototoxic dose 90*t*
Physician-patient relationship 200
Piclidenoson 118, 220
Pimecrolimus cream 77
Pioglitazone 144
Pitting 68
Pityriasis
  lichenoides chronica 38
  rosea 38
  rubra pilaris 42
Placebo 160-163
Placental transfer 177
Planned pregnancy 207
Plaque
  psoriasis 7
    chronic 7, 65, 66
    variants of chronic 8, 8*t*
  thickness 92

Plasma proteins 107
Polymorphonuclear leukocytes migration 74
Polysized erythematous plaques 204*f*
Ponesimod 118, 220
Porphyromonas gingivalis 25
Positive Mantoux reaction 204*f*
Post-translational modifications 256
Potential psoriasis treatment 237
Prebiotics, role of 51
Precision medicine 255, 259
Pregnancy 129
  and prepregnancy planning 177*t*
  flare during 207
  shifts maternal immune 206
Preterm birth 60
Probiotics 51
  role of 51
Profilin-1 247
Proinflammatory cytokines 52, 85, 114
Proinflammatory milieu 54
Protein
  degradation 241
  expression profiles 256
  microarrays 256
Protein-protein interaction networks 258
Proteomics 258
  methodologies in 256
Psolaren 90, 93, 94
  plus ultraviolet A 88
  treatment methodology of 89
Psoriasis 1, 23, 29, 36, 37, 51, 54, 57, 93*t*, 114-116, 122, 125*t*, 127*t*, 139, 183, 185, 186, 186*t*, 189, 194, 198, 203, 217, 234, 244, 256
  activation in 234
  adverse effects of drugs in 62*t*
  area and severity 52
  area, role of absolute 133
  assessment of 128
  bioinformatics in 257
  children 178
  chronic inflammation in 55*fc*
  classification of 123*t*
  clinical manifestations of 7

Index

clinical spectrum of 7b
comorbidities 61f
conventional systemic
    treatments for 100
diagnosis, applications of 203
differential diagnosis of 36,
    37t
disability index 65, 185
elderly 180
eligibility of 123
epigenetic biomarkers in 247
genetics 30
gut dysbiosis in 52
in pregnancy 205, 206f
increases oxidative stress 56
initial dose for 92
key cytokines in 32, 121
life stress inventory 65, 70,
    185
management of 82, 108, 139,
    177
mechanism 29t
medicine technologies in 248
moderate-to-severe 122
molecular pathogenesis 32f
newly reported mental
    comorbidity of 58
off-label in 77
pathogenesis of 24t, 29f, 237
pathophysiology of 23, 221
patients 153
    effective communication
        with 189
phototherapeutics for 84t
phototherapy for 94
pregnancy 175
proteomics in 256
recurrence of 24f
research 258
role in 247, 248
severity of 52, 66
    scoring of 65
specific 65
    quality of life scores 70
systemic drugs in 62
therapies for 65
topical treatments for 72
treatment of 75, 134, 175,
    217, 226, 244
treat-to-target approach in 133
use of biologics in 121

vulgaris 8f
    dermoscopy of 9f
    with hepatitis 208, 208f, 209f
    with latent tuberculosis 203
Psoriasis area and severity
    index 65, 66, 114
    calculation of 66
    high discrimination 67
    interpretation of 66t
    limitations of 66
    score 54, 66
Psoriasis management 175,
    194, 203
    clinical pearls in 192
    implications for 248
    treatment targets in 122
Psoriatic arthritis 59, 61, 65,
    69, 121, 128, 139, 143, 153,
    154, 157
    developing 153
    diagnosis of 154, 156
    disease activity index for 69
    extra-musculoskeletal
        features of 156
    management of 153, 157,
        160t, 164
    treatment of 158
Psoriatic disease, conditions
    of 154f
Psoriatic erythroderma 11, 12fc
Psoriatic lesions 74
Psoriatic march 57fc
Psychiatric comorbidities 184
Psychiatric disorders 183
Psychological stress 28
Pulsed dye laser 84
Purified protein derivative 104
Purpura 73
Pustular psoriasis 13, 14f, 65,
    69, 169, 215
    dermoscopy of 15f
    generalized 69, 169, 173
    treatment algorithm in 173fc
    types of 170
Pyrimidine dimers 83

Q

Quality of life 133, 169, 183, 184
    factors affecting 184
    improve 185
    measure, mix 65, 70

    measurement scales 66, 70
    pharmacological treatments
        in 186t
    psoriasis index of 65, 70, 185
    scores 70
Quantitative proteomics 256

R

Reactive oxygen species 55
Receptor-interacting protein 1
    kinase, inhibitor of 222
Receptors 238
Recommendations during
    pregnancy 177
    planning 177
Relapses, treatment of 90
Renal function, regular
    monitoring of 110
Renbök phenomenon 11
Renin–angiotensin–aldosterone
    system 56
Reproductive system 60
Resident memory T cells 33
Retinoic acid 219
    receptor 118
Rheumatoid arthritis 154
Ribonucleic acid
    circular 236
    interference 226, 237
    long noncoding 236, 248
    modulation of 225
    noncoding 234, 236
    role of noncoding 237
Risankizumab 123, 128, 246
Roflumilast 117
Rosacea 73
Rotational therapy 146
    with biologicals 147
    with cyclosporine A 146
Ruxolitinib 116, 224

S

S100 proteins 238, 256
Salford psoriasis index 65
Salicylic acid 76, 140
Saturated fatty acids 195
Scalp 244
    psoriasis 16, 16f
        dermoscopy of 17f
Schizophrenia 58

Index

Seborrheic dermatitis 43
Secukinumab 123, 127, 177, 179, 180
Sequential therapy 147
Severe acute respiratory syndrome coronavirus 2 26
Sex hormones, dysregulated 28
Shotgun proteomics 256
Signal transducer 227
Signaling pathways 256
Silvery-white scales 204f
Single nucleotide polymorphisms 246
Skin 60
   complaints 65
   diseases 56fc
   dysbiosis of 27
   trauma 23
   type 88, 88t, 89, 90
      photochemotherapy depending on 90t
SkinAtlas 249
Sleep disorders 27, 58
Small molecules 114, 144
Soluble biomarkers, role of 156
Special situations in psoriasis 62t
Specialized fluorescent tubes 83
Spesolimab 215
Sphingosine-1-phosphate 118
   lyase 1 227
   receptor agonist 219
Splinter hemorrhage 68
Staphylococcal colonization 59
Staphylococcus aureus 85
Steatotic liver disease 164
Stratum malpighii 9
Streptomyces tsukubensis 77
Stress 4
Sublight source 84
Sulci cutis 16f
Sulfasalazine 159
Sunlight 83
Sympathetic nervous system 56
Syndrome X 54
Syphilis, secondary 46
Systemic combination therapies 142
Systemic inflammation, abrogation of 133
Systemic Janus kinase inhibitors 114
Systemic therapies 178, 180
Systemic treatments 176

T

T cells 84
   regulatory 32
Tachyphylaxis 73
Tacrolimus 77, 140, 141
Tapinarof 117
Tazarotene 76, 140, 141, 148, 177
   sequential therapy of 148
T-cell mediated disorder 203
Th1 cytokines 247
Th17 cytokines 247
Therapeutic implications 255
Thymidine incorporation 74
Tildrakizumab 123, 128, 246
Tinea corporis 41
Tofacitinib 115, 116, 217
Topical agents 176
Topical calcineurin inhibitors 77, 178
Topical corticosteroids 72, 139
Topical crisaborole 78
Topical Janus kinase inhibitors 116
Topical roflumilast 78
Topical ruxolitinib 77
Topical therapies 178, 180, 223
Transcription, activator of 227
Transcriptomic profiling 257
Transforming growth factor-β 247
Trauma 3
Triethanolamine 75
Triggers 23
Triglycerides 52
Tuberculosis 130, 179
   infection, starting latent 203
Tumor necrosis factor 55, 62
   alpha 26, 32, 52, 62, 123, 148, 173, 183
      blockers 125, 125t
      inhibitor 145
   inhibitor 55, 128, 164
   receptor 123
   signaling, negative regulation of 235
Two-dimensional gel electrophoresis 256
Tyrosine kinase 2 inhibitors 146

U

Ubiquitin-proteasome system 241
Ulcerative colitis 59
Ultraviolet
   A 84
   B 83, 85, 87, 148
   C 83
   exposure 2
   radiation 75, 83
      artificial sources of 83
   spectrum 83
Unconventional medications 144
Unipolar depression 58
Unplanned pregnancy 207
Upadacitinib 115, 217
Upper respiratory tract infection 115
Uric acid levels 52
Ustekinumab 123, 129, 177, 179, 180

V

Variant annotation and prioritization 257
Varicella zoster virus 25
Vascular dementia 58
Vascular endothelial growth factor 227
Viruses 25
Vitamin
   A analogs 76
   D analogs 73, 176, 178

W

White blood cell 69
Whole-exome sequencing 254
Whole-genome sequencing 254
Woronoff's ring 7, 8f

Z

Zika virus 25